LIVING WELL WITH

Graves' Disease
and Hyperthyroidism

Also by Mary J. Shomon

Living Well with Hypothyroidism

The Thyroid Diet

**Living Well with Chronic Fatigue Syndrome
and Fibromyalgia**

Living Well with Autoimmune Disease

LIVING WELL WITH
Graves' Disease
and Hyperthyroidism

What Your Doctor

Doesn't Tell You . . .

That You Need to Know

MARY J. SHOMON

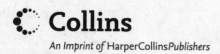

Collins

An Imprint of HarperCollins*Publishers*

HarperCollins books may be purchased for educational, business, or sales
promotional use. For information please write: Special Markets Department, HarperCollins Publishers, 10 East 53rd Street, New York, NY 10022.

FIRST EDITION

Designed by Joy O'Meara

Printed on acid-free paper

Library of Congress Cataloging-in-Publication Data

Shomon, Mary J.
    Living well with Graves' disease and hyperthyroidism : what your
doctor doesn't tell you . . . that you need to know / Mary J. Shomon.—
1st ed.
        p.   cm.
    Includes bibliographical references.
    ISBN-10: 0–06–073019–6
    ISBN-13: 978–0–06–073019–2
    1. Graves' disease—Popular works.   2. Hyperthyroidism—Popular
works.   I. Title.

RC657.5.G7.S566   2005
616.4'43—dc22

                                                            2005040402

05 06 07 08 09 WBC/RRD 10 9 8 7 6 5 4 3 2 1

For Daniel,
my dream baby

The secret of health for both mind and body
is not to mourn for the past,
not to worry about the future,
or not to anticipate troubles,
but to live the present moment wisely and earnestly.

—*The Buddha*

ACKNOWLEDGMENTS

I must always start by thanking my sweet husband, Jon, who doesn't always know how much a part of my books he truly is. I could never do this without him, and I wouldn't be a writer and patient advocate without him in my life. And to Julia, who is my dearest little inspiration. She is the future and she is always in my mind as I look for answers to help us all live well. Thanks to my best and dearest friend and sister, Jeannie Yamine, who is always, always there for me. I can never thank her enough.

Special thanks to my agent, Carol Mann, who is a wonderful advocate and mentor. And my editor at HarperCollins, Sarah Durand, who suggested this book, and as always, made it better with her incredible insights and understanding of our readers. Thanks, too, to Jeremy Cesarec at HarperCollins for all his top-notch help.

I owe a special debt to Richard Shames, MD, and Karilee Shames, PhD, RN, who are smart, caring practitioners, wonderful advocates for thyroid patients, good friends, and tireless supporters of my work.

Special thanks to the doctors at the Shiley Eye Center at the University of California–San Diego, David B. Granet, MD, Don O. Kikkawa, MD, and Leah Levi, MD, who spent a great deal of time sharing their insights on thyroid eye disease. They are a caring group who are helping people deal with a difficult aspect of this disease with grace and compassion.

Many other doctors, practitioners, and experts contributed to this book, and I appreciate their generosity of time and the caring and compassion they bring to their work with patients. So with gratitude I thank: Ridha Arem, MD; Dr. Edward Bauman; Herbert Benson, MD; Kenneth Blanchard, PhD, MD; David Brownstein, MD; Hyla Cass, MD; David Derry, MD; Phylameana Lila Desy; Barry Durrant-Peatfield, MD; Dr. Mike Fitzpatrick; Ted Friedman, MD; Hossein Gharib, MD; Dr. Ann Louise Gittleman; Dr. Leonard Holmes; Dr. Gina Honeyman-Lowe; Nadia Krupnikova, MD; Steve Langer, MD; Kate Lemmerman, MD; Dr. John Lowe; Joseph Mercola, DO; Dr. Viana Muller; Pat Rackowski; Swami Rameshwarananda; Dr. Byron Richards; Carol Roberts, MD; Noel Rose, MD; Glenn Rothfeld, MD; Marie Savard, MD; Dr. Sherrill Sellman; Dr. Brian Sheen; Jacob Teitelbaum, MD; Dr. Shasta Tierra-Tayam; Cynthia White; and Ken Woliner, MD.

To the patient advocates and experts on Graves' disease and hyperthyroidism, I owe much gratitude. In particular, thanks to John Johnson of ithyroid.com, who so generously shared his innovative nutritional protocols so that readers could benefit from his knowledge and experience. I would also like to acknowledge the wonderful work of Elaine Moore, Kelly Hale, and Kate Flax, who are such committed advocates for thyroid patients. I also need to recognize Virginia Ladd and Patricia Barber and the wonderful work they do with the American Autoimmune Related Diseases Association, a group I greatly admire.

As always, thanks to the docs and experts who keep me going personally, including Kate Lemmerman, MD, of the Kaplan Clinic in Arlington, Virginia; osteopath Dr. Scott Kwiatkowski of Bethesda, Maryland; my trainer, Silvia Treves; and my "smart friend," Dr. Bob Umlauf.

More thanks to my unofficial health news bureau—Rose Apter, Kim Carmichael Cox, Sherry Leu, Dottye Howard, and James Scheer—for always making sure I don't miss any breaking medical or health announcements!

And to the friends who bring joy and inspiration to my life: Mohammed Antabli and Franca Fiabane, Faris Bouhafa and Abla Majaj, Ric and Diane Blake, Wendy Sobey and Jim Strick, and Gen Piturro and Demo DeMartile. And my dear "Aunties" friends and their DHs—Jane and Joe Frank, Cynthia and David Austin, Laura and Tom Horton, and Kim and Cary Conley—as well as all the Momfriends, and my comrade in "living well," Teri Robert.

Many thanks to everyone in the family who is so supportive of my work, including my dad, Dan Shomon; brother, Dan Shomon Jr.; in-laws, Rus and Barbara Mathis; my inspiring aunt Rita Kelleher; and my dear cousins Ellen Blaze and Joan Kelleher. A special hello to my cousin Kate, who knows firsthand what it's like to go through this. And thanks to my mom, Patricia Rita Shomon. Pat is always with me.

Finally, I am forever grateful to the many thousands of people with Graves' disease and/or hyperthyroidism or hypothyroidism who told me their stories, sent e-mails detailing their experiences, generously shared their success stories, and contributed their joys and sorrows to this book. While there isn't space to list every one of you or include every story you shared, you are the heart and soul of this book, without a doubt.

May you all live well!

CONTENTS

INTRODUCTION

I've been a thyroid patient advocate for nearly 10 years, and I've received many e-mails from patients throughout this time. Sometimes the notes are despondent. Sometimes they are adamant. But almost always they tell a story like Audrey's:

> I was very tired. As time passed, I got more and more tired, where I couldn't keep my eyes open. First, the muscles in my legs and then the muscles in my arms became very painful. I couldn't raise my legs 2 inches off the floor or raise my arms straight up! My eyes bulged; I lost hair; I lost weight; I had jaundice; I had tremors. Finally, a lump appeared on my throat. Writing this out for you, I have tears in my eyes. Through all this, not one doctor picked up on the problem. I was told I was a hypochondriac. Finally, after seeing the lump, my doctor sent me for an ultrasound test and then nuclear testing. Finally, I was diagnosed with Graves' disease. Imagine the shock on my doctor's face and his embarrassment.

Lorrie's experience is also quite common:

> I felt kind of off. Nothing so serious that I was suffering terribly, but just not feeling myself. I started a job and soon was plagued by anxiety, stomach problems, heart palpitations, mood swings, and hot flashes. The doctors—I was sent to a gastroenterologist, a psychologist, a general practitioner, a

gynecologist, and an allergist—did not have a clue what was wrong with me. They wrote it off to stress and having a sensitive stomach. I continued enduring the symptoms and hoping that they would go away.

I tried to change things about my life in hopes that it would help. But five years after making dietary changes, lifestyle changes, changing my career, and moving cross-country, things were worse. I had even worse heart palpitations, achy joints, breathing problems, and I could not keep weight on. I ate enormous amounts of food that barely allowed me to maintain my weight. So I started the doctor circuit again. The allergist claimed I had asthma and gave me an inhaler. That inhaler nearly killed me one day while exercising because it sent my already skyrocketing heart rate into the stratosphere. Finally, all my symptoms and the fact that my hands were shaking violently clicked with my general practitioner and she gave me a thyroid blood test. I was suffering with severe hyperthyroidism that had gone undetected for years.

Unfortunately, Audrey and Lorrie are not alone. Millions of people in the United States, the majority of whom are women, are suffering from Graves' disease and hyperthyroidism—conditions that seriously disrupt quality of life and can be fatal if left untreated over time.

I wrote this book to help you determine if you have the symptoms of Graves' disease and hyperthyroidism. Then you'll find information to help you get the proper diagnosis, and perhaps most importantly, how to navigate the confusion of treatment options that range from antithyroid drugs to permanent, irreversible treatment such as radioactive iodine to the thyroid or surgery. Finally, the end result for most people treated for Graves' disease and hyperthyroidism is the opposite condition, hypothyroidism, which means living with an underactive thyroid. You'll learn how to manage that part of the disease as well, along with common and persistent symptoms such as weight gain, fatigue, depression, and hair loss. You'll also learn how to have a healthy pregnancy.

This book is for you if

- You strongly suspect you have Graves' disease and/or hyperthyroidism but are having difficulty getting a diagnosis by conventional means.
- You aren't sure if your various symptoms point to hyperthyroidism and you need to find out.
- You've been diagnosed with Graves' disease and/or hypothyroidism and have been told that you need to have a particular treatment right away. You want more information before you commit to decisions that may affect your health for the rest of your life.
- You have in the past or are currently being treated for Graves' disease or hyperthyroidism and are still struggling to feel well.
- You are receiving what your doctor feels is sufficient treatment, yet you still don't feel well.
- You're an open-minded health practitioner looking for innovative ways to understand and help your patients with Graves' disease and hyperthyroidism.
- You want to learn about living well with Graves' disease and hyperthyroidism from the perspective of empowered patients and caring practitioners.

Before I go any further, I think it might be useful to explain my own background. I'm not a doctor. I'm not a health professional. I have a degree in international studies from Georgetown University. In 1997, my battle with my own health led me to start and manage a popular patient-oriented Web site on thyroid disease as well as launch the only monthly report on conventional and alternative thyroid-related health news and treatments. Ultimately, this has turned into my mission as a patient advocate and health writer for books, Web sites, newsletters, and magazines.

As a Hashimoto's thyroiditis patient myself, I've had periods of Hashitoxicosis, or Hashimoto's-induced hyperthyroidism. Truly, I thought I was going mad. I felt agitated; my skin felt hot; my eyes were spasming, jumpy, and twitching. My eyes got so dry that everything was blurry and I couldn't drive at night. I could barely concentrate or focus on anything. I was exhausted, but I was restless and anxious when I tried to sleep. Everything I ate went right through me. And I consider myself fortunate because these miserable periods of hyperthyroidism—among the worst times in my life healthwise—were temporary flares in a disease that otherwise has caused me to have an underactive, underfunctioning thyroid.

I have written this book for the millions for whom Graves' disease and hyperthyroidism is not a temporary flare—it's a permanent, debilitating condition that can force you to live in a chronic state of poor health if untreated. If you have yet to be diagnosed, you may be mistakenly told that you have panic disorder or bipolar disease. Your friends and family may even accuse you of being anorexic. And you may be going from doctor to doctor looking for answers. I hope you'll find the answers you need here.

I've also written this book for those who have been diagnosed and are looking for ways to understand the various treatments. It's not enough that radioactive iodine is the standard of care in the United States. You want to know whether there are options that are less drastic and less permanent, or even natural/alternative medicine options. Again, I hope you'll find the answers and support you need here. Finally, by bringing you the stories of the gracious patients who have shared their own experiences, as well as the innovative and compassionate doctors who have taken the time to provide input on their treatment approaches, I want you to have hope—hope in the realization that you are not alone and hope in a future of living well with Graves' disease and hyperthyroidism.

PART ONE

Understanding Graves' Disease and Hyperthyroidism

1

Your Thyroid, Graves' Disease, and Hyperthyroidism

■ What Is the Thyroid?

The word *thyroid* comes from the Greek word *thyreoeides,* meaning "shield-shaped." The two lobes of the thyroid are known as the "wings of the butterfly" and the area connecting the two lobes is known as the "isthmus." Generally speaking, a gland is a discrete and separate soft body made up of a large number of vessels that produce, store, and release—or secrete—some substance. The thyroid is a small gland normally weighing only about an ounce. It is located in the lower part of the neck in front of the windpipe. You'll know where the thyroid is if you think of it as sitting behind your Adam's apple.

Glands that secrete their products inside the body, and more specifically those that secrete hormonal and metabolic substances, are known as endocrine glands. This makes your thyroid an endocrine gland, along with the parathyroids, the adrenal gland, the pancreas, and the pituitary gland. Diabetes, like thyroid disease, is considered an endocrine disorder. A doctor who specializes in treating patients with endocrine problems is called an endocrinologist.

Hormones are internal secretions carried in the blood to various organs. Your thyroid's main purpose is to produce, store, and release two key thyroid hormones: triiodothyronine (T3) and thyroxine (T4). The numbers refer to the amount of iodine molecules attached to each hormone. Thyroid cells absorb iodine. The thyroid obtains iodine through food, iodized salt, and supplements, then combines it with the amino acid tyrosine, converting the iodine/tyrosine combination into T4 and T3.

A healthy, functioning gland produces about 80 percent T4 and 20 percent T3. T3 is, however, the biologically active hormone that is used by the cells and is several times stronger than T4. The body converts the inactive T4 it produces to active T3 by removing one iodine molecule. This process is sometimes referred to as T4 to T3 conversion, or by the more scientific term monodeiodination. This conversion can take place in organs other than the thyroid, including the hypothalamus, a part of your brain.

T4 and T3 exist in two forms: free/unbound and bound. Free or unbound T4 or T3 is biologically active, and the bound part is bound to the thyroxine-binding globulin (TBG) protein. When measured in the blood, the free or unbound T4 and T3 levels tend to be most representative of the actual hormone available for use by the body.

The role of thyroid hormones is to control your metabolism—the process by which oxygen and calories are converted to energy for use by your cells and organs. There's not a single cell in your body that doesn't depend on thyroid hormones for regulation and for energy in some form. Thyroid hormones have a number of functions as they travel through the bloodstream:

- Thyroid hormones help cells convert oxygen and calories into energy.
- Thyroid hormones help you properly process carbohydrates.

- Thyroid hormones aid in the proper functioning of your muscles.
- Thyroid hormones help your heart pump properly and effectively.
- Thyroid hormones help you breathe normally.
- Thyroid hormones help your intestinal system properly digest and eliminate food.
- Thyroid hormones help strengthen your hair, nails, and skin.
- Thyroid hormones help your brain function properly.
- Thyroid hormones help with proper sexual development and functioning.
- Thyroid hormones help with normal bone growth.

Now that you have some idea of what the thyroid is and its location and function, let's look in more detail at how it fits into the overall functioning of the body.

The Thyroid Gland: Setting the Pace

When your thyroid works normally, it produces and secretes the amount of T4 and T3 necessary to keep various bodily functions moving at their proper pace. However, the thyroid does not do this alone. It works as part of a bigger system that includes the pituitary gland—an endocrine gland located at the base of your brain—and the hypothalamus.

Here's how the system works. The hypothalamus constantly monitors the pace of many of the body's functions. It also observes and reacts to a number of other factors, including environmental conditions such as heat, cold, and stress. If the hypothalamus senses that certain adjustments are needed to react to any of these factors, it produces thyrotropin-releasing hormone (TRH).

TRH is sent from the hypothalamus to the pituitary gland. The pituitary gland then produces a substance called thyrotropin, better known as thyroid-stimulating hormone (TSH). The pituitary gland also monitors the body and can release TSH based on the thyroid hormones circulating in your blood. TSH is sent to the thyroid gland, where it causes your gland to produce, store, and release more T3 and T4.

Released thyroid hormones are carried through the bloodstream by a plasma protein known as thyroxine-binding globulin (TBG). Now in the bloodstream, the thyroid hormone travels throughout the body, carrying orders to various organs. Upon arriving at a particular tissue in the body, thyroid hormones interact with receptors located inside the nucleus of your cells. Interaction of the hormone and the receptor will trigger a certain function, giving directions to that tissue regarding the rate at which it should operate.

When the hypothalamus senses that the need for increased thyroid hormone production has ended, it reduces production of TRH, which causes the pituitary to decrease production of TSH, which then slows production of thyroid hormone. This system keeps many of the body's organs working at the proper pace.

Think of the entire feedback loop as resembling the thermostat in your house. It's set to maintain a particular temperature, and when it detects that your house has become too hot, it signals the heating system to stop blowing heat. Similarly, when the house becomes too cold, the heat will kick on (or the air conditioning will turn off). Like a thermostat set to a particular temperature, your body is wired to maintain a certain level of circulating thyroid hormone function. When thyroid disease or conditions interfere with the system and the feedback process doesn't work, thyroid problems can develop.

▌ The Prevalence of Thyroid Problems

Thyroid problems are widespread. It's estimated that more than 200 million people worldwide have thyroid disease. Thyroid problems are particularly common in areas covered at one time by glaciers, where iodine is not present in the soil and in foods. In many of these countries, an enlarged thyroid known as goiter is seen in as many as one in five people, and it is usually due to iodine deficiency. An estimated 8 percent of the world population has goiter, mostly women. Thyroid problems, including autoimmune thyroid disease and thyroid cancer, are also more common in the areas around and downwind of the 1986 Chernobyl nuclear accident.

There are a minimum of 25 million people in the United States with thyroid disease, and as many as half of them are undiagnosed. In the United States, thyroid disease prevalence increases with age: one in five women may develop a thyroid problem. Generally, women are seven times more likely than men to develop thyroid conditions.

It's thought that Graves' disease and hyperthyroidism affect slightly less than 1 percent of the U.S. population, or slightly less than 2.9 million people. Some experts believe, however, that as many as 4 percent of Americans, or 11.8 million people, may have mild, subclinical Graves' disease, with little or no symptoms but with blood test evidence of slight hyperthyroidism.

The prevalence of Graves' disease is similar among Caucasians and Asians, and it is slightly lower among African-Americans. Graves' disease and hyperthyroidism affect women eight times more often than men. Graves' disease accounts for more than 95 percent of childhood hyperthyroidism, so it's thought that the prevalence of Graves'/hyperthyroidism in children is approximately 0.02 percent. Children make up only 5 percent of all Graves' and hyperthyroidism patients.

The mortality rate for untreated Graves' disease and hyperthyroidism is as high as 11 percent. In the United States, however, going without treatment is extremely rare, and when death is associated with these conditions, it's primarily in the elderly and is typically due to related heart problems.

∎ Thyroid Conditions

There are a number of conditions that can affect the function and structure of the thyroid.

Hypothyroidism/Underactive Thyroid

Hypothyroidism means there is too little thyroid hormone. This can be due to a thyroid that is not producing enough hormone, treatment with radioactive iodine, drugs or nutritional deficiencies, or dysfunction due to nodules, infection, or atrophy. When the thyroid is partially or totally removed as a treatment for cancer, nodules, goiter, Graves' disease, or hyperthyroidism, the vast majority of patients become permanently hypothyroid. A small number of infants are born with congenital hypothyroidism—that is, either without a thyroid or with a nonfunctioning thyroid. Hypothyroidism is treated with thyroid hormone replacement drugs to provide the body with the thyroid hormone that the gland isn't able to produce.

Hyperthyroidism/Overactive Thyroid (Thyrotoxicosis)

Thyrotoxicosis refers to the various effects of exposure to too much thyroid hormone. Hyperthyroidism implies that this excess of hormones originated in the thyroid gland itself and not, for example, by taking too many thyroid hormone drugs. Hyperthyroidism can be caused by a number of thyroid problems, including autoimmune thyroid disease, nodules that produce thyroid hormone, overdosage of thyroid hormone replacement drugs, infection, and other causes. Hyperthyroidism is typically treated with drugs to reduce the thyroid's ability to produce hormones, by radioactive iodine treatment to chemically deactivate the thyroid (a treatment known as ablation), or by surgery.

Goiter/Enlargement

Goiter refers to an enlargement of the thyroid gland. The gland can grow as a response to deficiencies of iodine, thyroid inflammation or infection, or autoimmune disease. Particularly large goiters may be cosmetically unattractive and can compromise breathing and swallowing, so they are often surgically removed. Smaller goiters may respond to drug treatment.

Nodules/Lumps

Many people have nodules in the thyroid, but few are palpable (capable of being felt externally). In some cases, nodules on the thyroid exist without any disease and cause no symptoms. A very small percentage of nodules are cancerous, in which case the entire thyroid is usually surgically removed. The vast majority of nodules are benign; however, they may impair the thyroid's ability to function properly and may cause hypothyroidism, or they may themselves emit excess thyroid hormone and cause hyperthyroidism. Particularly large nodules that compromise breathing or swallowing are usually surgically removed. Smaller nodules frequently respond to drug treatment.

▎ Thyroid Diseases

A variety of diseases affect the thyroid and trigger thyroid conditions.

Autoimmune Thyroid Disease

There are two different autoimmune diseases in which an immune system dysfunction targets the thyroid: Graves' disease and Hashimoto's disease. In the United States, the vast majority of thyroid patients are either hypothyroid or hyperthyroid due to an autoimmune disease. Graves' disease—sometimes referred to as diffuse toxic goiter because of the usual presence of a goiter—typically causes hyperthyroidism. In Graves' disease, autoantibodies bind to the gland, which causes hyperthyroidism. Treatment usually involves antithyroid drugs, radioactive iodine ablation, or surgical removal of the thyroid, with the goal being euthyroidism—normal thyroid function—or hypothyroidism. Most Graves' disease patients end up hypothyroid over time, requiring lifelong thyroid hormone replacement.

Hashimoto's disease is the most common form of thyroiditis—an inflammation of the thyroid—so the condition is often referred to as Hashimoto's thyroiditis. It is far more common than Graves' disease and is the cause of most hypothyroidism in the United States. In Hashimoto's, antibodies react against proteins in the thyroid, causing gradual destruction of the gland itself. Before the thyroid is destroyed, it has occasional thyrotoxic periods known as Hashitoxicosis during which the thyroid overproduces thyroid hormone. Eventually, however, the gland's attack on itself destroys the ability to produce thyroid hormones. Typically, treatment involves lifelong thyroid hormone replacement.

Toxic Multinodular Goiter/Toxic Adenoma/Plummer's Disease

Toxic multinodular goiter, also known as toxic adenoma or Plummer's disease, describes a condition where the thyroid is enlarged and contains nodules that produce thyroid hormone, causing hyperthyroidism. Treatment usually involves antithyroid drugs, radioactive iodine ablation, or surgical removal of the thyroid. Most patients end up hypothyroid, requiring lifelong thyroid hormone replacement.

Thyroid Cancer

Thyroid cancer is one of the least common cancers in the United States. It is characterized by malignant nodules of the thyroid. Most cases are treatable with surgical removal of the gland, and patients have excellent long-term survival rates. Because the entire thyroid is usually removed, almost all thyroid cancer patients end up hypothyroid and need thyroid hormone replacement for the rest of their life.

Thyroiditis

While Hashimoto's disease is by far the most common form of thyroiditis, there are other forms that also involve inflammation of the thyroid gland:

- De Quervain's thyroiditis, granulomatous thyroiditis, painful thyroiditis, subacute thyroiditis: a viral-induced thyroiditis that can have a thyrotoxic phase
- Painless thyroiditis, silent thyroiditis, lymphocytic thyroiditis: a temporary thyroid condition that may involve mild hyperthyroidism during its thyrotoxic phase followed by a period of hypothyroidism before returning to normal
- Postpartum thyroiditis: a form of painless or "silent" thyroiditis that affects as many as 5 to 9 percent of women within a year of giving birth and typically starts with a thyrotoxic period of hyperthyroidism
- Acute suppurative thyroiditis: a rare situation where the thyroid is infected with bacteria and abscessed

▋ Thyrotoxicosis and Hyperthyroidism

Most doctors, except perhaps endocrinologists who specialize in thyroid treatment, tend to use the terms *hyperthyroidism* and *thyrotoxicosis* interchangeably, but this is not technically correct. Thyrotoxicosis refers to the various symptomatic and biochemical effects of exposure to too much thyroid hormone. In thyrotoxicosis, it doesn't matter whether the thyroid gland is the main source of that excess hormone or not.

In contrast, hyperthyroidism—which is a type of thyrotoxicosis—implies that the excess of thyroid hormone comes from overactivity of the thyroid gland itself. In hyperthyroidism, the thyroid synthesizes and releases thyroid hormone more quickly than normal. Dr. Glenn Rothfeld describes the idea of hyperthyroidism well in his book, *Thyroid Balance*, when he says that it's "like having a stuck accelerator in your car, continually flooding the engine with gasoline."

Causes of Thyrotoxicosis

Hyperthyroidism causes 85 to 90 percent of all thyrotoxicosis cases. Subsequently, almost all hyperthyroidism is caused by Graves' disease (also known as diffuse toxic goiter). The causes of hyperthyroidism and thyrotoxicosis are listed in the following table, and are explained in this chapter.

CAUSES OF THYROTOXICOSIS

Hyperthyroidism
(causes 85–90% of all thyrotoxicosis)

Thyrotoxicosis Causes Not Induced by Gland Overproduction
(cause 10–15% of all thyrotoxicosis)

- Graves' Disease (the primary cause of most hyperthyroidism)

- Toxic Multinodular Goiter/Toxic Adenoma/Plummer's Disease

- Toxic Adenoma/Autonomous Nodule

- De Quervain's Thyroiditis/Granulomatous Thyroiditis/Painful Thyroiditis/Subacute Thyroiditis

- Painless Thyroiditis/Silent Thyroiditis/Lymphocytic Thyroiditis

- Postpartum Thyroiditis

- Hashimoto's Disease/Hashitoxicosis

- Transient Hyperthyroidism of Hyperemesis Gravidarum (THHG)

- Trauma to the Thyroid

- Factitious Thyrotoxicosis/Thyrotoxicosis Faclitia/Iatrogenic Thyrotoxicosis

- Iodide-Induced Thyrotoxicosis/Jod-Basedow Syndrome

- Drugs

- Organ Donations

- Struma Ovarii

- Follicular Thyroid Cancer

- Pituitary Adenoma

- Molar Pregnancy/Choriocarcinoma/Human Chorionic Gonadotropin Elevation

▮ Graves' Disease and Other Causes of Hyperthyroidism

Graves' Disease/Diffuse Toxic Goiter

Graves' disease goes by a variety of names. In addition to diffuse toxic goiter, because goiter is almost always present in the condition, it's also known as toxic diffuse goiter and as exophthalmic goiter, in recognition of exophthalmos, an eye condition characterized by protrusion of the eyeballs and a characteristic staring expression, which is sometimes seen in Graves' disease patients.

Graves' disease was first identified by the British Dr. Caleb Parry in the 1780s, but it was named after the Irish doctor Robert Graves in the 1830s. Occasionally, however, you may see the condition referred to as Parry's disease in recognition of the earlier doctor's work. Dr. Baron Carl Adolph von Basedow studied the condition at length in the 1840s. Thus, in the non-English-speaking world, the names von Basedow's disease, Basedow's disease, or Graves-Basedow disease are more common, particularly in Germany as well as some other European and African countries.

Graves' disease is an autoimmune disease in which hyperthyroidism—an excess of thyroid hormone—is triggered by the presence of antibodies known as thyroid-stimulating immunoglobulins (TSIs). TSIs are sometimes called thyrotropin receptor antibodies (TRAb). These TSIs attach or bind themselves to and activate the gland's receptors for thyroid-stimulating hormone (TSH). In essence, they mimic the effects of TSH and cause the entire thyroid gland to enlarge (diffuse goiter). The thyroid follicles themselves increase their ability to synthesize and release thyroid hormone, so too much thyroid hormone is produced and circulates in the bloodstream.

TSH levels drop to low or undetectable levels because the pituitary and the hypothalamus sense that there is enough thyroid hormone circulating. But because TSI production is not part of the overall feedback loop, the thyroid is continually stimulated to produce more hormone. Therefore, T4 and T3 levels become extremely high and lead to thyrotoxicosis.

The antibodies seen in Graves' disease can also attack the eyes and the skin, causing two related conditions:

1. Infiltrative ophthalmopathy, also known as Graves' ophthalmopathy or thyroid eye disease, which can cause a protrusion or bulging of the eyeball, discomfort in the

eyes, and severe vision disturbances in the most serious cases

2. Infiltrative dermopathy (also known as Graves' dermopathy or pretibial myxedema), the primary symptom being a thickened patch of skin on the shins

The typical treatments for Graves' disease can include drugs such as antithyroid drugs, beta blockers, corticosteroids, blockade drugs, and in some cases, an antithyroid/thyroid hormone combination known as block replace therapy. Another treatment frequently used in the United States is thyroid ablation with radioactive iodine 131, a procedure known as RAI. Partial or complete surgical removal of the thyroid is also a treatment for Graves' disease that resolves the condition quickly. Ultimately, though, there is no cure. Like other autoimmune diseases, the exact cause is still being researched, so treatments focus on eliminating the symptoms, including hyperthyroidism.

Toxic Multinodular Goiter/Plummer's Disease

In the United States, toxic multinodular goiter (or multinodular toxic goiter) is the second most common cause of hyperthyroidism after Graves' disease. In areas where iodine deficiency is a problem, it is often the primary cause of hyperthyroidism. Because the condition was initially described by Henry Plummer in 1913, it is also referred to as Plummer's disease. Toxic multinodular goiter involves multiple nodules that have usually developed over many years, and once the nodules reach a certain size, the follicles begin to produce thyroid hormone on their own. The condition is more common in older people, particularly those with a longstanding goiter. Because of the slow onset of symptoms, it may be harder to diagnose, and subtle development of symptoms may be overlooked or attributed to other causes.

Toxic multinodular goiter can be treated with antithyroid drug therapy, but lifelong treatment may be required. Surgery can be immediately effective in resolving the condition. Some doctors also recommend RAI, but a higher dose than is typically given for Graves' disease patients may be needed.

Toxic Adenoma/Autonomous Nodule

A toxic adenoma is also known as an autonomously functioning thyroid nodule (AFTN). It is typically a single palpable nodule that gets to a point where it produces thyroid hormone on its own separate from the thyroid's own production. When the nodule produces enough thyroid hormone to suppress TSH levels, it is labeled toxic. Nodules that are toxic are rarely cancerous; rather, they are almost always benign adenomas.

Toxic nodules rarely go away on their own. Antithyroid drugs can be used as a treatment, but they may have to be taken for the rest of the patient's life. Surgery can be immediately effective in resolving the condition. Some doctors also recommend RAI. Finally, ablation of the nodule with percutaneous ethanol injection (PEI) is a safe and effective treatment, although it is not widely used. One or two injections of alcohol are given per week for a total of three to six injections per nodule. Many doctors in the United States are not familiar with this easy-to-perform technique. Research has shown that PEI is an appropriate therapy for most toxic adenomas less than 13 milliliters in volume. The size of the nodule is the primary determinant of PEI's success.

De Quervain's Thyroiditis/Granulomatous Thyroiditis/Painful Thyroiditis/Subacute Thyroiditis—Thyrotoxic Phase

De Quervain's thyroiditis, also known as granulomatous thyroiditis or painful thyroiditis, results from a viral infection of the thyroid gland. Sometimes also called subacute thyroiditis, this condition was first reported in 1825, but it was recorded in detail by De

Quervain in the early 1900s. De Quervain's thyroiditis usually starts out as a flu, cold, or upper respiratory infection, which then shifts to pain, tenderness, and swelling in the neck, jaw, and thyroid area, along with fever. Initially, it often triggers a 4- to 10-week period of hyperthyroidism as excess thyroid hormone is released into the bloodstream after the virus attacks the thyroid. Later, the thyroid may return to normal or shift into another 4- to 10-week period of hyperthyroidism.

De Quervain's thyroiditis is most common in temperate climates and occurs more often during the summer and fall. The condition tends to follow viral epidemics, including mumps, measles, influenza, adenovirus, mononucleosis, myocarditis, cat scratch fever, and Coxsackie virus.

Some patients with mild pain and few symptoms do not require any treatment. Those with some hyperthyroid-related symptoms are usually treated with beta blockers, nonsteroidal antiinflammatory drugs (NSAIDs) such as aspirin or ibuprofen, and in severe cases, a short course of corticosteroids to reduce inflammation may be given. Thyroid hormone may be prescribed to help the gland rest.

Painless Thyroiditis/Silent Thyroiditis/Lymphocytic Thyroiditis—Thyrotoxic Phase

Painless thyroiditis, also known as silent thyroiditis or lymphocytic thyroiditis, is fairly rare and involves a slight enlargement of the thyroid gland. The symptoms are similar to Graves' disease, but they do not involve any eye symptoms and the thyroid is usually only slightly enlarged. The thyroid is not tender to the touch or painful. Periods of slight hyperthyroidism may be followed by hypothyroidism, but usually the thyroid returns to normal function within 3 months.

Painless thyroiditis usually needs no treatment. It is estimated that 80 percent of patients return to normal thyroid function fairly quickly. During the hyperthyroid phase, however, beta blockers may be given to help alleviate heart rate and anxiety-like symptoms. The second phase is typically a hypothyroid phase that may last several months. Treatment for this stage is with thyroid hormone replacement drugs. Typically, patients are taken off the drugs after a few months to see if thyroid function has returned to normal, which it will for most patients. A small percentage of patients become permanently hypothyroid and need to be on lifelong thyroid hormone replacement.

Postpartum Thyroiditis—Thyrotoxic Phase

Postpartum thyroiditis is a form of silent thyroiditis that develops in 5 to 9 percent of women within a year of having given birth. The condition usually follows a pattern similar to painless thyroiditis, with a period of hypothyroidism followed by hyperthyroidism, followed by a return to normal function within 6 months. This condition is often mistaken for postpartum anxiety or depression.

As with painless thyroiditis, postpartum thyroiditis doesn't typically require treatment unless symptoms are particularly problematic. In that case, beta blockers may be given during the thyrotoxic phase and thyroid hormone replacement may be prescribed during the hypothyroid phase. Patients should be taken off the drugs after a few months to see if thyroid function has returned to normal, which it will for the majority of people with postpartum thyroiditis. A small percentage of patients, however, do become permanently hypothyroid and need to remain on lifelong thyroid hormone replacement.

Hashimoto's Disease—Thyrotoxic Phase/Hashitoxicosis

Hashitoxicosis occurs when someone with the autoimmune condition Hashimoto's disease experiences sporadic periods of hyperthyroidism. As thyroid cells are destroyed in the autoimmune process, stored supplies of thyroid hormone may be rapidly released into the bloodstream, triggering these periods of hyperthyroidism.

They are often followed by a return to the more common hypothyroidism of Hashimoto's disease. Patients with this disease can go in and out of these hyperthyroid periods over the course of months or even years as their thyroid is slowly destroyed.

According to holistic physician Dr. Richard Shames, author of *Thyroid Power,*

> *Some people who are diagnosed with Graves' disease instead are in the temporary "hyper" phase of Hashimoto's hypothyroidism. These folks should be treated very differently than the typical Graves' hyperthyroidism patients. It's amazing how many medical doctors don't make this distinction, not realizing that Hashimoto's can be a cause of hyperthyroidism.*

Hashitoxicosis is frequently mistaken for Graves' disease because some doctors diagnose and treat hyperthyroidism without running antibody tests that could establish underlying Hashimoto's disease.

Transient Hyperthyroidism of Hyperemesis Gravidarum (THHG)

Some women who are pregnant and have severe morning sickness (hyperemesis gravidarum) develop hyperthyroidism. Usually, this happens only when vomiting is severe and substantial weight loss occurs. This short-term hyperthyroidism, known as transient hyperthyroidism of hyperemesis gravidarum (THHG), is accompanied by nausea and vomiting, along with other typical hyperthyroidism symptoms such as rapid heart rate and anxiety. Weight loss is usually noticeable, and due to dehydration these women may need to be hospitalized to receive intravenous fluids. Antithyroid drugs are usually given to treat this temporary hyperthyroidism. They can often be discontinued, since thyroid levels will probably return to normal before delivery.

Trauma to the Thyroid

Trauma to the thyroid can trigger a transient inflammatory reaction that results in a temporary period of hyperthyroidism. Trauma can include vigorous manipulation of the thyroid, strong palpation, surgery to the surrounding area, biopsy of the thyroid, and neck injury such as whiplash or injury from an automobile seat belt after a crash.

Many practitioners are not aware of trauma-induced hyperthyroidism. But the thyroid should be checked whenever there are hyperthyroidism symptoms after trauma. Because this problem would likely be fairly transient and quickly resolved, treatment may not be required. If symptoms are troublesome, treatment would typically include beta blockers, nonsteroidal antiinflammatory drugs (NSAIDs) such as aspirin or ibuprofen, and a short course of corticosteroids to reduce inflammation in severe cases.

■ Other Causes of Thyrotoxicosis

Factitious Thyrotoxicosis/Thyrotoxicosis Factitia/ Iatrogenic Thyrotoxicosis

This type of thyrotoxicosis results from taking too much prescription thyroid medication; or taking natural thyroid found in over-the-counter energy or diet supplements or over-the-counter glandular and thyroid support supplements; or consuming actual thyroid gland of animals.

Some patients accidentally take too much prescription thyroid medications due to physician or pharmacist error or mistakes in their own self-administration of drugs. Some patients deliberately take too much thyroid hormone in an effort to resolve symptoms or to lose weight. Others take over-the-counter pills or supplements without being aware of their thyroid content.

There are rare cases of factitious thyrotoxicosis developing from overexposure to improperly butchered meat and game. Meat from the thyroid gland and thyroid area may be accidentally mixed in to ground meat. This condition is sometimes referred to as hamburger thyrotoxicosis.

Treatment for factitious thyrotoxicosis is usually quite simple. The prescription thyroid drug dosage is calibrated to maintain normal thyroid levels. Of course, patients should stop taking the suspect supplements and stop eating any suspect meat. If symptoms are severe, antithyroid medications and beta blockers may be necessary for a short time until the excess iodine in the system has been eliminated.

Iodide-Induced Thyrotoxicosis/Jod-Basedow Syndrome

Iodide-induced thyrotoxicosis is also known as Jod-Basedow syndrome. This condition involves thyrotoxicosis triggered by an overdose of iodine that is usually due to a medical test using iodine contrast dye, exposure to topical antiseptics such as povidone-iodine, use of the heart drug amiodarone, overconsumption of iodine drops or supplements, or herbal remedies and foods that contain iodine such as kelp, bladder wrack, and seaweeds. In these situations, the thyroid is for some reason unable to adapt to the excess of iodine. This condition is more common in people who have an autonomous nodule or adenoma. Treatment consists of stopping excess iodine intake. Antithyroid medications and beta blockers may be necessary for a short time until iodine levels return to normal.

▌ Miscellaneous Causes

Drugs

The following drugs may cause thyrotoxicosis and hyperthyroid symptoms:

- Immunosuppressants
- Antiretroviral therapy for AIDS
- Interferon beta-1b and interleukin-4 (when used therapeutically, they may cause Graves' disease)
- Monoclonal antibody treatment for multiple sclerosis

Organ Donations

There are sporadic reports in the medical literature of people receiving donor organs from people with Graves' disease who then later develop the disease themselves.

Struma Ovarii

Struma ovarii is thyroid tissue located outside the thyroid that is linked to benign tumors in the skin or ovary. While rare, struma ovarii can give off excess thyroid hormone and cause thyrotoxicosis.

Follicular Thyroid Cancer

While it's not common, metastatic follicular thyroid cancer tissue can in some cases produce thyroid hormone and can cause thyrotoxicosis in patients with larger tumors.

Pituitary Adenoma

Pituitary adenomas are benign tumors of the pituitary gland that secrete TSH. While the thyroid is overproducing thyroid hormone, TSH remains high because it's being secreted by the adenoma. These tumors are quite rare, but they can be fairly aggressive and invasive. Diagnosis is usually made by blood testing, magnetic resonance imaging (MRI), and a computerized tomography (CT) scan of the pituitary without and with contrast agents. The treatment is almost always transsphenoidal surgical removal. This type of surgery goes through the sphenoid sinus in the space behind the nose. The incision may be made in the back of the nose, the front of the nasal septum, or under the lip and through the upper gum to enter the nasal cavity and sphenoid sinus. Particularly invasive and/or very large tumors may require further treatment, including radioactive iodine (RAI) to ablate the thyroid and/or stereotactic radiation therapy to the pituitary gland. In stereotactic radiation (or radiosurgery), a relatively high dose of focused radiation is delivered precisely to the pituitary adenoma in one surgical treatment session.

Molar Pregnancy/Choriocarcinoma/Human Chorionic Gonadotropin Elevation

In a molar pregnancy, sometimes called a hydatidiform mole, the sperm fertilizes an empty egg. Although no baby is formed, the placenta still grows and produces the pregnancy hormone human chorionic gonadotropin (HCG). Choriocarcinoma is a cancer that originates in cells of the placenta; these cells also typically produce HCG. The high levels of HCG associated with molar pregnancy and choriocarcinoma can activate the TSH receptor to the extent that thyrotoxicosis may occur. A positive pregnancy test and/or history of molar pregnancy may be signs of this condition. Typically, the thyrotoxicosis will resolve with complete treatment of the molar pregnancy or choriocarcinoma.

▌ Related Conditions

Graves' Ophthalmopathy

Graves' ophthalmopathy is an inflammatory autoimmune eye disorder often seen in conjunction with Graves' disease. (Besides Graves' disease patients, it can develop in a small percentage of people with Hashimoto's disease and in some people with normal thyroid function but with Graves' antibodies.)

Graves' ophthalmopathy is also known by a variety of other names, including thyroid eye disease (TED), thyroid-associated ophthalmopathy (TAO), thyroid-associated orbitopathy, orbital dystrophy (OD), dysthyroid orbitopathy, thyroid ophthalmopathy, exophthalmos, immune exophthalmos, Graves' orbitopathy, and Graves' eye disease.

Graves' ophthalmopathy is most likely to develop within the first 18 months after the onset of Graves' disease, but in some people it develops years later. Smoking increases the risk of Graves' ophthalmopathy. It may also cause symptoms to become more severe, the condition to become more resistant to treatment, and the chance of relapse after treatment to increase.

Some 75 to 90 percent of people with Graves' ophthalmopathy have a milder form of the disease, so treatment primarily involves comfort measures such as lubricating the eyes, wearing sunglasses, and using prism lenses. Among those with Graves' ophthalmopathy, an estimated 5 percent have particularly severe symptoms. The more severe the case, the more likely it is that corticosteroid drugs, radiation, immunosuppressant drugs, and surgery will be required in order to resolve vision problems, restore appearance, or in rare cases, preserve sight. Graves' ophthalmopathy is discussed at greater length in chapter 7.

Thyroid Storm

Thyroid storm is a rare complication of Graves' disease and/or hyperthyroidism, affecting only 1 to 2 percent of patients who are hyperthyroid. Thyroid storm, which is also known as thyrotoxic crisis or thyrotoxic storm, is a life-threatening condition in which the effects of thyroid hormone suddenly become extremely potent and cause a variety of dangerous temperature, heart, and blood pressure fluctuations in the body. It can be triggered by a variety of situations, including:

- Infection: lung infection, throat infection, or pneumonia
- Blood sugar changes: diabetic ketoacidosis, insulin-induced hypoglycemia

- Surgery to the thyroid
- Abrupt withdrawal of antithyroid medications
- Radioactive iodine (RAI) ablation of the thyroid
- Excessive palpation of the thyroid
- Severe emotional stress
- Thyroid hormone overdose
- Toxemia of pregnancy and labor

Thyroid storm can involve life threatening high fever, high heart rate, and elevated blood pressure that often comes on quickly. If not treated, it can result in death within hours.

With treatment, the condition has a 60 to 70 percent survival rate. Without treatment, the mortality rate is higher than 50 percent. Treatment for thyroid storm usually involves intravenous antithyroid drugs to help calm the thyroid, beta blockers and other drugs to help stabilize the heart and blood pressure, and drugs for fever (but not aspirin, because it can increase thyroid hormone levels). Intravenous fluids are commonly given to treat dehydration.

2

Risks, Signs, and Symptoms

In addition to some of the causes of thyrotoxicosis, Graves' disease, and hyperthyroidism that were discussed in the previous chapter, it's important to take a look at the more specific risk factors, triggers, and symptoms of these conditions. Having one or even many of these risk factors, triggers, or symptoms does not necessarily mean you have Graves' disease and/or hyperthyroidism now or will develop it in the future. But if you suspect you might have a thyroid condition, a review of the various risk factors can be an important diagnostic clue. Or if you have been diagnosed and are trying to manage your condition, you may find some helpful information to help minimize your risks and triggers or recognize unexpected symptoms. This information is also summarized in an easy-to-use checklist in chapter 3 that you can photocopy and fill out to bring to your doctor to aid in diagnosing and managing your condition.

∎ Risk Factors

Gender

The main risk factor for Graves' disease is being female. As noted earlier, Graves' disease and hyperthyroidism affect women eight times more often than men.

Personal History

Having any past history of thyroid problems, autoimmune disease, or endocrine disease puts you at greater risk for developing Graves' disease and hyperthyroidism. In the case of thyroid disease, doctors may have told you that they were monitoring your thyroid because blood test results were inconclusive or borderline. Your doctor might have diagnosed a goiter or nodule but decided it didn't warrant treatment. You may not even remember that years ago you took thyroid hormone for a short period. Many people have a brief episode of thyroid trouble after a pregnancy or an illness, with a diagnosis of transient, or temporary, thyroiditis. Past thyroid problems increase your chances of eventually developing Graves' disease and hyperthyroidism.

If you currently have or had any other autoimmune disease, you are at greater risk for Graves' disease and hyperthyroidism. There is no fail-safe statistic that determines your increased risk, but having an autoimmune disease tends to cause further imbalances, leaving you at greater risk of developing Graves' disease or other conditions that lead to hyperthyroidism.

A past history of endocrine diseases raises your risk of developing Graves' disease and hyperthyroidism. Some of the most common endocrine conditions besides thyroid disease include:

- Adrenal diseases such as Addison's, Cushing's, Turner's syndrome, adrenal insufficiency, and pheochromocytoma
- Pancreatic diseases such as diabetes, hypoglycemia, insulin resistance, metabolic syndrome, and juvenile diabetes

- Pituitary diseases such as acromegaly and prolactinoma
- Parathyroid conditions such as hyperparathyroidism
- Bone conditions such as osteoporosis
- Sex hormone–related conditions such as polycystic ovary syndrome, premature menopause, infertility, and menstrual disorders
- Growth hormone–related conditions such as dwarfism

Family History

Research has found that if an identical twin has Graves' disease, there is about a 50 percent chance that the other twin will also develop the condition. In fraternal twins, the risk drops to 30 percent. If your brother or sister has Graves' disease, you have a 4 to 13 percent chance of also developing this condition.

Any past or present history of thyroid conditions in your family also raises your risk for a thyroid condition. Approximately 15 percent of people with Graves' disease have a close relative with it. And 40 percent of those with first-degree relatives (parents, siblings, children) with Graves' disease who themselves test positive for thyroid antibodies will go on to develop various thyroid conditions.

If you are a woman, your risk is greater if you have family members with thyroid conditions. One study found that among those with first-degree female relatives with Hashimoto's and Graves' diseases, 30 to 50 percent had thyroid autoantibodies. The presence of these antibodies increases the risk of developing autoimmune thyroid conditions.

If you have first-degree relatives or grandparents with a history of autoimmune conditions, you are at greater risk of developing autoimmune disease as well, including Graves' disease, which is one of the most prevalent autoimmune conditions. There isn't a direct cause and effect relationship between genetics and autoimmune disease. There is no way to directly calculate the risk of having a child with a particular autoimmune disease, for example. A family history means that you are more likely to also have an autoimmune disease, but rather than inheriting a specific condition, you inherit a higher risk of developing autoimmune diseases in general.

There are eight core autoimmune diseases that appear to have strong genetic interrelationships with each other and are being extensively studied: rheumatoid arthritis, juvenile rheumatoid arthritis, systemic lupus, multiple sclerosis, autoimmune thyroid disease (including Graves' disease), type 1 diabetes, psoriasis, and inflammatory bowel disease.

Age

While the conditions can occur anytime, the riskiest ages for developing Graves' disease and hyperthyroidism are between 20 and 40. These diseases are rare in children, who make up only 5 percent of those with these conditions.

Pregnancy

Pregnancy is a risk factor for Graves' disease and hyperthyroidism for several reasons. First, transient hyperthyroidism of hyperemesis gravidarum (THHG) can occur in some women who have severe vomiting and weight loss in pregnancy. Next, having had a baby in the past 12 months means that you are at risk of a variety of thyroid conditions, including postpartum thyroiditis and Graves' disease. Some doctors estimate that up to 8 percent of women have postpartum thyroiditis that causes hyperthyroidism. Most of these women have never had a thyroid problem in the past.

Five weeks after having delivered her third child at age 33 and having felt great since the delivery, Karla said she woke up and couldn't raise her body from the bed:

I felt like a truck had run me down. My husband had to pull me up into a sitting position. I had no energy or strength. I could not lie down during the day, as I could not gather any

*strength to get myself up. The following week, I went to my
OB-GYN for my 6-week checkup. When I described my
symptoms, he ordered a thyroid test. The tests came back in
the hyperactive range.*

Finally, suspected pregnancy, as evidenced by a positive pregnancy test, may be a risk factor for hyperthyroidism. If you are not
pregnant, the elevated HCG level that the test is picking up as evidence of pregnancy may be a sign of either a molar pregnancy or a
type of placental cancer known as choriocarcinoma. In both situations, the high level of HCG pregnancy hormone can trigger periods
of hyperthyroidism.

Smoking

If you are or were a smoker, you have an increased risk of
Graves' disease and hyperthyroidism, particularly, Graves' ophthalmopathy. Smokers with Graves' ophthalmopathy tend to have more
severe symptoms that are more resistant to treatment.

Researchers analyzed studies on the connections between smoking and thyroid disorders. They found that cigarettes contain thio-
cyanate, a chemical that adversely affects the thyroid gland. The
health risks are greater for women. Smoking cessation decreases the
risk for Graves' disease.

Excessive Intake of Thyroid Hormone

As described in chapter 1, excessive intake of thyroid hormone
can trigger thyrotoxicosis. You can end up with too much thyroid
hormone via a number of ways. First, you may be taking too much
prescription thyroid hormone replacement medicine. This can be
due to an error by you, your physician, or pharmacist. Some people,
however, intentionally self-medicate in an attempt to relieve symptoms or lose weight. Access to offshore pharmacies that do not require prescriptions also means that some people purchase and take

prescription thyroid medications without a doctor's oversight and may run the risk of overmedicating themselves.

Next, you may take an excess of over-the-counter energy supplements, diet supplements, glandular supplements, or thyroid support supplements, not realizing that some of these products contain actual animal thyroid glandular derivatives. This animal thyroid can act like prescription thyroid medication. The actual amounts of thyroid in these substances is usually unknown and is not indicated on labels, so you can easily take too much.

In the 1980s, there was an epidemic of thyrotoxicosis in the Midwest because a batch of hamburger meat had been contaminated with cow thyroid glands during butchering by a process called gullet trimming, where meat is taken from the area around the animal's larynx, which can include thyroid tissue. Eating the hamburgers delivered high amounts of thyroid, resulting in some consumers coming down with symptoms of hyperthyroidism. There are other cases where improperly butchered game such as deer has been associated with thyrotoxicosis when thyroid tissue was inadvertently included in the butchered meat.

Doctors in Canada were puzzled by one woman who had periods of hyperthyroidism over an 11-year period. She did not have thyroid antibodies and did not take thyroid medications or supplements. The mystery was explained, however, when it was discovered that her husband periodically slaughtered a cow on the farm where they lived and their butcher was unaware of prohibitions against gullet trimming. The woman made hamburgers from the stored ground meat, and over time, she became hyperthyroid. Although gullet trimming has been prohibited in all cattle and pork processing plants, it is still possible to develop thyrotoxicosis by eating improperly butchered farm animals or game from hunting.

Exposure to or Excess of Iodine/Iodine Drugs

Being exposed to or ingesting an excess of iodine can sometimes trigger thyrotoxicosis. This condition is occasionally referred to as Jod-Basedow syndrome or Jod-Basedow phenomenon.

You may have a history of thyroid disease, thyroid nodules, or no thyroid history at all, but for some reason exposure or overexposure to iodine triggers an episode of hyperthyroidism. Sometimes medical tests are the trigger; you may have had an x-ray or a scan that used iodine contrast dye, or you may have had a medical procedure where a topical antiseptic such as povidone or iodine was used. These situations might trigger a hyperthyroid episode fairly quickly after the test or procedure.

Judith, a woman in her 30s going through a period of thyrotoxicosis, discovered her thyrotoxicosis was triggered by iodine:

My first symptoms showed up about two weeks after a gynecological procedure where an iodine solution was used to cleanse the vagina. I did not associate the two until much later.

One particularly well-known link is the risk of iodine-induced hyperthyroidism from the drug amiodarone, which contains iodine and is used to treat heart arrhythmia. Amiodarone therapy is known to cause thyroid problems, including thyrotoxicosis, in 14 to 18 percent of people taking it. Before starting amiodarone, you should ideally have baseline thyroid function tests. If you take the drug, you should have thyroid testing done every 4 to 6 months. Some practitioners recommend discontinuing amiodarone if you beome hyperthyroid, but in some cases doctors will have you continue amiodarone while also prescribing antithyroid drugs and glucocorticoids. Once your thyroid is normalized, if you need to continue taking amiodarone or you need to restart it, the majority of doctors recommend that you have RAI to ablate the thyroid and to prevent recurrence of thyrotoxicosis.

In addition to straight iodine supplementation, which you can get via iodine tablets or solution, you can also get too much iodine from a variety of supplements. Be on the lookout for these ingredients in thyroid support supplements, diet and weight-loss formulas, energy formulas, fat fighters, carb blockers, cellulite remedies, and other formulas:

- Bladder wrack *(Fucus vesiculosus)*
- Bugleweed
- Kelp
- Norwegian kelp
- Kelp fronds
- Irish moss
- Seaweed

Cellasene, a discontinued dietary supplement that included iodine-rich bladder wrack extract, was touted as a solution for cellulite. The warning label for Cellasene indicated that it shouldn't be used by thyroid patients. I received a number of reports from people who said they had taken the prescribed dosage for 8 weeks as recommended on the packaging, then developed symptoms of Graves' disease and hyperthyroidism. One woman said her doctor had seen several people who developed Graves' within weeks or several months of starting Cellasene. Most of the patients I heard from used antithyroid drugs for several months and returned to normal thyroid function.

Eating large amounts of seaweed has occasionally been known to trigger hyperthyroidism in some people.

Medical/Drug Treatments

Some of the medical treatments known to trigger Graves' disease and/or thyrotoxicosis include:

- Interferon beta-1b and interleukin-4.
- Immunosuppressant therapy.
- Antiretroviral treatment for AIDS.
- Monoclonal antibody (Campath-1H) therapy for multiple sclerosis—a third of patients receiving this treatment develop Graves' disease within 6 months.
- Organ donation—receiving a donated organ or a bone marrow transplant can be a risk factor for Graves' disease, as the antibodies and lymphocytes can potentially be transferred with the organ or marrow.
- Lithium—although lithium is usually linked to hypothyroidism, some patients become hyperthyroid.

Drugs that cause increased TSH production and may cause hyperthyroidism include:

- Amphetamines.
- Cimetidine/ranitidine (Tagamet/Zantac) for ulcer treatment.
- Clomiphene (Clomid) for fertility treatments.
- L-dopa inhibitors such as chlorpromazine (Thorazine) and haloperidol (Haldol) for psychotic disorders.
- Metoclopramide (Reglan) and domperidone (Motilium) for nausea/vomiting.
- Glucocorticoids/adrenal steroids such as prednisone and hydrocortisone.
- Propranolol, a beta blocker.
- Aminoglutethimide for breast and prostate cancer treatment.

- Ketoconazole, an antifungal.
- Para-aminosalicylic acid, a tuberculosis drug.
- Sulfonamide drugs, including sulfadiazine, sulfisoxazole, and acetazolamide, which have been used as diuretics and antibiotics.
- Sulfonylureas, including tolbutamide and chlorpropamide, which are used to treat diabetes.
- Raloxifene (Evista) for osteoporosis.
- Carbamazepine, oxcarbazepine, and valproate for epilepsy.

Recent History of Hyperthyroidism-Inducing Conditions

As discussed in chapter 1, a number of conditions and diseases can cause thyrotoxicosis or hyperthyroidism, and a recent diagnosis of any of these conditions should be considered a risk factor:

- Struma ovarii
- Follicular thyroid cancer
- Pituitary adenoma
- Molar pregnancy
- Choriocarcinoma

Nuclear Exposure

Nuclear plants can accidentally release radioactive materials that are damaging to the thyroid. If you lived in or were visiting the area near the Chernobyl plant during or in the weeks after the nuclear accident on April 26, 1986, then you are at an increased risk for thyroid problems. The main countries at risk include Belarus, the Russian Federation, and the Ukraine. There is a reduced risk to Poland, Austria, Denmark, Finland, Germany, Greece, and Italy. You may have also been exposed to potentially thyroid-damaging radioactive materials if you lived near or in the area downwind from the former nuclear weapons plant at Hanford in south central Washington State during the 1940s through 1960s, particularly

1955 to 1965. Hanford released radioactive materials that can cause autoimmune thyroid disease.

During the 1950s and 1960s, approximately one hundred nuclear bomb tests were conducted at the Nevada nuclear test site northwest of Las Vegas. The fallout from the tests was most concentrated in counties of western states located east and north of the test site, such as Utah, Idaho, Montana, Colorado, and Missouri. Exposure to this fallout increases the risk of thyroid cancer, particularly in the Farm Belt, where children drank fallout-contaminated milk. There are also cases of autoimmune thyroid problems in the United States that may be due to the iodine-131 released during these nuclear tests.

In the late 1990s, the newspaper the *Tennessean* presented the results of an effort to investigate a mysterious pattern of illnesses including autoimmune thyroid problems that seem to have been concentrated around the Oak Ridge nuclear facility in eastern Tennessee. According to the newspaper, this same pattern was evident at other nuclear facilities in Tennessee, Colorado, South Carolina, New Mexico, Idaho, New York, California, Ohio, Kentucky, Texas, and Washington State.

Infection

Viral infection has been implicated as a trigger for various types of thyroiditis that can cause thyrotoxicosis. The viral illnesses most often identified as triggers include upper respiratory infections, colds, influenza, mumps, measles, adenovirus, mononucleosis, myocarditis, cat scratch fever, and Coxsackie virus. Symptoms of infection frequently include right-sided abdominal pain and fever, and a small percentage of people will have skin rash, joint pains, and arthritic-like symptoms.

There is a strong relationship between *Yersinia enterocolitica* infection and thyroiditis. *Yersinia enterocolitica* bacteria are found in the fecal matter of livestock, domesticated animals, and wild animals. You can be exposed to these bacteria via contaminated meats, especially raw or undercooked products, poultry, unpasteurized milk and dairy products, seafood (particularly oysters) from sewage-contaminated waters, and produce fertilized with raw manure. Foods can also be contaminated by food handlers who have not properly washed their hands before touching food or utensils. Improper storage can contribute to contamination.

Measuring antibodies against the bacteria, one research study found that evidence of *Yersinia enterocolitica* infection in thyroid patients was highest in Graves' disease patients, followed by Hashimoto's thyroiditis patients. The researchers concluded that this bacterial infection may be a trigger of Graves' disease.

Trauma

Some research has suggested that trauma to the thyroid or neck area can result in thyrotoxicosis or thyroiditis. Researchers speculate that this may be due to injury to and subsequent inflammation of the thyroid tissues themselves. The types of trauma that have been linked to thyrotoxicosis include:

- Recent vigorous manipulation of the thyroid
- Recent vigorous palpation of the thyroid
- Recent surgery to the thyroid, parathyroids, or the area surrounding the thyroid
- Recent biopsy of the thyroid
- Recent neck injury such as whiplash or a seat belt injury from a car accident
- Recent injection to the thyroid—for example, percutaneous ethanol injection (PEI)

Allergies/Sensitivities

Allergies are a risk factor and may be a trigger for Graves' disease. One study looked at a group of patients with Graves' disease in remission, evaluating a smaller group among them who had seasonal allergies to tree pollen. After exposure to the pollen, the patients with allergies all developed allergic rhinitis, which was then followed by notable increases in levels of two types of antibodies: antithyroid peroxidase and antithyroglobulin autoantibodies. Those patients without allergies did not have fluctuations in these antibodies. Researchers concluded that seasonal allergies could worsen and aggravate Graves' disease.

Another risk factor is sensitivity or full intolerance to gluten, which is found in most wheat and many grain products. The condition is known as celiac disease or gluten intolerance. Gluten is a known trigger of autoimmune diseases and is linked to autoimmune thyroid problems in particular. Interestingly, people with autoimmune disease are 10 to 30 times more likely than the general public to also have celiac disease or gluten intolerance, and it's thought that having celiac disease increases the risk of developing other autoimmune disorders such as type 1 diabetes, autoimmune thyroid, and other endocrine diseases. In some patients, treating the celiac disease with a gluten-free diet has actually restored thyroid antibody levels to normal, eliminating the resulting thyroid problem.

In addition to gluten, other food allergies and sensitivities are thought to create a propensity for autoimmune disease development, including Graves' disease. It's believed that the constant irritation caused by exposure to an allergen inflames the intestinal lining. Ultimately, that lining becomes permeable and a condition known as leaky gut develops. With leaky gut, the inflammation permits larger molecules and proteins that normally would not be antigenic to pass through the intestinal lining and directly into the bloodstream, where they are perceived as invaders and trigger an autoimmune reaction.

Toxic/Environmental Exposures

According to Dr. Noel Rose, the nation's leading expert on autoimmunity, overexposure to mercury, gold, cadmium, and other heavy metals can induce autoantibodies and has been linked to autoimmune disease. Some practitioners point to mercury exposure in particular—via mercury dental fillings and consumption of mercury-contaminated fish—as a potent trigger for autoimmune conditions including Graves' disease.

While there is agreement that consumption of mercury-laden fish should be limited, the issue of mercury toxicity from dental fillings is controversial because conventional dentists maintain that these fillings are entirely safe. Dental amalgam containing mercury is used extensively in tooth fillings. According to the American Dental Association, up to 76 percent of dentists in a 1995 survey said they use it as their primary restoration material.

Aspartame

Nutritionist Edward Bauman, PhD, is an expert in food/disease interactions. Dr. Bauman is particularly concerned about the artificial sweetener aspartame. He feels that aspartame is a particular problem for thyroid health and can specifically contribute to hyperthyroidism.

The aspartame concerns are definitely controversial. While the Food and Drug Administration (FDA) and manufacturers maintain that the product is safe, there are accusations that accurate data have not been made available to the public regarding testing and side effects. H. J. Roberts, MD, FACP, FCCP, has studied aspartame extensively and published research on the topic. According to Dr. Roberts:

> The consumption of products containing aspartame (Nutra-Sweet) by health-conscious persons, coupled with a marked decrease of caloric intake and excessive physical activity, may trigger primary hyperthyroidism (Graves' disease). The cases of two biologically unrelated step-sisters are reported, along with another patient. These individuals also complained of other symptoms frequently experienced by aspartame reac-

tors. Comparable complaints occurred in four additional persons previously treated for Graves' disease who then consumed aspartame. Physicians should interrogate patients with recent Graves' disease about aspartame consumption. They ought to be observed for a possible spontaneous remission after stopping these products before recommending radioiodine treatment or surgery. Similarly, the occurrence of unexplained palpitations, tachycardia, "anxiety attacks," headache, weight loss, hypertension, and other features in patients with prior Graves' disease warrants specific inquiry about aspartame use when entertaining the diagnosis of recurrent hyperthyroidism.

After firefighter Janet Starr Hull collapsed on the job, she was told she had life-threatening Graves' disease. Searching for the cause of her illness, Hull discovered what she felt was the culprit—aspartame:

> *I was diagnosed with an "incurable" case of Graves' disease. . . . I never really had Graves' disease, but my doctors were convinced I did. I had aspartame poisoning. . . . Aspartame poisoning is commonly misdiagnosed because aspartame symptoms mock textbook disease symptoms such as Graves' disease.*

After Janet stopped consuming aspartame, her Graves' symptoms disappeared. She is now a nutritionist and health care practitioner. She told her story in her book, *Sweet Poison: How the World's Most Popular Artificial Sweetener Is Killing Us.*

Other toxins may increase the risk of Graves' disease and thyrotoxicosis or they may be triggers. The study of how long-term exposure to toxins affects the thyroid is really just beginning. Scientists are studying the effect of certain chemicals on our endocrine glands and the thyroid in particular. There's strong evidence that exposure to certain toxic chemicals may increase the risk of developing thyroid disease. Some chemicals of concern include dioxins; methyl tertiary butylether (MTBE), an oxygenate added to gasoline; and other chemicals that act as endocrine disrupters.

One concern has been with various insecticides, including those used to treat airplanes and popular insecticides used against the West Nile virus–carrying mosquitoes. Some of these pesticides include resmethrin, which goes by the brand name Scourge, and sumithrin, which goes by the name Anvil. Resmethrin and sumithrin, synthetic pyrethroid insecticides, are registered with the Environmental Protection Agency for use in mosquito control. Allergic responses to pyrethroids have been reported. There are also indications that pyrethroids may interfere with the immune and endocrine systems. Other adverse chronic effects, including effects on the liver and thyroid, have been reported in toxicology testing.

Stress

Many people have reported that various stressful events occurred before their symptoms began, and it's thought that stress can activate the immune system and provide a more conducive environment for the development of autoimmune diseases. One study found that stress actually increased the occurrence of Graves' by almost eightfold. In one analysis, severe emotional stress was seen as the primary precipitating factor in the development of Graves' disease in 14 percent of the patients studied.

What sorts of events are considered major stressors that might be triggers? The Holmes and Rahe Life Change Scale is the famous ranking of the stress value of various life events. Among the scale's most stressful events are death of family or friends, marrriage/divorce/separation, jail, personal injury or illness, getting fired, and retiring from your job.

Marie, a thyroid patient in her forties, has weathered the ups and downs of her condition for a decade. Marie is certain that stress was a trigger in her case:

> *I do believe that our bodies respond to our thoughts and emotions. Each time I have had a change in thyroid condition, it has been preceded by a strong emotional shock or a period of extreme stress.*

Other Risk Factors

Left-handedness, ambidextrousness, and prematurely gray hair are all considered signs of increased risk for Graves' disease, as well as autoimmune disease in general. It's theorized that the genes for these traits may share some similarities with genes that pass on Graves' and/or autoimmune disease susceptibility.

■ Conditions That Raise the Suspicion of Graves' Disease and Hyperthyroidism

Polyglandular Autoimmune Syndrome

Graves' disease can sometimes be part of a syndrome of a number of autoimmune conditions known as polyglandular autoimmune syndrome. This condition is sometimes referred to as autoimmune polyglandular syndrome, autoimmune endocrine failure syndrome, autoimmune polyendocrine syndrome, or immuno-endocrinopathy syndrome. There is a type I and type II variation of this disorder, and each involves development of several different conditions. Having one or more of the conditions in type I or type II polyglandular autoimmune syndrome means you are at higher risk for developing Graves' disease.

Type I Polyglandular Autoimmune Syndrome

Pituitary gland failure
Candidiasis
Malabsorption syndrome
Chronic active hepatitis
Type 1 diabetes
Vitiligo
Premature menopause
Addison's disease
Pernicious anemia
Hyperthyroidism, thyroiditis, hypothyroidism
Parathyroid gland failure
Alopecia

Type II Polyglandular Autoimmune Syndrome

Myasthenia gravis
Parkinson's disease
Celiac disease
Type 1 diabetes
Vitiligo
Premature menopause
Addison's disease
Pernicious anemia
Hyperthyroidism, thyroiditis, hypothyroidism
Parathyroid gland failure
Alopecia

Mental Health Diagnoses

Various mental health diagnoses may be risk factors for Graves' disease and hyperthyroidism or may be more common in people with these disorders. Diagnoses can include:

- Clinical depression
- Panic disorder/panic attacks
- Phobias
- Generalized anxiety disorder

Other Conditions

There are a variety of other conditions that make you more likely to have Graves' disease or hyperthyroidism. A complete list is included in the checklist in chapter 3.

▌ Signs and Symptoms

There are numerous symptoms of Graves' disease, hyperthyroidism, and thyrotoxicosis. One common symptom is simply to feel under the weather. You may feel fluish and achy, have a low-grade fever, or have a persistent headache. Some people find it hard to catch their breath and may feel dizzy or light-headed at times.

Goiter and Other Throat/Neck Changes

The most common symptom of Graves' disease and a frequent symptom in other thyrotoxic conditions is goiter, which is an enlargement of the thyroid. Graves' patients make up the majority of people who are hyperthyroid or thyrotoxic. Among them, 90 percent of younger patients have goiter, and about 75 to 80 percent of older patients have goiter.

In some cases, you can see the goiter easily. Your neck may be enlarged or swollen, or you or your doctor may be able to feel the enlarged thyroid. It is also possible to feel a smaller nodule or lump in your thyroid, or enlarged or tender lymph nodes in your neck.

However, even in the absence of a goiter or swelling, you may have strange feelings in the neck or throat. These feelings have been described as fullness; discomfort with neckties, necklaces, turtlenecks, or scarves; and a sense of neck or throat pressure. Some patients describe a peculiar "buzzy" feeling in the neck/thyroid area, as if a low current of electricity were running through it, or as if the thyroid were vibrating.

You may have a choking sensation, a feeling that something is stuck in your throat, making it difficult to swallow. Your tongue may even feel thick or it may tremble. A chronic or persistent sore throat not associated with a cold, flu, or allergies may also be a symptom.

Weight and Appetite Changes

One of the most common symptoms reported by people with Graves'/hyperthyroidism and thyrotoxicosis is an increased metabolism. This can show up in a number of ways. Some people constantly feel thirsty and hungry. Other people don't eat less and haven't changed their exercise habits, but they lose weight fairly rapidly or even dramatically. Some actually eat substantially more and also lose weight quickly. Another symptom is an inability to gain weight even with increased caloric intake. When your body is in a thyrotoxic state, the excess thyroid hormones enhance your ability to break down fat and muscle, which may contribute to weight loss.

Weight loss during pregnancy, especially when accompanied by nausea and/or vomiting, is a symptom. Some patients with postpartum thyroid conditions also have rapid weight loss after pregnancy.

Some people actually stop eating or eat very little and may be considered anorexic. Women, especially teenagers, have actually been misdiagnosed as anorexic.

Rene was in her early twenties and was very thin at the time her thyroid problem became apparent. Her friends incorrectly accused her of being anorexic:

They constantly told me, "You're too thin, quit working out so much, eat more—you must be anorexic." It honestly hurt my feelings because I knew I was eating probably more than I ever had before, but I just didn't gain weight. . . . I figured my friends were jealous because they are all overweight.

When a teenager experiences rapid weight loss, it's common for parents, teachers, and friends to assume that the teen is suffering from anorexia. But psychiatrist Dr. Nadia Krupnikova says,

Teenagers who are experiencing rapid weight loss should always be thoroughly evaluated for a thyroid condition before the mental health diagnosis of anorexia is made.

One unique change is an increased appetite for carbohydrates. Researchers have documented that brain chemistry changes actually increase the appetite for carbohydrates but not for protein and fat. Hyperthyroidism apparently has the ability to change the neurophysiology of how we choose the food we eat.

While it seems contradictory, 10 percent of patients actually gain weight. This symptom is more common in teenagers. The appetite and caloric intake increase, but metabolism is not sufficient to burn off the extra calories even though it also increases.

If you become thyrotoxic while diabetic, you may find yourself having more symptoms of uncontrolled diabetes, including hunger, shakiness when hungry, and dizziness. Hyperthyroidism causes an insulin-resistant state, and your body becomes increasingly insensitive to the effects of insulin as in type 2 diabetes. Diabetics may need increased insulin and may have to make changes to other medications.

Temperature

Because of the increase in metabolism, you may find yourself feeling warm or hot when others are cold. You may be running a low-grade fever and may feel very intolerant of warm or hot temperatures. Some people like Carla, a patient in her thirties, experience hot flashes or excessive sweating:

> *I was so hot I could hardly stand it! In the middle of winter, I was wearing shorts and a T-shirt and no shoes. I turned off the heat register in my office and turned on the fan when it was below zero outside!*

Heart and Blood Pressure Changes

Heart and blood pressure changes may be symptomatic of Graves' disease and hyperthyroidism. You might feel that your heart is racing and pounding. If you take your pulse, it may be over 100 beats per minute. You may feel like you can "hear" your heartbeat in your head. You may have flutters, noticeable skipped beats, or a strange pattern or rhythm to your heart rate. You may have a headache and feel breathless or even dizzy. Some people feel a twinge of pain or more specific pain in the chest area.

Jennifer was only in her late twenties when she began to experience pain and trembling in her chest:

> *I did not just have hand tremors, but it was like all the muscles in my body were slightly trembling, so when you added that to my shortness of breath and other cardiovascular symptoms, it really felt like my chest was the center point for most of my symptoms and all the muscles of my body were on the verge of exploding out of my body via my chest.*

Conditions set off by thyrotoxicosis include atrial fibrillation, in which the upper chambers of your heart (atria) and the lower chambers (ventricles) are out of sync. The atria beat faster than the ventricles and not in a consistent rhythm. Ventricular tachycardia is a rapid heartbeat. Atypical sinus rhythm, also known as sinus tachy-cardia, is a disruption in the heart's natural rhythms.

Diana had heart-related symptoms that helped her get diagnosed:

I started experiencing a rapid heartbeat. It continued all day and night and somehow I managed to sleep a few hours. When I awoke early the next morning, I was still having the racing heart, and whenever I stood up, I wanted to faint. I told my husband to take me to the emergency room because something strange was happening. I thought I was having a stroke or heart attack because I also had chest pain. I spent two days in ICU because of an irregular heartbeat. Sometimes it got as high as 160 beats per minute.

Gastrointestinal System Changes

It's common for people to report having more frequent bowel movements and they may be looser than normal. Some people have diarrhea, although this is more common with more severe states of thyrotoxicosis and thyroid storm. You may find that you have to urinate more frequently. A smaller percentage of people experience nausea and/or vomiting. Excessive vomiting in pregnancy can be a symptom as well. Finally, some people report pain in the upper right abdominal area.

Energy Level, Muscle, and Joint Changes

Changes in energy level, muscles, and joints are common in Graves', thyrotoxicosis, and hyperthyroidism. You may feel generally fatigued, exhausted, and weak. Some people find they feel weak in their muscles. Thyrotoxicosis can rapidly reduce muscle mass, which can bring on weakness quickly.

You may experience leg muscle weakness. It may be more difficult to climb stairs or to go from a sitting to a standing position. Some people have a similar weakness in their upper arms.

Sherry, a mother of two in her mid-thirties, experienced dramatic weight loss before the muscle weakness set in:

I had started out at 159 pounds and went down to 98 pounds! I looked like I had anorexia. The worst part was I could not stand at the stove long enough to cook hamburger meat for tacos without sitting down. I had to get a grocery cart when I went shopping even if it was only to get milk because it was such a task to walk that far and also carry the milk. There was no way I could pick up my daughters. I remember that it was also a real task to get the wet clothes out of the washer into the dryer. Simple things that I had taken for granted were really a challenge for me!

For Barb, one of the worst symptoms was the leg pain and weakness:

I had been very tired and had trouble with the muscles in my legs. In December of 2001, I woke up in a lot of pain, but tried to go about my business. I hobbled out to the mailbox to get the mail and I wasn't able to walk back! It took me about 45 minutes to get back into the house. My legs were in so much pain that I just couldn't make them work! All kinds of horrible thoughts went through my head. I thought I might have polio or some other horrible disease that would leave me unable to walk for the rest of my life.

Some people find that they develop exercise intolerance—that is, they don't recover quickly after exercise and are more easily fatigued. A more rare symptom is periodic paralysis, which is a rapid onset of extreme weakness. Some patients find they cannot walk during these temporary attacks. (For some unknown reason, periodic paralysis is more common in Asian men.)

In contrast, some people actually have a lot of energy because the increased metabolic rate revs them up. Some patients report dramatic increases in their level of exercise, having little need for sleep, and feeling highly energetic.

Skin Changes

Changes to the skin are common. Interestingly, because increased metabolism causes more rapid turnover of skin cells, you may find your skin is smoother, younger-looking, even velvety. More often, however, a variety of skin problems are reported, including worsening acne, bruising, spider veins on the face and neck, blister-like bumps on the forehead and face (called miliaria bumps), a flushed appearance to the face, throat, palms, and elbows, and sometimes a yellowish cast to the skin.

Hives and itching are frequent symptoms of Graves' disease and thyrotoxicosis. A loss of skin pigmentation known as vitiligo may also occur. One unusual skin condition seen in people with Graves' disease is called pretibial myxedema, dermopathy, infiltrative dermopathy, or sometimes Graves' dermopathy. If you develop pretibial myxedema, you may get waxy, red-brown lesions on your shins and lower legs that are itchy and inflamed. These lesions typically heal into rough, leathery patches. Occasionally pretibial myxedema can affect the tops of your feet, toes, arms, face, shoulders, or trunk.

Hair, Hand, and Feet Changes

Graves' disease and thyrotoxicosis may cause hair loss, typically from the head and from various spots on the body (known as axillary hair loss). There is moderate hair loss in about 40 percent of patients. Hair may also become thinner, finer, softer, and you may find that it can't hold a curl or a perm.

One study found that about 25 percent of the people who have the autoimmune disease alopecia, which can cause varying degrees of hair loss, have elevated thyroid antibodies or thyroid problems. Thus, hair problems are quite common in thyroid patients.

Nails may be more shiny than usual and break easily because they are either softer or more brittle. Hands and palms may be warm and moist. Two more unusual conditions can be seen in some patients. In the first, acropachy, or thyroid acropachy, the fingertips and toes swell and become wider, sometimes even clubbed. This can be accompanied by arthritic damage to the joints in the fingers and/or toes. In the second condition, onycholysis, also called Plummer's nails, the underlying nail bed separates from the skin.

Eye Changes

The eyes are a frequent target for symptoms. Some studies have shown that nearly everyone with Graves' disease has some form of eye involvement, even if it is minor. You don't have to have a full case of Graves' ophthalmopathy in order to experience various eye-related symptoms.

One of the symptoms most commonly associated with Graves' disease is proptosis or exophthalmos, a bulging or protrusion of the eyeballs. When proptosis is severe, it may be difficult to completely close the eyes during sleep, which makes them dry and the cornea more susceptible to damage.

Your eyes may feel uncomfortable, including dryness, a gritty feeling, the sensation that there's something in your eye, excessive tearing and watering. You may feel an achiness or pain behind your eyes, or even a headache in the eye area.

The appearance of the eyes can change. They may appear bloodshot, with visible blood vessels. The upper and lower eyelids may look irritated and puffy, and you may have a noticeable "stare." Your upper eyelids may retract, giving you a wide-eyed, startled look.

Eye movement can be affected. One of the characteristic eye changes is called lid lag, in which your upper eyelid doesn't smoothly follow along when you look down. You may have tics or twitching, infrequent blinking, tremor in the eyelids when your eyes are closed, and your eyes may feel jumpy. Shifting your gaze quickly may make you feel dizzy or disoriented.

In more severe cases of Graves' ophthalmopathy, your vision may be blurred or diminished. Colors and brightness may be lessened. Many people with more severe eye disease have diplopia—that is, double vision. Most diplopia is binocular, meaning if you cover one eye, you don't see double. Poor night vision, light sensitivity (known as photosensitivity), and an aversion to light are also symptoms. Finally, some people report seeing flashing lights or floaters.

Thinking/Cognition Changes

Changes in thinking are common in Graves' disease and thyrotoxicosis. Some of the most commonly reported symptoms include difficulty concentrating, difficulty making decisions, confusion, and feeling as if your thinking is disorganized. You may have dyslexia, or difficulty with reading, calculating, and thinking. You may have memory problems, find yourself forgetting things more frequently, or feel that your mind is going blank all the time. You may feel as if your mind is always racing and you can't shut your thoughts off. Some people with Graves' disease and hyperthyroidism also have attention deficit hyperactivity disorder (ADHD) or may be misdiagnosed as having ADHD.

Mood/Feelings Changes

Most patients with Graves' disease or hyperthyroidism experience some changes to mood and feelings. Many people experience symptoms of depression: a constant sad or empty feeling, hopelessness or pessimism, guilty feelings, and a sense of helplessness. You may withdraw emotionally and lose interest or pleasure in activities and hobbies that you once enjoyed, including sex. In more extreme depression, you may have thoughts of death or suicide.

Patients report major swings in mood and emotions, even to the extent that they feel they are behaving erratically or overemotionally. Some people report feelings of uncontrollable anger, irrational anger, or aggressiveness.

Hayley, a woman in her forties, describes the mood swings she experienced when hyperthyroid:

> Within 2 or 3 seconds, my mood would swish from being normally buoyant down into a chasm. So intense was the swing that I would need to get up and walk around. I began to have crying and sobbing episodes . . . howling my eyes out . . . but at the same time I didn't feel sad! I would walk into the kitchen and make myself a cup of tea, bawling my eyes out and surprising myself at the intensity of the crying and the tears that flowed but not feeling particularly sad or upset about anything. . . . If my teenage son annoyed me, I became aggressive with him, which was totally out of character for me. I would shriek at him and want to hit him. He thought I was going insane.

Leonor found herself going through a divorce in her late forties, before she was finally diagnosed.

> I couldn't handle my life. Everything was a burden to me, so I had to get rid of something. . . . Unfortunately, I picked my husband, as I was being mean to him and aggressive and panicking without understanding why and saying to me the whole time, "What are you doing to him? You love him so much and you are being awful. . . . That's not you!" But I couldn't stop my behavior.

Anxiety is perhaps even more common, given the elevated heart rate, blood pressure, and overall hypermetabolic condition. Symptoms can include feeling restless, irritable, on edge, nervous, or inexplicably frightened. You may be worrying all the time and find that you can't stop.

Physically, people become hyperreflexive and hyperkinetic. You may find yourself jumpy and easily startled, have fast reflexes, tremors, or shaky hands. You may find that you can't sit still and are always moving, jiggling, tapping a foot, or drumming your fingers.

I'll always remember a Graves' disease patient who told me that before she was diagnosed, she was sitting on the examining table and the doctor stood behind her and clapped loudly. After she nearly jumped off the table, he told her that he was pretty certain she was hyperthyroid because of her reaction. (Effective, but perhaps not the most sensitive way for a doctor to evaluate a symptom.)

Some people start having panic attacks, including the full list of symptoms such as palpitations, sweating or chills, difficulty breathing, terror, nausea, feeling as if you are going to die, tingling or numbness, dizziness or faintness. Some patients are actually incorrectly diagnosed as having panic disorder. It is possible to become manic, psychotic, or delirious with hyperthyroidism. Symptoms include an unusual sense of elation, unusual self-confidence, hallucinations, hearing voices, and other extreme symptoms.

Sleep Problems

Problems with sleep are fairly common in people with an overactive thyroid. Symptoms can include difficulty falling asleep. Even after you do fall asleep, you may wake up frequently and find it hard to fall back asleep. You may have insomnia and not be able to sleep at all. Because you are not reaching a deep sleep, you may wake up feeling tired and unrefreshed, or even oversleep, leaving you exhausted all the time, like Genevieve, a 28-year-old woman.

I know some individuals claim to be very productive or have increased energy with Graves', but I never had that. I was dead on my feet and had an increasingly muddled mind, and once I finally got to sleep at night, I would sleep for 12 to 14 hours and it was impossible to wake me up.

Especially in Men

Some men who are hyperthyroid report a decrease in their sex drive or a low sex drive. Men may also have fertility problems. Hyperthyroidism raises their testosterone levels, which artificially speeds up the maturation of sperm. Sperm that are immature and incapable of fertilizing an egg can be released. One study found that men who had Graves' disease or hyperthyroidism and went off their antithyroid drugs had a significant drop in the concentration of their sperm, had reduced sperm motility, and some actually had an almost nonexistent sperm count. The sperm count and quality improved dramatically or returned completely to normal with sufficient treatment.

Gynecomastia, an enlargement or tenderness in the breasts, is also a well-recognized but rare symptom in men.

Especially in Women

Infertility is more common in thyroid patients than in the general population. Studies have shown a linkage between hyperthyroidism and increased rates of anovulation (failure to release an egg), implantation failure, donor egg failure, and in vitro fertilization failure.

Infertility and recurrent miscarriage can be associated with the presence of thyroid antibodies. Some researchers estimate that the risk of miscarriage is twice as high when a woman is positive for various thyroid antibodies.

Some women report a lower sex drive, but the opposite can also be true. There are reports of raging libido and even sexually obsessive behavior associated with hyperthyroidism. Women can also experience a constant state of excessive vaginal lubrication.

Hormonal problems are quite common with thyroid problems. These can include worsening of premenstrual syndrome (PMS) and more difficult symptoms during perimenopause and menopause. In younger girls, the start of menstruation may be delayed entirely. Those who have already begun to menstruate may find that their periods stop. Some women have unusually light and/or short menstrual periods known as oligomenorrhea and longer time between cycles. Less commonly, some patients report menorrhagia, or unusually heavy menstrual periods.

Especially in Newborns/Babies

Newborns who are hyperthyroid are more likely to be premature and have a low birth weight. They may have a smaller head in comparison to the body, a yellowish cast to the skin, a visible goiter or enlarged neck, and prominent eyes. These babies may also have an elevated heart rate and body temperature. They may be irritable, restless, hyperactive, and appear to be anxious or unusually alert.

Hyperthyroid babies may have an appetite but frequent diarrhea and vomiting. They may gain too much weight or even lose weight, and they are at risk of failure to thrive.

Especially in Children

Children almost always have a goiter and many of the other standard symptoms of Graves' disease and hyperthyroidism. They may have sudden growth spurts, an unusually large appetite, or periods of rapid weight loss.

School may be a place where the symptoms become evident. Poor handwriting, poor school performance, and difficulty concentrating are all possible. Children can feel weak, especially in the thigh and shoulder muscles, which may become particularly evident during playtime, sports, or physical education classes.

Children may often be fatigued and exhausted, appearing moody and lacking motivation. Sometimes parents suspect their child may be taking illegal drugs. Behavioral changes may include hyperactivity, frequent emotional outbursts, temper tantrums, crying easily, and irritability. Children may have trouble sleeping or may wet the bed.

Anxiety symptoms most common in children include restlessness, tremors, and hyperactive-like movements such as leg swinging and finger tapping. Heart-related symptoms tend to be similar to those in adults.

One symptom that is unique to children and is a complication of thyrotoxicosis is craniosynostosis, in which two or more cranial bones mesh to form a single bone. The various eye symptoms can affect children, but they are less common and usually less severe than in adults.

Especially in Teenagers

Identifying Graves' disease and hyperthyroidism in teenagers can be difficult because symptoms such as moodiness, increased appetite, and emotional changeability are fairly common in many healthy teenagers. It's especially important to note that unexplained rapid or sudden weight loss may be seen in teenagers, but it can be mistaken for anorexia. A diagnosis of anorexia should not be made until a complete thyroid assessment is done. Occasionally, because the increased appetite may be greater than the increase in metabolism, teenagers may have unexplained weight gain.

Teenagers may have unusual nervousness, ADHD-like symptoms, and other behavioral changes. Graves' disease and hyperthyroidism can delay puberty. Facial hair and pubic hair may be less developed and genitals less enlarged in boys. In girls there's often a delay in both the start of menstruation and growth of underarm and pubic hair. Muscle weakness in teenagers may show up as poor performance in athletics.

Callie's symptoms started when she was 14 and she found that being a teen made it all the more difficult to get diagnosed:

The symptoms were subtle at first but were always pawned off as a symptom of being a teenager. Losing weight, eating more, sleeping more, being moody—all were pegged as normal teenage fare. From 14 to 16, it did not cause any extreme problems, but around my 17th birthday I really started to severely crash. I missed all or partial school days for over a month and a half straight before I was taken to the doctor. Graves' disease has had a definite impact on my life. I never finished out my junior year of high school. I had missed too many days and was not getting any better, so I had to take a medical leave of absence. I had to take summer school and repeat some classes as a senior.

Especially in the Elderly

While weight loss and the other classic symptoms of Graves' disease and hyperthyroidism are seen in seniors, they may not be as easily recognizable. Goiter is seen in 90 percent of younger patients with Graves' disease, whereas only 75 to 80 percent of older patients have a goiter.

Many older people exhibit apathetic hyperthyroidism, which may actually resemble an underactive thyroid condition. Seniors might feel withdrawn, depressed, weak, lacking in energy, confused, forgetful, even constipated. They may not lose weight. Some seniors experience more frequent falls and injuries as well as shaking.

Older people with thyrotoxicosis are more likely to experience atrial fibrillation and other irregular heart rhythms as well as congestive heart failure. Some people are more susceptible to dementia, confusion, and even delirium. Again, because symptoms such as fatigue, weakness, falls, and dementia are sometimes expected in the elderly, a thyroid diagnosis may be overlooked.

■ Thyroid Storm Risks and Symptoms

Although it's fairly rare, some people with Graves' disease or hyperthyroidism develop thyroid storm, in which heart rate, blood pressure, and body temperature can become uncontrolled. If thyroid storm is suspected, the patient should immediately go to a hospital emergency room, since this condition is life-threatening. It can develop and worsen quickly, and it requires treatment within hours to avoid fatal complications such as stroke or heart attack. Thyroid storm is more common in the elderly.

Risks for thyroid storm include:

- Untreated Graves' disease and/or hyperthyroidism
- Infection: lung infection, throat infection, or pneumonia
- Blood sugar changes: diabetic ketoacidosis, insulin-induced hypoglycemia
- Recent surgery to the thyroid
- Abrupt withdrawal of antithyroid medications
- Radioactive iodine (RAI) treatment of the thyroid
- Excessive palpation of the thyroid
- Severe emotional stress
- Thyroid hormone overdose
- Toxemia of pregnancy and labor

Common symptoms of thyroid storm include:

- Fever of 100°F to as high as 106°F
- High heart rate that can be as high as 200 beats per minute
- Palpitations, chest pain, and shortness of breath
- High blood pressure
- Confusion, delirium, and even psychosis

- Extreme weakness and fatigue
- Extreme restlessness, nervousness, and mood swings
- Exaggerated reflexes
- Difficulty breathing
- Nausea, vomiting, and diarrhea
- Recent dramatic weight loss
- Profuse sweating and dehydration
- Stupor or coma

3

Risks, Signs, and Symptoms Checklist

Chapter 2 covers a variety of factors that can increase your risk of having thyrotoxicosis, Graves' disease, and hyperthyroidism. There are also a number of factors that may trigger the conditions. Finally, a variety of symptoms are associated with these conditions. I urge you to make a copy of this checklist and fill it out. You can bring it to your physician for help in getting an initial evaluation and diagnosis. If you've already been diagnosed but are having continued symptoms, the checklist is a helpful tool to use in communicating with your doctor.

RISK FACTORS

Gender
___ Female

Personal History
___ I have a past history of thyroid problems.
___ I have a past history of autoimmune disease.

___ In particular, I have one or more of the other seven core-related autoimmune diseases:

   ___ *Rheumatoid arthritis*

   ___ *Juvenile rheumatoid arthritis*

   ___ *Systemic lupus*

   ___ *Multiple sclerosis*

   ___ *Type 1 diabetes*

   ___ *Psoriasis*

   ___ *Inflammatory bowel disease*

___ I have a past history of endocrine disease:

   ___ *Adrenal problems (Addison's, Cushing's, Turner's syndrome, adrenal insufficiency, pheochromocytoma, other adrenal problems)*

   ___ *Pancreatic diseases (diabetes, hypoglycemia, insulin resistance, metabolic syndrome, juvenile diabetes)*

   ___ *Pituitary diseases (acromegaly, prolactinoma, others)*

   ___ *Parathyroid conditions (hyperparathyroidism, others)*

   ___ *Osteoporosis*

   ___ *Sex hormone imbalances (polycystic ovary syndrome, premature menopause, infertility, menstrual disorders)*

   ___ *Growth hormone imbalances (dwarfism, deficiency, others)*

Family History

___ I have a first-degree relative (parent, child, sibling) with Graves' disease or hyperthyroidism.

___ I have a first-degree relative (parent, child, sibling) with another thyroid condition.

___ I have a first-degree relative (parent, child, sibling) who has tested positive for thyroid antibodies.

___ I have a female relative (mother, grandmother, sister, daughter) with a thyroid condition, or who has tested positive for thyroid antibodies.

___ I have a first-degree relative (parent, child, sibling) or grandparent with an autoimmune disease.

__ In particular, I have a first-degree relative (parent, child, sibling) or grandparent with one or more of the other seven core-related autoimmune diseases:

    __ *Rheumatoid arthritis*
    __ *Juvenile rheumatoid arthritis*
    __ *Systemic lupus*
    __ *Multiple sclerosis*
    __ *Type 1 diabetes*
    __ *Psoriasis*
    __ *Inflammatory bowel disease*

Age
__ I am between the ages of 20 and 40.

Pregnancy
__ I am currently pregnant.
__ I had a baby in the last 12 months.
__ I have tested positive on a pregnancy test.
__ I have just been diagnosed with a molar pregnancy.
__ I have just been diagnosed with choriocarcinoma.

Smoking
__ I am currently a smoker.
__ I was formerly a smoker.

Excessive Intake of Thyroid Hormone
__ I recently refilled my thyroid hormone medication prescription, or filled it at a different pharmacy, or changed my prescription.
__ I am taking more thyroid hormone medication than has been prescribed.
__ I am taking thyroid hormone medication that has not been prescribed to me by a doctor.
__ I am taking over-the-counter energy supplements.

___ I am taking over-the-counter diet supplements.

___ I am taking over-the-counter thyroid support supplements.

___ I am regularly eating meat that has been privately butchered from slaughtered farm animals.

___ I am regularly eating game meat from hunting.

Exposure to or Excess of Iodine/Iodine Drugs

___ I recently had an x-ray or scan that used iodine contrast dye.

___ I recently had a medical procedure where a topical antiseptic (povidone-iodine) was used.

___ I take the heart drug amiodarone.

___ I take iodine supplements in pill or liquid form.

___ I take the following supplements or combination supplements that include as an ingredient:

    ___ *Bladder wrack* (Fucus vesiculosus)

    ___ *Bugleweed*

    ___ *Kelp*

    ___ *Norwegian kelp*

    ___ *Kelp fronds*

    ___ *Irish moss*

    ___ *Seaweed*

___ I use(d) Cellasene or other iodine-rich cellulite remedies.

___ I eat large amounts of seaweed.

Medical/Drug Treatments

___ I am currently or have recently been treated with interferon beta-1b.

___ I am currently or have recently been treated with interleukin-4.

___ I am currently or have recently been treated with immunosuppressant therapy.

___ I am currently being treated with antiretroviral treatment for AIDS.

___ I am currently or have recently been treated with monoclonal antibody (Campath-1H) therapy for multiple sclerosis.

___ I have recently received a donated organ.

___ I have recently received a bone marrow transplant.
___ I am taking the following drugs:
  ___ *Lithium*
  ___ *Amphetamines*
  ___ *Cimetidine/ranitidine (Tagamet/Zantac) for ulcer treatment*
  ___ *Clomiphene (Clomid) for fertility treatments*
  ___ *L-dopa inhibitors such as chlorpromazine (Thorazine) and haloperidol (Haldol) for psychotic disorders*
  ___ *Metoclopramide (Reglan) and domperidone for nausea/ vomiting*
  ___ *Glucocorticoids/adrenal steroids such as prednisone and hydrocortisone*
  ___ *Propranolol, a beta blocker*
  ___ *Aminoglutethimide for breast and prostate cancer treatment*
  ___ *Ketoconazole, an antifungal*
  ___ *Para-aminosalicylic acid, a tuberculosis drug*
  ___ *Sulfonamide drugs, including sulfadiazine, sulfisoxazole, and acetazolamide, which have been used as diuretics and antibiotics*
  ___ *Sulfonylureas, including tolbutamide and chlorpropamide, which are used to treat diabetes*
  ___ *Raloxifene (Evista) for osteoporosis*
  ___ *Carbamazepine, oxcarbazepine, and valproate for epilepsy*

Recent History of Hyperthyroidism-Inducing Conditions
___ I have recently been diagnosed with struma ovarii.
___ I have recently been diagnosed with follicular thyroid cancer.
___ I have recently been diagnosed with pituitary adenoma.
___ I have recently been diagnosed with molar pregnancy.
___ I have recently been diagnosed with choriocarcinoma.

Nuclear Exposure
___ I lived near or was visiting the area near or downwind from the Chernobyl nuclear plant on or after April 26, 1986. (Areas at risk include Belarus, the

Russian Federation, and the Ukraine. Reduced-risk areas are Poland, Austria, Denmark, Finland, Germany, Greece, and Italy.)

___ I lived near or in the area downwind from the former nuclear weapons plant at Hanford in south central Washington State during the 1940s through 1960s, particularly 1955 to 1965.

___ I live(d) near or work(ed) at a nuclear facility.

Infection

___ I have or recently have had the following viral infection(s):

    ___ *Upper respiratory infection*

    ___ *Cold*

    ___ *Influenza*

    ___ *Mumps*

    ___ *Measles*

    ___ *Adenovirus*

    ___ *Mononucleosis*

    ___ *Myocarditis*

    ___ *Cat scratch fever*

    ___ *Coxsackie virus*

___ I have recently been diagnosed with *Yersinia enterocolitica* infection.

___ I have recently eaten raw or undercooked poultry.

___ I have recently consumed unpasteurized milk and/or dairy products.

___ I have recently eaten seafood, particularly oysters, from potentially contaminated waters.

Trauma

___ I recently had my thyroid or neck area vigorously manipulated or palpated.

___ I recently had surgery to the thyroid, parathyroids, or the area surrounding the thyroid.

___ I recently had a biopsy of the thyroid.

___ I recently had an injection to the thyroid—that is, percutaneous ethanol injection (PEI).

___ I recently injured my neck—for example, whiplash or a seat belt injury from a car accident.

Allergies/Sensitivities
___ I have seasonal allergies, especially to pollen and trees.
___ I have food allergies.
___ I have been diagnosed with gluten intolerance or celiac disease.

Toxic/Environmental Exposures
___ I frequently eat the kind of fish that contain higher levels of mercury, including:

    ___ *Swordfish*
    ___ *Shark*
    ___ *Mackerel*
    ___ *Tuna*

___ I have mercury dental fillings.
___ I am exposed through work or other means to higher than usual levels of heavy metals such as gold, cadmium, and others.

Aspartame
___ I regularly use aspartame.
___ I regularly eat foods or drink diet drinks that contain aspartame.
___ I am exposed to insecticides and pesticides.

Stress
___ In the last year, I have experienced one or more of the following high-stress events:

    ___ *Death of spouse*
    ___ *Divorce*
    ___ *Marital separation*
    ___ *Jail term*
    ___ *Death of close family member*
    ___ *Personal injury/illness*

___ *Marriage*
___ *Fired from work*
___ *Marital reconciliation*
___ *Retirement*
___ *Change in family member's health*
___ *Pregnancy*
___ *Sex difficulties*
___ *Addition to family*
___ *Business readjustment*
___ *Change in financial status*
___ *Death of close friend*
___ *Change in number of marital arguments*
___ *Taking out a mortgage/loan greater than $10,000*
___ *Foreclosure of mortgage/loan*

Other Risk Factors
___ I am left-handed.
___ I am ambidextrous.
___ I am prematurely gray-haired.

CONDITIONS THAT RAISE THE SUSPICION OF GRAVES' DISEASE AND HYPERTHYROIDISM

Polyglandular Autoimmune Syndrome
___ I have one or more of the conditions associated with type I polyglandular autoimmune syndrome:
___ *Pituitary gland failure*
___ *Candidiasis*
___ *Malabsorption syndrome*
___ *Chronic active hepatitis*
___ *Type 1 diabetes*
___ *Vitiligo*
___ *Premature menopause*

___ *Addison's disease*

___ *Pernicious anemia*

___ *Hyperthyroidism, thyroiditis, hypothyroidism*

___ *Parathyroid gland failure*

___ *Alopecia*

___ I have one or more of the conditions associated with type II polyglandular autoimmune syndrome:

___ *Myasthenia gravis*

___ *Parkinson's disease*

___ *Celiac disease*

___ *Type 1 diabetes*

___ *Vitiligo*

___ *Premature menopause*

___ *Addison's disease*

___ *Pernicious anemia*

___ *Hyperthyroidism, thyroiditis, hypothyroidism*

___ *Parathyroid gland failure*

___ *Alopecia*

Mental Health Diagnoses

___ I have recently been diagnosed with clinical depression.

___ I have panic attacks.

___ I have recently been diagnosed with panic disorder.

___ I have phobias or have recently been diagnosed as having a phobia.

___ I have recently been diagnosed with generalized anxiety disorder.

Other Conditions

I have the following condition(s):

___ *Acquired immune deficiency syndrome (AIDS)*

___ *Acromegaly*

___ *Addison's disease*

___ *Adrenal insufficiency*

___ *Allergies*

___ *Alopecia*

___ *Alzheimer's disease*

___ *Ankylosing spondylitis*

___ *Anxiety*

___ *Atrial fibrillation*

___ *Attention deficit hyperactivity disorder (ADHD)*

___ *Autoimmune disease, any*

___ *Autoimmune hypoparathyroidism*

___ *Autoimmune oophoritis*

___ *Bipolar disease/manic depression*

___ *Breast cancer*

___ *Candidiasis/Candida infections of skin or mucous membranes*

___ *Cardiomyopathy*

___ *Celiac disease/gluten intolerance*

___ *Choriocarcinoma*

___ *Chronic active hepatitis*

___ *Chronic fatigue syndrome (CFS)/chronic fatigue immune dysfunction syndrome (CFIDS)*

___ *Clinical depression*

___ *Congestive heart failure*

___ *Crohn's disease*

___ *Delirium*

___ *Depression*

___ *Down syndrome*

___ *Dyslexia*

___ *Fibromyalgia*

___ *Follicular thyroid cancer*

___ *Generalized anxiety disorder*

___ *Guillain-Barré syndrome*

___ *Gynecomastia*

___ *Hashimoto's thyroiditis*

___ *Hyperparathyroidism*

___ *Hypoglycemia*

__ Infertility
__ Insulin resistance
__ Juvenile arthritis
__ Lupus
__ Malabsorption syndrome
__ Mania
__ Ménière's disease
__ Menstrual disorders
__ Metabolic syndrome
__ Mitral valve prolapse
__ Molar pregnancy
__ Multiple sclerosis
__ Myasthenia gravis
__ Osteoporosis
__ Panic disorder
__ Paranoia
__ Parathyroid gland failure
__ Parkinson's disease
__ Pernicious anemia
__ Pheochromocytoma
__ Phobias
__ Pituitary adenoma
__ Pituitary gland failure
__ Polycystic ovary syndrome
__ Polyglandular autoimmune syndrome
__ Premature menopause
__ Premature ovarian failure
__ Prolactinoma
__ Psoriasis
__ Psychosis
__ Raynaud's phenomenon
__ Recurrent miscarriage
__ Reiter's syndrome

___ *Rheumatic fever*
___ *Rheumatoid arthritis*
___ *Sarcoidosis*
___ *Scleroderma*
___ *Sjögren's syndrome*
___ *Struma ovarii*
___ *Turner's syndrome*
___ *Type 1 diabetes*
___ *Ulcerative colitis*
___ *Urticaria*
___ *Vitiligo*

▌ Signs and Symptoms

There are numerous symptoms of Graves' disease, hyperthyroidism and thyrotoxicosis. You may simply feel under the weather. You may feel fluish and achy, have a low-grade fever, or have a headache. Some people find it hard to catch their breath and feel dizzy or light-headed. Here is a more specific list of symptoms by category.

GOITER AND OTHER THROAT/NECK CHANGES

___ I have a goiter.
___ My thyroid/neck is enlarged.
___ I can feel a lump in my neck or thyroid area.
___ I have enlarged and/or tender lymph nodes.
___ My throat and neck feel full.
___ I find neckties, turtlenecks, necklaces, and/or scarves around my neck uncomfortable.
___ I have a feeling of neck or throat pressure.
___ I have a strange buzzy feeling in my neck/thyroid area.
___ I sometimes feel like I am choking or have something stuck in my throat.

___ It's hard to swallow.
___ My tongue feels thick.
___ My tongue trembles.
___ I have pain and tenderness in my neck and/or thyroid area.

WEIGHT AND APPETITE CHANGES

___ I feel thirsty much of the time.
___ I am unusually hungry.
___ I am losing weight even though I haven't changed my diet and exercise.
___ I have experienced rapid and/or dramatic weight loss without dieting.
___ I am able to eat substantially more and not gain weight.
___ I am able to eat more and am still losing weight.
___ I can't gain weight even if I eat more.
___ I am losing weight during pregnancy.
___ I am having excessive vomiting and nausea accompanied by weight loss during pregnancy.
___ I have had a baby in the last year and experienced a rapid and/or dramatic weight loss without dieting.
___ I have no appetite.
___ I have recently been diagnosed as anorexic.
___ I am craving and/or eating more carbohydrates (bread, rice, pasta, sweets, fruits, sugary foods, etc.).
___ I am gaining weight.
___ I'm a diabetic and have symptoms of poor blood sugar control (hunger, shakiness when hungry).

TEMPERATURE

___ I feel warm or hot when others are cold.
___ I feel warm or hot all the time.
___ I have a low-grade fever.
___ I am very intolerant of any warm or hot temperatures.

___ I'm experiencing hot flashes.
___ I'm sweating excessively.
___ I'm frequently thirsty.

HEART AND BLOOD PRESSURE CHANGES

___ I feel like my heart is racing or pounding.
___ My pulse rate is high (insert beats per minute here: _____ bpm).
___ I feel like I can hear my heartbeat in my head.
___ I feel palpitations or fluttering in my heart.
___ I notice my heart skipping beats.
___ My heart rate has a strange pattern or rhythm.
___ I have frequent headaches.
___ I often feel breathless.
___ I frequently feel dizzy.
___ I have occasional chest pain.

GASTROINTESTINAL SYSTEM CHANGES

___ I have more frequent bowel movements.
___ My bowel movements are looser than normal.
___ I have diarrhea.
___ I have to urinate more frequently.
___ I am experiencing nausea and/or vomiting.
___ I am pregnant and vomiting excessively.
___ I have pain in the upper right abdominal area.

ENERGY LEVEL, MUSCLE, AND JOINT CHANGES

___ I feel fatigued and exhausted.
___ I feel weak.
___ My muscles feel weak.
___ My legs feel weak.

___ My arms and/or shoulders feel weak.

___ I have aches and pains in my muscles and/or joints.

___ I am more fatigued and sore than normal after exercise.

___ I have experienced one or more episodes of extreme weakness—for example, difficulty walking.

___ I have had an unusual increase in energy.

___ I'm feeling a need to exercise far more than usual.

___ I need very little sleep.

SKIN CHANGES

___ My skin is smoother, younger-looking, and/or velvety.

___ I have worsening acne.

___ I'm bruising easily.

___ I have prominent spider veins on my face and/or neck.

___ I have blister-like bumps on my forehead and/or face.

___ My face, throat, palms, and/or elbows have a flushed appearance.

___ My skin is yellowish.

___ I'm having hives frequently.

___ I'm experiencing itching.

___ I'm getting patches of unpigmented skin/vitiligo.

___ I have waxy, red-brown lesions on my lower legs, feet, toes, arms, face, shoulders, and/or trunk.

HAIR, HAND, AND FEET CHANGES

___ I'm losing hair from my head.

___ I'm losing body hair.

___ My hair has become thinner.

___ My hair has become finer.

___ My hair has become softer.

___ My hair can no longer hold a perm.

___ My hair can no longer hold a curl.

___ My nails are more shiny than usual.

___ My nails break more easily.

___ My nails are softer.

___ My nails are more brittle.

___ My hands and palms are warm and moist.

___ My fingertips and/or toes are swelling and becoming wider.

___ I have pain in the joints of my fingers/toes.

___ My nail bed is separating from my finger.

EYE CHANGES

___ My eyeballs are bulging or protruding.

___ I can't completely close my eyes during sleep.

___ My eyes feel uncomfortable.

___ My eyes feel dry.

___ I have a gritty feeling in my eyes.

___ It feels as if there is something in my eye.

___ My eyes are tearing and watering frequently.

___ I feel an achiness or pain behind my eyes.

___ I frequently have a headache in the eye area.

___ My eyes appear red.

___ There are visible blood vessels in my eyes.

___ My upper and lower eyelids look irritated and puffy.

___ I have a noticeable stare.

___ My upper eyelids are retracting.

___ I have a wide-eyed, startled look.

___ I have tics, twitches, and/or tremor in my eyes and/or eyelids.

___ I don't blink frequently.

___ My eyes feel jumpy.

___ When I shift my gaze quickly, I feel dizzy or disoriented.

___ My vision is blurred.

___ My vision is worsening.

___ Colors are less vivid.

___ Brightness is diminishing.
___ I have double vision.
___ I have poor night vision.
___ I'm light sensitive.
___ I see flashing lights or floaters.

THINKING/COGNITION CHANGES

___ I'm having difficulty concentrating.
___ I find it difficult to make decisions.
___ I'm feeling confused.
___ My thinking is disorganized.
___ I have dyslexia.
___ I'm having difficulty with reading.
___ I'm having difficulty calculating.
___ I have memory problems and forget things more frequently.
___ I feel like my mind is going blank regularly.
___ My mind is always racing; I can't shut my thoughts off.

MOOD/FEELINGS CHANGES

___ I feel sad or empty.
___ I feel hopeless or pessimistic.
___ I feel guilty and/or helpless.
___ I am withdrawing emotionally.
___ I've lost interest or pleasure in activities and hobbies that I once enjoyed.
___ I've lost interest or pleasure in sex.
___ I have thoughts of death or suicide.
___ I have mood swings.
___ I feel that sometimes I am behaving erratically or overemotionally.
___ I inappropriately feel uncontrollable and/or irrational anger or aggressiveness at times.

___ I feel anxious or nervous.

___ I feel restless.

___ I'm irritable and on edge.

___ I feel inexplicably frightened at times.

___ I'm frequently worrying and I find it hard to stop worrying.

___ I'm jumpy.

___ I'm easily startled.

___ My reflexes are particularly fast.

___ I have tremors.

___ My hands are shaky.

___ I can't sit still.

___ I'm always moving, jiggling, tapping a foot, or drumming my fingers.

___ I'm having panic attacks.

___ I'm feeling unusually elated.

___ I'm feeling unusually self-confident.

___ I'm having hallucinations.

SLEEP PROBLEMS

___ I find it hard to fall asleep.

___ After I've fallen asleep, I frequently wake up.

___ When I wake up in the middle of the night, I find it hard to fall back asleep.

___ I have insomnia and can't sleep.

___ I wake up feeling tired and unrefreshed.

___ I frequently oversleep.

___ I am frequently exhausted.

ESPECIALLY IN MEN

___ I have a reduced sex drive.

___ I have a low sex drive.

___ I am having fertility problems.

___ I have enlarged or tender breasts.

ESPECIALLY IN WOMEN

___ I'm unable to get pregnant.

___ I'm showing signs that I'm not ovulating.

___ I've had donor egg failure.

___ I've had in vitro fertilization failure.

___ I've had a miscarriage or multiple miscarriages.

___ My sex drive is low or nonexistent.

___ I have a suddenly raging libido/very high sex drive.

___ I'm behaving in a sexually obsessive way.

___ I'm having constant excessive vaginal lubrication.

___ My premenstrual syndrome (PMS) seems to have gotten worse.

___ My perimenopause symptoms seem to have gotten worse.

___ My menopause symptoms seem to have gotten worse.

___ I'm 13 or older and have not started menstruating.

___ My menstrual periods have stopped.

___ My menstrual periods have become unusually light.

___ My menstrual periods have become unusually short.

___ My menstrual periods are coming less frequently.

___ I'm having unusually heavy menstrual periods.

ESPECIALLY IN NEWBORNS/BABIES

___ My newborn or infant was born prematurely.

___ My newborn or infant had a low birth weight.

___ My newborn or infant has a smaller head in comparison to his/her body.

___ My newborn or infant has a yellowish cast to the skin.

___ My newborn or infant has a visible goiter or enlarged neck.

___ My newborn or infant has prominent eyes.

___ My newborn or infant has an elevated heart rate.

___ My newborn or infant regularly runs a fever.

___ My newborn or infant is irritable and restless.

___ My newborn or infant appears hyperactive.

___ My newborn or infant appears anxious.

___ My newborn or infant is unusually alert.

___ My newborn or infant has frequent diarrhea and/or vomiting.

___ My newborn or infant is not gaining weight.

___ My newborn or infant is losing weight.

ESPECIALLY IN CHILDREN

___ My child has a goiter and/or enlarged neck area.

___ My child has had a recent sudden growth spurt.

___ My child has developed an unusually large appetite.

___ My child has had a period of rapid weight loss.

___ My child has recently developed poor handwriting.

___ My child is experiencing poor school performance.

___ My child is having difficulty concentrating at school.

___ My child is weak in the legs or arms.

___ My child is often fatigued and exhausted.

___ My child appears moody and lacks motivation.

___ I worry that my child may be taking illegal drugs.

___ My child has emotional outbursts.

___ My child is having more temper tantrums.

___ My child is crying easily.

___ My child is more irritable than usual.

___ My child is having trouble sleeping.

___ My child is wetting the bed.

___ My child is restless.

___ My child has tremors.

___ My child can't sit still and exhibits hyperactive-like movements, including leg swinging, finger tapping, etc.

ESPECIALLY IN TEENAGERS

__ My teenager is moody.

__ My teenager has an increased appetite.

__ My teenager is emotionally changeable.

__ My teenager has had unexplained, rapid, or sudden weight loss.

__ My teenager may be anorexic.

__ My teenager is suddenly gaining weight rapidly.

__ My teenager is particularly nervous or anxious.

__ My teenager's puberty is delayed.

__ My teenager shows signs of muscle weakness.

ESPECIALLY IN THE ELDERLY

__ I feel withdrawn.

__ I feel depressed.

__ I feel weak and tired, lacking in energy.

__ I feel confused.

__ I am forgetful.

__ I am experiencing constipation.

__ I'm experiencing more frequent falls and injuries.

__ I'm experiencing more shaking.

__ I'm noticing more abnormal heart rhythms and palpitations.

▌ Thyroid Storm Risks and Symptoms

If you have the following symptoms of this rare but potentially fatal condition, seek emergency medical treatment immediately.

RISKS FOR THYROID STORM

__ I have Graves' disease and/or hyperthyroidism.

__ I recently had an infection—for example, lung infection, throat infection, or pneumonia.

__ I've had recent blood sugar changes such as diabetic ketoacidosis or insulin-induced hypoglycemia.

__ I recently had surgery on my thyroid.

__ I just went cold turkey off antithyroid medication.

__ I just had radioactive iodine (RAI) treatment.

__ My thyroid was excessively palpated recently.

__ I have recently been under severe emotional stress.

__ I have taken an overdose of thyroid hormone.

__ I am experiencing or have been experiencing toxemia of pregnancy and labor.

SYMPTOMS

__ I have a fever of 100°F to as high as 106°F.

__ My heart rate is high, even up to 200 beats per minute.

__ I'm having heart palpitations.

__ I'm feeling chest pain.

__ I'm experiencing shortness of breath.

__ I'm experiencing confusion, delirium, or psychosis.

__ I feel extremely weak and fatigued.

__ I feel extremely restless or nervous.

__ I'm having mood swings.

__ My reflexes are exaggerated.

__ I'm having difficulty breathing.

__ I'm experiencing nausea, vomiting, and/or diarrhea.

__ I've had a recent dramatic weight loss.

__ I'm sweating profusely.

__ I'm in a stupor.

4

Getting Diagnosed

As part of your regular physical examination, your doctor should feel your neck area, palpating your thyroid to detect any enlargement and/or lumps. Many experts feel that the thyroid-stimulating hormone (TSH) test, one of the most basic blood tests to detect thyroid dysfunction, should be part of standard blood workups and should be run regularly on women of childbearing age and on both women and men after age 50. It's possible that your diagnosis of Graves' disease or hyperthyroidism may be picked up inadvertently. For others, however, getting diagnosed begins with either the doctor or patient suspecting that something may be wrong with the thyroid. This chapter talks about the various steps in getting a proper diagnosis.

▮ Clinical Signs

Diagnosis starts with a complete clinical evaluation involving an examination of the thyroid by a knowledgeable professional. Your practitioner should feel for thyroid enlargement, nodules, and masses. The doctor should also listen to your thyroid using a stethoscope. Your reflexes will be checked because hyperresponsive reflexes can be a sign of hyperthyroidism. Your skin, hair, and eyes will be examined for classic signs. Your heart rate, rhythm, and blood pressure will be checked. You should be weighed. The doctor should also evaluate your lymph node areas (neck, underarm, groin) and your spleen. Blood tests should be run and additional tests such as ultrasounds or scans may be ordered. Other clinical details will be observed and family history will be discussed. In combination with symptoms, the clinical observation plus the results of tests should be considered to make a careful, thorough, and accurate diagnosis.

There are many clinical signs that your practitioner should look for in making a diagnosis of Graves' disease or hyperthyroidism.

Thyroid-Specific Signs

- Goiter: The most common sign of Graves is goiter/thyroid enlargement, which occurs in 90 percent of younger patients and 75 to 80 percent of older patients. A goiter may be visible, palpable, or seen on imaging tests.
- Nodules: the doctor may be able to feel or even see nodules or lumps in your thyroid.
- "Thrill" on palpation: the practitioner can "feel" increased blood flow in the thyroid.
- Bruit on palpation: when listening with a stethoscope, the practitioner can hear the sound of increased blood flow in the thyroid.

Liver Irregularities

- Enlarged liver: may be felt by the practitioner or observed on imaging tests
- Jaundice: observable in skin tone or via blood tests

Reflexes
- Exaggerated reflexes

Heart and Circulation Irregularities
- High blood pressure
- Fast heart rate known as atypical sinus rhythm or sinus tachycardia: a fast but regular heartbeat, over 100 (normal heart rate is 70 to 80)
- Ventricular tachycardia: rapid heartbeat felt as palpitations and sometimes pounding
- Atrial fibrillation: upper chambers of the heart (atria) and lower chambers (ventricles) not functioning properly; atria beating faster than ventricles with an inconsistent rhythm
- Mitral valve prolapse: felt as palpitations and heart flutters

Skin, Hair, and Nails
- Smooth, young-looking skin
- Swollen fingertips (acropachy)
- Loss of skin pigmentation (vitiligo)
- Warm, moist hands and palms
- Hives
- Lesions on the shins (pretibial myxedema/dermopathy)
- Increased acne
- Flushing or ruddiness of face/throat
- Blister-like bumps of the forehead and face (known as miliaria bumps)
- Spider veins in face and neck area
- Onycholysis: distal separation from underlying nail bed, also called Plummer's nails
- Thinning, finer hair
- Hair loss

Eyes

- Bulging or protrusion of the eyes
- Red, inflamed, and/or bloodshot eyes
- Dry eyes
- Watery eyes
- Stare in the eyes
- Retraction of upper eyelids, resulting in a wide-eyed look
- Infrequent blinking
- Lid lag: when the upper eyelid doesn't smoothly follow downward movements of the eyes when you look down
- Swelling of upper eyelids
- Twitching in the eyes
- Uneven motion of upper eyelid
- Uneven pupil dilation in dim light
- Tremor of closed eyelids
- Eyelid puffiness
- Inflamed cornea

Miscellaneous

- Tremors
- Shaky hands
- Hyperkinetic movements: table drumming, tapping feet, jerky movements (often more severe in children)
- Fever
- Weight loss
- Low bone density
- Enlarged tonsils
- Enlarged lymph nodes

In Men

- Gynecomastia (breast enlargement or tenderness)
- Low sperm count
- Lower sperm motility

In Fetuses, Via Fetal Monitoring

- Fetal goiter
- Elevated fetal heart rate
- Increased fetal movement
- Poor fetal body growth
- Abnormally rapid fetal bone growth

In Newborns

- Yellow color to skin
- Increased bilirubin levels
- Smaller head
- Low birth weight
- Prominent eyes

In Children

- Craniosynostosis: condition in which two or more cranial bones mesh to form a single bone; complication of thyrotoxicosis in children
- Hyperkinetic movements: table drumming, tapping feet, jerky movements

■ Thyroid Blood Tests

Interpreting blood tests to diagnose Graves' disease and various types of hyperthyroidism and thyrotoxicosis is a complicated process. The first step is understanding the blood tests that may be done as part of your diagnosis.

In some cases, I've included normal ranges and values associated with different tests, but keep in mind that normal ranges can vary from lab to lab and may be expressed quite differently in various countries. So be sure to get a printout of your lab tests, along with information from your practitioner on what the normal range is for each test. Most lab reports will provide this information along with the results so that you can review where your tests fall according to your particular lab's values.

TSH Test (Ultrasensitive)

The ultrasensitive thyroid-stimulating hormone (TSH) test (also known as a second-generation or third-generation TSH test) measures the amount of TSH in your bloodstream. The test is sometimes called the thyrotropin-stimulating hormone test. Typically the TSH level remains in the normal range only when the thyroid gland is healthy and functioning normally.

Perceived thyroid normal ranges are in tremendous flux right now. Throughout the 1980s and 1990s in North America, the normal TSH range was from about 0.3–0.5 at the bottom end to 5.0–6.0 at the high end. At the lab where they sent my blood, for example, a TSH of over 5.5 was considered hypothyroid, and under 0.5 was hyperthyroid. Anywhere in between was considered normal, or euthyroid.

Values below the bottom end of the TSH normal range usually indicate hyperthyroidism. In more severe hyperthyroidism, this level may even be undetectable, or zero. Nonexistent or nearly undetectable TSH levels are also referred to as suppressed levels. The lower the TSH, the more suppressed the thyroid is considered to be and the more hyperthyroid you may be.

Values above the top of the normal range can indicate hypothyroidism—an underactive thyroid. The higher the number, the more hypothyroid/underactive your thyroid is considered to be.

In November 2002, the National Academy of Clinical Biochemistry (NACB), part of the American Association for Clinical Chemistry (AACC), issued revised laboratory medicine practice guidelines for the diagnosis and monitoring of thyroid disease. Of particular interest were the following statements in the guidelines:

[More than] 95% of rigorously screened normal euthyroid volunteers have serum TSH values between 0.4 and 2.5 mIU/L. . . . A serum TSH result between 0.5 and 2.0 mIU/L is generally considered the therapeutic target for a standard L-T4 replacement dose for primary hypothyroidism.

Based on these findings, the American Association of Clinical Endocrinologists (AACE) made an important announcement in January 2003:

Until November 2002, doctors had relied on a normal TSH level ranging from 0.5 to 5.0 to diagnose and treat patients with a thyroid disorder who tested outside the boundaries of that range. Now AACE encourages doctors to consider treatment for patients who test outside the boundaries of a narrower margin based on a target TSH level of 0.3 to 3.0. AACE believes the new range will result in proper diagnosis for millions of Americans who suffer from a mild thyroid disorder, but have gone untreated until now.

In the years since the original NACB guidelines were released, many laboratories have still not adopted these new guidelines. In addition, many physicians are either unaware of the AACE announcement or refuse to change their procedures until the labs revise their standards, creating a catch-22 situation. Thus, for patients who test below 0.5 or above 3.0, whether they get diagnosed and treated for a thyroid condition may depend on their laboratory and practitioner being up-to-date with AACE recommendations.

■■

	Hyperthyroidism (Numbers below range are considered hyperthyroid/overactive.)	TSH ("Normal" Range Euthyroid/thyroid is neither hyperthyroid nor hypothyroid.)	Hypothyroid (Numbers above range are considered hypothyroid/ underactive.)
Former guidelines*	Below 0.5	0.5 to 5.0–6.0	Above 5.0–6.0
New guidelines per NACB and AACE as of 2003	Below 0.3	0.3–3.0	Above 3.0

*Many laboratories and practitioners are still using these outdated guidelines as of late 2004, and all evidence indicates that this will continue.

Total T4/Total Thyroxine/Serum Thyroxine

Total T4 measures the total amount of circulating thyroxine in your blood: T4 that is bound to protein and T4 that is free and unbound. A high value can indicate hyperthyroidism. Total T4 levels can be artificially high, however, because pregnancy and estrogen (such as in hormone replacement drugs or birth-control pills) raise thyroid-binding globulin, which elevates total T4, even when the levels circulating in your bloodstream are normal.

Free T4

Free T4 measures the free, unbound thyroxine levels circulating in your bloodstream. It is typically elevated in hyperthyroidism. Free T4 is considered a more accurate and reliable test than total T4.

Total T3/Total Triiodothyronine/Serum Triiodothyronine

Total T3 is a measure of the T3 that is bound to protein as well as the T3 that is free and unbound. The total T3 level is typically elevated in hyperthyroidism. (Elevation is above 180–200, whereas normal range is 60–180 at some labs.)

Free T3

Free T3 measures free, unbound triiodothyronine in your bloodstream. Again, the "free" level is considered more accurate than the total T3.

You may have a low or even normal TSH and free T4 but an elevated free T3 level. In that situation, your thyroid gland is producing very high levels of T3, but it is still producing normal levels of T4. So measuring free T3 gives more accurate information on which to base a diagnosis, which in this case would confirm hyperthyroidism. At some labs, the normal range for free T3 is 2.2–4.0.

Thyroglobulin/Thyroid-Binding Globulin/TBG

When the thyroid is injured or inflamed, it produces a protein known as thyroglobulin, sometimes called thyroid-binding globulin (TBG). The thyroglobulin produced by the thyroid ends up in the bloodstream. A normal thyroid produces low or no thyroglobulin, so undetectable thyroglobulin levels usually mean normal thyroid function.

Thyroglobulin is typically elevated in Graves' disease, thyroiditis, and thyroid cancer. It is not elevated, however, if too much thyroid hormone is being taken and is causing thyrotoxicosis. This test can, therefore, help determine the cause of thyrotoxicosis in some patients.

T3 Resin Uptake (T3RU)/T7

When performed with a T3 and T4 test, the T3 resin uptake (T3RU) test is sometimes referred to as the T7 test. This test can help assess whether your thyroid is actually dysfunctional, or whether hormones are binding in the bloodstream, causing abnormal results. Conditions causing hyperthyroidism typically increase T3RU.

Other Blood Tests

Besides thyroid tests, other blood test results that point to but are not diagnostic of hyperthyroidism include:

- High sedimentation ("sed" rate)
- Abnormal (high or low) cholesterol
- Abnormal (high or low) triglycerides
- Abnormal (high or low) iron or ferritin
- Elevated serum calcium
- Elevated alkaline phosphatase
- Elevated sex hormone–binding globulin levels
- Elevated blood sugar/poor glucose tolerance
- Elevated hemoglobin A1C
- Elevated bilirubin
- Elevated aminotransferases
- Decreased free testosterone levels

▍Antibodies Tests

Thyroid antibodies are proteins made by your immune system. These proteins typically affect you in several ways:

- Antibodies may stimulate your thyroid to work harder.
- Antibodies may block your thyroid's receptors for thyroid hormone or TSH.
- Antibodies may trigger swelling and nodules.
- Antibodies may trigger inflammation, which slowly destroys your thyroid tissue.
- Antibodies may target your eyes and/or skin, causing Graves' ophthalmopathy or Graves' dermopathy.

Typically, antibody testing may be used to help firm up a diagnosis, but the majority of practitioners don't monitor antibodies during treatment. Their reasoning is simple: since antibodies are evidence of autoimmune disease and since they don't really know much about treating the autoimmune aspect of Graves' disease, the antibody levels are of no use to them clinically.

Some practitioners regularly monitor antibody levels, however, because they recognize that these levels can reflect and even anticipate changes in the activity and severity of thyroid dysfunction. In particular, lower antibody levels may indicate improvement, and an absence of antibodies may point to remission.

Thyroid Peroxidase (TPO) Antibodies (TPOAb)/Antithyroid Peroxidase Antibodies

One of the most common antibody tests is thyroid peroxidase or TPO antibodies, also known as antithyroid peroxidase antibodies. This test is often done as a first step in determining if you have autoimmune thyroid disease. These antibodies work against thyroid peroxidase, an enzyme that plays a part in the T4 to T3 conversion and synthesis process. TPO antibodies (TPOAb) frequently show up as a sign that thyroid tissue is being destroyed, such as in Hashimoto's disease and in some other types of thyroiditis.

If you have these antibodies, you definitely have an autoimmune thyroid condition. But the test is not definitively diagnostic for Graves' disease. Among patients with confirmed Graves' disease, studies have shown that only 50 to 60 percent will test positive for TPO antibodies. Thus, it's not a reliable stand-alone test for diagnosing Graves' disease.

Antithyroid Microsomal Antibodies/Antimicrosomal Antibodies

In some cases, antithyroid microsomal antibodies are measured, but the TPO antibody test is now considered more state of the art. Antimicrosomal antibodies are typically elevated when you have Hashimoto's thyroiditis. It's thought that as many as 80 percent of Hashimoto's patients have elevated levels of these antibodies.

Thyroglobulin Antibodies/Antithyroglobulin Antibodies

If you have already been diagnosed with Graves' disease, having high levels of thyroglobulin antibodies means that you are more likely to eventually become hypothyroid.

Thyroid Receptor Antibodies (TRAb)/Thyroid-Stimulating Immunoglobulin (TSI)

Perhaps the most conclusive but controversial antibodies tracked in Graves' disease and hyperthyroidism are the thyroid receptor antibodies (TRAb), which are also referred to as thyroid-stimulating immunoglobulins (TSIs). These antibodies bind to the TSH receptor and stimulate the thyroid to become more active.

Some practitioners believe—incorrectly—that the tests aren't accurate; however, the newest generations of these tests are, in fact, quite accurate. This antibody testing is somewhat expensive at a cost of approximately $200 per sample, without additional markups often added by practitioners.

The TRAb/TSI test can confirm Graves' disease. Although experts can't agree, it's thought that from 75 to 95 percent of all Graves' patients will test positive for these antibodies. But practitioners do agree that the presence of TRAb/TSI is considered diagnostic for Graves' disease. The higher the levels, the more active the Graves' disease is thought to be. These higher levels are often seen in patients with larger goiters, Graves' ophthalmopathy, and Graves' dermopathy.

TRAb/TSI monitoring is considered useful by some practitioners for a variety of purposes, including:

- To determine the cause of the hyperthyroidism and accurately diagnose Graves' disease if a diagnosis is not easily made.
- To predict remission, since declining TRAb/TSI during antithyroid therapy may point to remission in the majority of

patients. Some patients may have a decline with no remission, however.

Everyone agrees that it's important to measure levels of these antibodies during pregnancy. Elevated TRAb/TSI levels during pregnancy, particularly early on and during the third trimester, are a risk factor for fetal or neonatal thyroid dysfunction because the mother's antibodies can transfer to her unborn baby via the placenta, making her baby hyperthyroid in utero or at birth. Research has shown that as many as 10 percent of pregnant women with elevated TRAb/TSI deliver hyperthyroid babies.

∎ Imaging/Evaluation Tests

A variety of imaging and evaluation tests are sometimes used to make a more conclusive diagnosis.

Nuclear Scan/Radioactive Iodine Uptake (RAI-U)

Radioactive iodine uptake (RAI-U) is a test to help differentiate between Graves' disease, toxic multinodular goiter, and thyroiditis. A small dose of radioactive iodine-123 is administered as a pill. Several hours later, the amount of iodine in your system is measured, often accompanied by an x-ray that views how iodine is concentrated in your thyroid.

Intake of high amounts of iodine in your diet can interfere with the test results, so your doctor will typically recommend that you fast before the test. Ask how long you should fast. Be sure you tell your doctor about any medications or supplements you are taking, particularly those that contain iodine, such as multivitamins, kelp, bladder wrack, and seaweed. Also keep in mind that if you've had medical tests that used iodine contrast dyes, this may skew your RAI-U results for weeks or months and make the test results less accurate. Be sure to mention any tests using contrast to your doctor before having RAI-U.

An overactive thyroid usually takes up higher amounts of iodine than normal, and that uptake is visible in the x-ray. A thyroid that takes up iodine is considered hot or overactive versus a cold or underactive thyroid.

- In Graves', RAI-U is elevated. You can see that the entire gland becomes hot. (In contrast, in Hashimoto's thyroiditis, the uptake is usually low, with patchy hot spots in the gland.)
- If you have thyroid nodules, RAI-U can show them and determine whether they are hot. If you are hyperthyroid due to a hot nodule, not Graves' disease, the nodule will show up as hot, and the rest of your thyroid will be cold. Hot nodules may overproduce thyroid hormone, but they are rarely cancerous. An estimated 10 to 20 percent of cold nodules are cancerous, however.

Dr. Ted Friedman relies on careful examination and RAI-U nuclear medicine testing to help differentiate the causes of hyperthyroidism. Dr. Friedman explains:

In Graves' disease, the thyroid gland will be diffusely enlarged and smooth and exophthalmos will be present. The thyroid uptake and scan will show high uptake in all parts of the gland. In toxic multinodular goiter, the thyroid gland will be enlarged with multiple nodules. Thyroid uptake and scan will show a high uptake with a patchy distribution. In a single hot nodule, only one nodule will be felt, and the thyroid uptake and scan will show a high uptake in one nodule with suppression of uptake in the rest of the gland. In subacute thyroiditis, the gland will be enlarged but tender. Thyroid uptake will be low.

Almost all forms of hyperthyroidism show higher radioactive iodine uptake. In rare cases, you can have a cold scan with low uptake but still be hyperthyroid. That situation is typically only if you are thyrotoxic due to overexposure to thyroid hormone.

Many doctors like to do the RAI-U test because they can frequently perform the test in their own office—and charge for it—and they can get results quickly, versus sending blood work to a lab, which requires several days to process results. Some practitioners believe this test is not, however, as accurate or safe for diagnosing Graves' disease as blood tests.

Radioactive iodine-131 (the type of iodine used for ablation of the thyroid and cancer treatment) is not used in this scan. This scan uses radioactive iodine-123, which is considered better and safer for testing because it has a shorter half-life and gives off a very low level of radiation. With a half-life of approximately 13 hours, an accurate RAI-U scan can be done in as little as 20 minutes after an intravenous administration, or from 1 to 24 hours after taking RAI orally. At a typical oral dose of 100 to 300 millicuries, the best timing for an accurate scan is after 6 hours. In some cases, technetium 99M is used instead of iodine. The half-life of technetium is 6 hours. Technetium is sometimes preferred in women who are breastfeeding because the radioactivity dissipates more quickly, so a nursing mother can get back to nursing her infant more quickly. Because this test involves radioactivity, it is not performed on pregnant women under any circumstances.

Computerized Tomography (CT) Scan

A CT scan, or CAT scan, is a specialized type of x-ray that is infrequently used to evaluate the thyroid. CT scans cannot detect smaller nodules, but they can diagnose a goiter or larger nodules.

Magnetic Resonance Imaging (MRI)

MRI is done when the size and shape of the thyroid need to be evaluated. MRI can't tell anything about how your thyroid is functioning—that is, whether you are hyperthyroid or hypothyroid—but it can detect enlargement and may be diagnostically useful in conjunction with blood tests. It is sometimes preferable to x-rays or CT scans because it doesn't require any injection of contrast dye and doesn't involve radiation.

Orbital CT Scan or MRI

A CT scan or MRI of the eye orbit is sometimes done to diagnose Graves' ophthalmopathy if you have Graves' disease antibodies but normal thyroid hormone levels.

Thyroid Ultrasound

Ultrasound of the thyroid is done to evaluate nodules, lumps, and gland enlargement. Ultrasound can also determine whether a nodule is a fluid-filled cyst or a mass of solid tissue. It cannot tell whether a nodule or lump is benign or malignant, however.

In Graves' disease, the thyroid is usually enlarged. A reduction in the size of your thyroid is one of the first signs that you are responding to antithyroid drug treatment. If you are on antithyroid drugs, therefore, your doctor may use ultrasound to monitor the success of your treatment.

Needle Biopsy/Fine-Needle Aspiration (FNA)

This technique helps to evaluate lumps or cold nodules. A thin needle is inserted directly into the lump to withdraw cells. In some cases, ultrasound is used to help guide the needle into the correct position. Pathology assessment of the cells can often reveal Hashimoto's thyroiditis as well as cancerous cells. Definitive information is available in 75 percent of biopsied nodules.

▮ Self-Testing

Symptoms of Graves' disease and hyperthyroidism should never be viewed casually. A health care professional should be consulted as soon as possible for evaluation and diagnosis. It can be helpful, however, to use self-checks and testing as a way to stay on top of your health and benefit from early detection.

The Thyroid Neck Check

One self-test that can potentially detect thyroid abnormalities is a thyroid neck check. Hold a mirror so that you can see your neck just below the Adam's apple and above the collarbone. This is the general location of your thyroid gland. Tip your head back while keeping this view of your neck and thyroid area in the mirror. Take a drink of water and swallow. As you swallow, look at your neck. Watch carefully for any bulges, enlargement, protrusions, or unusual appearances in this area. Repeat this process several times. If you see any bulges, protrusions, lumps, or anything that appears unusual, see your doctor right away. You may have a goiter (an enlarged thyroid) or a thyroid nodule. Be sure you don't get your Adam's apple confused with your thyroid gland. The Adam's apple is at the front of your neck; the thyroid is farther down and closer to your collarbone. Remember this test is by no means conclusive and cannot rule out thyroid abnormalities. It's just helpful to identify a particularly enlarged thyroid or masses in the thyroid that warrant evaluation.

Home Finger-Prick Blood Test

If you don't have insurance or prefer to start with self-testing, you can do a home TSH test. A company called Biosafe received FDA approval for an affordable (less than $50) home TSH test. Biosafe's test kit requires an almost painless finger prick using a finger lancet. All you need is a couple of drops of blood, which you put into a collection device and send to Biosafe's labs for analysis. Results are mailed back to you quickly. For information or to order a test kit, you can call Biosafe at 800-768-8446, extension 123, or find out more at this book's Web site: http://www.thyroid-info.com/biosafe.

Order Your Own Lab Tests

Another option is more conventional blood testing. A blood draw from a laboratory is required, but a doctor and prescription for the blood work are not needed for testing. HealthCheckUSA offers online and telephone ordering of three different test options: (1) a standard TSH test; (2) the Comprehensive Thyroid Profile, which includes T3 uptake, total T4, T7, and TSH; and (3) the Comprehensive Thyroid Profile II, which includes free T3, free T4, and TSH. The tests are priced extremely affordably, and HealthCheckUSA doctors sign off on blood work requests. You receive the results directly, online, or by mail. You can order tests by calling 800-929-2044 or by visiting the Web site at http://www.thyroid-info.com/healthcheckusa.

▌ Graves' Disease Diagnosis

Getting the right diagnosis can be complicated. Hyperthyroidism results in a below normal TSH level except in those rare situations where TSH is being produced, as in a TSH-releasing pituitary adenoma. For this reason, the sensitive TSH assay is considered the best test for hyperthyroidism.

While TSH can be useful in screening, it can't be relied on entirely because there's a lag in time (approximately 6 weeks) between changes in thyroid hormone status in the blood and the resulting changes in TSH levels. In people who are in a state of thyroid flux, such as those who have been recently treated for hyperthyroidism or those who may be taking too much thyroid hormone replacement medicine, TSH is giving a picture of what the individual thyroid blood levels looked like 6 weeks ago. This isn't always effective for picking up subtle situations or for monitoring hyperthyroidism treatment in progress.

You can have elevated TSH levels—which most would think are indicative of hypothyroidism—and still be thyrotoxic. It's not common, but it can happen in the case of various pituitary problems, including a pituitary secreting adenoma, pituitary resistance to thyroid hormone, or antibodies that the pituitary incorrectly recognizes as TSH.

If a TSH test comes back low, a free T4 should be the next test done. If blood tests are being done because hyperthyroidism is already suspected, free T4 should be done right along with the TSH, since it will help to confirm the hyperthyroidism diagnosis. (Some practitioners still measure total T4; however, free T4 is considered more accurate.)

If free T4 comes back high, then you are diagnosed as hyperthyroid. If free T4 comes back normal, free T3 should be tested, since it's possible, although rare, for patients to have an excess of only T3 that is causing the hyperthyroidism. Once diagnosed with hyperthyroidism, the next challenge is to determine why.

If you have obvious Graves' ophthalmopathy symptoms such as bulging eyes or obvious dermopathy symptoms such as pretibial myxedema, some doctors will make a diagnosis of Graves' disease without further testing. In the absence of any of these obvious Graves' disease symptoms, the next step is for your doctor to attempt to diagnostically confirm Graves' disease. How your doctor does this depends on his or her style and preferred process. Some doctors will run antibody tests, looking for TRAb/TSI. Some will order RAI-U. Others will request both.

Elevated TRAb/TSI or high RAI-U is diagnostic evidence of Graves' disease.

Without testing to confirm Graves' disease, there is a small chance that your autoimmune thyroid disease symptoms—even the Graves' ophthalmopathy—may actually be Hashimoto's disease, not Graves'. Thyroid expert Dr. Richard Shames, author of *Thyroid Power*, urges patients not to accept a diagnosis of Graves' disease without blood work and an RAI-U scan:

> *Get a scan or ultrasound—if there's anything lumpy about that gland, you're more likely dealing with Hashimoto's. In Graves', the gland is homogeneous and uniform, it lights up all over. If it's Hashimoto's, it's lumpier.*

To recap, a classic Graves' disease patient profile would include:

- TSH—low or suppressed
- Free T4—elevated and/or elevated free T3
- Elevated TRAb/TSI
- High RAI uptake

The following table summarizes the various hyperthyroidism diagnoses and the test results typically associated with them.

	TSH	Free T4	Free T3	Antibodies	RAI-U
Graves' disease	Usually low to undetectable	Normal to high	Normal to high	Elevated TRAb/TSI	Elevated
Hyperthyroidism due to pituitary disorder (i.e., TSH-secreting adenoma)	Normal to high	High	Normal to high	Normal	Normal

	TSH	Free T4	Free T3	Antibodies	RAI-U
Hyperthyroidism due to overexposure to thyroid hormone	Usually low to undetectable	Normal to high	Normal to high	Normal	Normal
Hyperthyroidism, thyrotoxicosis due to other causes	Usually low to undetectable	Normal to high	Normal to high	Normal	Elevated

▮ Diagnosis Problems

Your Doctor or HMO Won't Test You

One challenge to diagnosis is getting past your doctor's resistance to your request for a thyroid test. A doctor may feel threatened by your introduction of medical information. In other cases, doctors may discourage testing because they are in a health maintenance organization (HMO) or managed care environment where their rating, reputation, or even income is affected by the number of tests they order. Some doctors simply don't have enough time to determine what's going on, much less order tests. According to Dr. Ken Woliner:

> HMOs and PPOs pay so poorly for "time with your physician" that medical practices run people through so quickly. If a health plan only pays $25 for a visit—whether 5 minutes or an hour—the practice has to see six to eight patients an hour. When a doctor (or sometimes a physician assistant or nurse practitioner) spends only 7 minutes per patient, they don't have time to listen to their complaints, and patients get blown off. There are studies that show that the average doctor cuts off their patient after only 7 seconds, finishes the visit in less than 7 minutes, and leaves behind an average of 2.3

*prescriptions—with the most common medications being an-
tidepressants and sleeping pills.*

When faced with a doctor who won't order tests for your thyroid, the best option is to find another doctor, even if you have to
pay yourself. But if you have no options, here are a few tips:

- Be persistent. Ask for a thyroid test. Show the doctor articles about hyperthyroidism that reflect your symptoms
  even if he or she won't read them. Ask again and again.
- Bring your Graves' Disease/Hyperthyroidism Risks, Signs,
  and Symptoms Checklist to an appointment and ask that it
  be included in your medical chart after the doctor signs it,
  dates it, and indicates that he or she has read the checklist
  and discussed it with you. Make sure you get a signed and
  dated copy for yourself. Send a copy to the HMO's or insurance company's ombudsman or consumer liaison along
  with your request that testing be approved.
- Write a simple letter stating that you have specifically re-
  quested tests for thyroid disease for the reasons listed and
  that your doctor has refused. Insist that the doctor sign it,
  place a copy in your records, and give you a copy. (You
  can then send a copy to the HMO to argue for testing or a
  referral to another doctor or an endocrinologist, if
  needed.)

I've frequently suggested these ideas to people who write to me,
and they work. Most doctors will order the test rather than officially
document their decision to refuse a patient's request. Apparently,
the concerns over malpractice or mismanagement charges made by
patients override doctors' reluctance to test. It may seem ridiculous
that you have to fight to get standard medical tests and treatment,
but it's your health that is at stake, so keep fighting.

Your Hyperthyroidism Is Subclinical or Borderline

Subclinical hyperthyroidism is defined as having a low TSH level (i.e., less than 0.1) but normal free T4 and T3 levels. Borderline hyperthyroidism means that your TSH level may be right on the edge of being too low and free T4 or T3/free T3 levels may be on the edge of being too high. In most cases, your doctor may not treat you if you fall into this category, believing that as long as hormone levels are still "normal"—even if TSH is low—it should not matter because all levels need to be abnormal in order to warrant treatment.

Unfortunately, subclinical hyperthyroidism and borderline hyperthyroidism mean that you are at greater risk to become overtly hyperthyroid, at greater risk for heart-related problems, and at greater risk for osteoporosis. These risks are particularly of concern in older patients. Seniors with subclinical hyperthyroidism, for example, face three times the risk of atrial fibrillation.

There is no agreement among experts regarding whether subclinical or borderline hyperthyroidism should be treated; however, the current standard of care is that treatment is not necessary. The American Association of Clinical Endocrinologists (AACE) recommends that if you have subclinical hyperthyroidism, you should be evaluated periodically. Some experts recommend that if you are subclinically hyperthyroid, you should be tested 8 weeks after the initial finding; if low TSH continues, a trial of antithyroid drugs should be considered.

Some studies have found, however, that subclinical hyperthyroidism presents such a risk of atrial fibrillation that it should be treated if the patient is over age 60. Dr. Hossein Gharib, a past president of AACE, believes that older patients with subclinical hyperthyroidism should be carefully and regularly monitored:

If TSH suppression is sustained, I prefer treatment in the elderly. Younger patients may be followed for a while.

Some practitioners believe that when thyroid hormone tests are irregular, the antibody tests should be conducted to determine if in fact there is evidence of autoimmune thyroid disease, particularly Graves' disease.

Diagnosis Is Difficult

Graves' and hyperthyroidism are difficult to identify. With symptoms that can seem vague, including anxiety, insomnia, moodiness, weight loss, and fatigue, many people don't suspect they have a thyroid problem; nor do their doctors. They may be treated on a symptom-by-symptom basis. On one visit, they get a drug to help them sleep; on another visit, they get an antidepressant; and so on.

Even when a thyroid problem is suspected, the vast majority of people go through testing and diagnosis with their general practitioners. Typically, these doctors just don't see many people with Graves' disease and hyperthyroidism, so they have no need or incentive to stay up on the latest diagnostic techniques. This lack of experience and a very limited education regarding thyroid disease during medical school mean that most doctors are ill-prepared to identify Graves' disease and hyperthyroidism. They may also find it particularly challenging to navigate the complexities of thyroid function, hormone and antibody blood work, and imaging tests. They may fail to order the various tests that can definitively identify the problem, or the antibodies that signal Graves' disease, or the blood work and imaging tests that point to other causes of hyperthyroidism.

Pat was suffering from palpitations, shortness of breath, anxiety, and other symptoms. Her doctor diagnosed panic attacks and put her on an antianxiety drug. Pat wasn't convinced, however, and still suffering the same symptoms a year later, she asked to be tested for a thyroid problem:

My doctor asked me if I was losing weight, and I said, "No, I'm gaining," so he told me to come back for retesting in a few months or if I started to lose a lot of weight. I never lost any weight, but within a few months I was very, very sick. I was running a body temperature of 101°, shaking so bad that I couldn't drive or write a check, couldn't walk to the mailbox because of the weakness and pain in my legs; lifting my arms to brush my hair was agonizing; and I had approximately ten loose bowel movements daily and my hair was falling out by the handfuls.

It wasn't until her symptoms dramatically worsened that Pat was finally diagnosed.

Carla explains that her symptoms went on for two years:

I was losing hair, having panic attacks, and two fingers on my left hand kept spasming. I told this to my family doctor, my gyno, and the rheumatologist who was treating me for fibromyalgia. From each, I got the same response, which was "hmmmm."

Carla was tested by a rheumatologist for autoimmune disease. She had very elevated nonspecific antibodies, but her doctor dismissed this information as well:

I then asked for another thyroid panel and was told, "No, you just had one two years ago and everything was fine." I insisted. When the test results came in, the doctor's office called me literally screaming, wanting to know who my pharmacist was. I asked why they would need this information and was told they had to get me on heart medication immediately! My T4 was at 16 and rising (it subsequently went to 22). I told each doctor how disappointed I was in them.

Finding the Right Practitioner

If you strongly suspect you have Graves' disease and/or hyper-thyroidism, you should consider bypassing your general practitioner and going straight to an endocrinologist or asking for a referral to one early on in your diagnostic process. Endocrinologists are doctors who specialize in diseases of the endocrine system. They typically have the initials FACE after their name—fellow, American College of Endocrinology. The two main issues endocrinologists typically deal with are diabetes and thyroid problems. Some endocrinologists, however, have subspecialties such as reproductive endocrinology (fertility), nuclear medicine, growth disorders, or osteoporosis.

Although an endocrinologist is usually a better choice for your Graves' and hyperthyroidism treatment, not just any endocrinologist will do. A key challenge is finding one who focuses on thyroid disease. A large majority of endocrinologists focus almost exclusively on diabetes and treat thyroid problems as a sideline, if at all. You should contact the doctor's office before making an appointment to find out if the specialist has expertise in dealing with thyroid problems, particularly Graves' disease and hyperthyroidism.

If you are having difficulty getting diagnosed and results have shown you as subclinical or borderline hyperthyroid, the fairly conventional focus of most endocrinologists may fall short of what you need. You should consider an osteopathic, holistic, or metabolically oriented physician with expertise in thyroid disease and hormonal medicine.

Deb, a physician and Graves' disease patient herself, feels that an endocrinologist is essential to getting the correct diagnosis and interpreting the often confusing blood test results:

Only endocrinologists understand how to interpret thyroid function tests. I had gotten thyroid function tests on myself 3 weeks before I was finally diagnosed but did not interpret

*them correctly. I assumed that I was normal because my T4
was normal. If the standard panel had tested for T3, it would
have shown that my T3 was sky high. But they didn't teach us
in medical school about the subtleties one can see in these test
results.*

Reluctance to Report Symptoms/Get Diagnosed

A subset of people don't go to the doctor to report Graves' and
hyperthyroidism symptoms because they have a positive view of
their symptoms. In the short run, it's hard to convince some people
who are experiencing dramatically increased energy, high produc-
tivity, and rapid weight loss that this is a problem. Some patients
don't want to be diagnosed because they suspect the problem and
know that treatment will likely cause them to regain the weight
they've lost. Behind the scenes, however, untreated hyperthyroidism
is taking its toll, and the risks of osteoporosis, heart problems, fertility problems, thyroid storm, and a host of other concerns rise
dramatically the longer you are untreated.

Of course, as hyperthyroidism worsens, people begin to get fatigued and weak due to chronic lack of sleep. Extreme weight loss
leaves them weak, dehydrated, and facing accusations of anorexia.
Eventually, other symptoms usually appear, including palpitations,
rapid heart rate, anxiety, mood swings, panic attacks, intestinal dis-
tress, hair loss, and weakness. A delay in seeking treatment can have
lifelong consequences and can even be life-threatening.

Tendency to Dismiss Symptoms as Mental Health Problems

Perhaps one of the biggest diagnostic challenges is that Graves'
disease and hyperthyroidism symptoms are often related to mood
and emotion. In the past, Graves' disease was actually considered a
mental illness, and that stigma lingers. All thyroid disorders, in fact,
suffer from this stigma because they frequently have mental health

symptoms and side effects. When your symptoms are anxiety, moodiness, depression, or panic attacks, it's far more likely that you will be diagnosed from a mental health perspective rather than a medical one.

Dr. Nadia Krupnikova is a psychiatrist and clinical assistant professor of psychiatry at George Washington University in Washington, D.C. Dr. Krupnikova explains the challenge that faces patients and their doctors:

In general, any disorder that is ill-defined and presents with mood- or behavior-related symptoms is automatically viewed by most physicians as nonmedical. For general practitioners, that means that they are likely to prescribe either antianxiety medications like benzodiazepines, or antidepressants, rather than search for a medical cause for the symptoms.

Dr. Krupnikova frequently sees patients referred to her by general practitioners who believe these patients need psychiatric help. She explains:

I've seen one case where a patient was having severe panic attacks and exhibiting extremely manic behavior—many doctors would have diagnosed bipolar disease. But it turned out the patient was actually severely hyperthyroid. Once the thyroid problem was corrected, the panic and mania was completely resolved.

Dr. Krupnikova says that unfortunately patients who complain about a wide variety of symptoms, especially when their complaints include behavioral or mood-related symptoms, are frequently assumed to have mental health problems. She has even heard colleagues derisively refer to these more complicated patients as "crackpots." According to Dr. Krupnikova, any patient with an onset of depression, mania, or panic attacks should have full blood work done to rule out thyroid disease and other health problems *before* any mental health problem is diagnosed.

On her long road to getting diagnosed, Tammy explains that at one point she was referred to a psychologist for counseling:

My husband encouraged me to go, saying counseling might help. At this time, I felt helpless. I could tell he now felt the doctors must be right . . . maybe I wasn't as sick as I seemed to be. This was a crushing blow . . . losing the support of my best friend and husband hurt more than I can ever describe. Once again wounded but determined to prove them wrong, I went to the appointments. . . . I talked with the counselor. . . . I tried using the breathing routines he felt would help control the heart palpitations and did my best. I still refused to take the antidepressants I was told would be the cure-all. I knew that would not be the case. Finally, after several sessions I was told that I didn't need to return for any more visits. The doctor felt I was fine . . . he had patients that needed him more than me— patients with severe mental reasons for being there. He said, "I don't see that I can help you. You seem to have a problem where the heart is triggered by an unknown cause, but anxiety is not the cause, but shows as a result." And so it went.

If you are having symptoms that may be Graves' disease or hyperthyroidism but your doctor is suggesting it's a mental health issue and recommends you see a psychologist, Dr. Krupnikova suggests that you push instead for a full psychiatric consultation:

If you have a referral to a psychiatrist, ideally a psychopharmacologist, you'll get a complete workup to rule out medical conditions—including thyroid disease—that can be causing the symptoms. Only then, if it's determined that you need an-

tianxiety drugs, antidepressants, or therapy, will they be rec-
ommended.

If you feel fairly certain that your symptoms are not evidence of a mental health problem, you need to find a physician who will run the tests you need or go to a psychopharmacologist. Psychopharmacologists focus entirely on the use of medications to treat symptoms; they don't do therapy. And psychopharmacologists pride themselves on being excellent detectives. As Dr. Krupnikova says,

> *A good psychopharmacologist does not want to put you on an antidepressant only to find out later that your symptoms were caused by a thyroid problem. They will almost always explore all the possible medical causes before they assume something is a mental illness.*

Ultimately, you need to trust your own instincts.

PART TWO

Conventional Treatment Options

5

Drug Treatments

Most people with an overactive thyroid will end up taking one or more drugs in order to control or treat the hyperthyroidism and its side effects. The majority of practitioners outside the United States consider drug treatment the primary way to manage Graves' disease and hyperthyroidism. These practitioners leave permanent options such as radioactive iodine and surgery as a last resort to be used when drug treatment fails or in extreme situations. The majority of doctors in the U.S. medical establishment, however, view drugs as useful to control Graves' disease and hyperthyroidism initially—but usually only as preparation for radioactive iodine (RAI), or in rare cases, surgery.

The most commonly used drugs for Graves' disease and hyper-thyroidism treatment are antithyroid drugs and beta blockers. These drugs help prevent the thyroid from releasing hormone, in some cases inhibit conversion of T4 to T3, and help calm down the symp-toms such as increased heart rate and blood pressure.

An innovative variation on antithyroid therapy has become popu-lar with some practitioners. The treatment, known as block-replace therapy, involves suppression of the thyroid using antithyroid drugs, combined with sufficient thyroid hormone replacement to restore thyroid levels to normal.

In rare cases, blockades, including iodine and lithium, are used to help slow thyroid hormone production down quickly, sometimes in preparation for surgery. Finally, corticosteroids and glucocorticoids, also known simply as steroid drugs, are sometimes used in acute cases of hyperthyroidism, particularly when ophthalmopathy is progressing rapidly and threatening eyesight.

▮ Antithyroid Drugs

Antithyroid drugs have been in use since the 1940s. They are given to help achieve a remission in hyperthyroidism and its symptoms. The two main antithyroid drugs are:

1. Methimazole (pronounced meth-IM-a-zole), brand name Tapazole (pronounced tap-UH-zole), sometimes also called thiamazole. It is used around the world. Carbimazole (pronounced car-BIM-a-zole), which metabolizes to methimazole and is known by its brand name Neo-Mercazole, is typically used in the United Kingdom and in some places in Europe.
2. Propylthiouracil (pronounced proe-pill-thye-oh-YOOR-a-sill), usually known as PTU, is not typically available as a brand-name drug. PTU is the drug of choice in the United States.

Antithyroid drugs work by making it more difficult for the body to use iodine to produce thyroid hormone. But an important point to note is that antithyroid drugs do not block the effects of thyroid hormone produced by the gland before starting the drug. So even after you begin taking an antithyroid drug, your thyroid will continue to release the hormone it has already formed, sometimes for as long as three months, causing continued hyperthyroidism symptoms.

Methimazole inhibits the thyroid from using iodine to produce thyroid hormone. PTU has two effects: it inhibits the thyroid from using iodine to produce thyroid hormone and it inhibits T4 to T3 conversion.

Initial Effects

PTU has a shorter half-life than methimazole and acts more quickly, so some people see the effects of PTU right away. Also, because PTU blocks T4 to T3 conversion, it may reduce T3 levels more quickly, resolving symptoms faster compared to methimazole. PTU, therefore, is sometimes given in thyroid storm or during severe hyperthyroidism because of its fast-acting characteristics. On either drug, achieving euthyroidism—normal thyroid levels—may require 3 weeks to as long as 3 months.

Beta blockers such as propranolol are typically used during the initial period of taking an antithyroid drug to help slow heart rate, calm palpitations, and lower blood pressure.

Talk to Your Doctor

Before you start antithyroid drugs, talk to your doctor about any history of liver problems such as hepatitis or jaundice, since they can affect your ability to process these drugs safely and your risk of side effects can be greater.

Be sure to tell your doctor if you have ever had a blood disease such as decreased white blood cells (leukopenia), decreased platelets (thrombocytopenia), or aplastic anemia. Tell your doctor if you are pregnant, plan to become pregnant, or are breastfeeding. If you become pregnant while taking antithyroid drugs, call your doctor immediately.

Finally, before you have any medical tests or surgical procedures, including dental surgery, inform your doctor that you are taking antithyroid medication.

Interactions

If your doctor prescribes antithyroid drugs, you should talk to him or her about any other medications you take. Antithyroid drugs may change the potency or effectiveness of certain drugs, or the effectiveness of your antithyroid drug may be affected. Drugs that may require adjustment include:

- Amiodarone
- Iodinated glycerol
- Potassium iodide
- Anticoagulants (blood thinners) such as warfarin (Coumadin)
- Beta-adrenergic blocking agents—for example, propranolol (Inderal), metoprolol (Lopressor, Toprol XL)
- Digitalis glycosides
- Digoxin (Lanoxin)
- Diabetes medications
- Theophylline (Theo-Dur, Theochron, Elixophyllin, others)
- Acebutolol (Sectral)
- Carvedilol (Coreg)
- Labetalol (Normodyne, Trandate)
- Penbutolol (Levatol)
- Pindolol (Visken)
- Timolol

Dosing

The dose of antithyroid drugs will differ based on your particular case. Follow your doctor's orders and the directions on the label. Typically, most doctors will start you on an initial loading dose.

When euthyroidism is achieved, you will drop to a maintenance dose to keep you in the normal euthyroid range.

The following table shows some typical doses of PTU and methimazole. Again, note that you should follow your doctor's orders for your own treatment.

PTU

	Initial Dose	Maintenance
Mild hyperthyroidism	300 mg 1–3 times/day	100–150 mg total/day, in 1–3 divided doses
Moderate hyperthyroidism	600 mg 1–3 times/day	150–200 mg total/day, in 1–3 divided doses
Severe hyperthyroidism	900 mg 1–3 times/day	200–250 mg total/day, in 1–3 divided doses

METHIMAZOLE

	Initial Dose	Maintenance
Mild hyperthyroidism	5 mg 3 times/day	5–10 mg/day
Moderate hyperthyroidism	10 mg 3 times/day	10–20 mg/day
Severe hyperthyroidism	20 mg 3 times/day	20–40 mg/day

Antithyroid drugs work best when you can keep a constant amount in your bloodstream. To maintain that constant level, it's important to take your doses at the proper times, and if you are taking more than one pill a day, evenly space your doses. The shorter half-life of PTU compared to methimazole means that it must be taken more frequently in order to maintain consistent blood levels. Generally, methimazole is taken once a day (or twice a day for those on larger doses) and PTU is taken three times per day.

Since food in your stomach may change the absorption of your antithyroid drug, be sure that you are consistent in how you take it—either always take it with meals or always on an empty stomach. Methimazole may cause an upset stomach, so you may want to consistently take it with food.

If you miss a dose of your antithyroid drug, take the missed dose as soon as you remember it. However, if it is almost time for the next dose, skip the missed dose and continue your regular dosing schedule. Do not take a double dose to make up for a missed one.

For those who can't take oral medications, rectal suppositories are available.

Storage

You should store your antithyroid drugs tightly closed, at room temperature, away from heat and away from direct light. Don't store antithyroid drugs near a bathroom or kitchen sink or any other area where there is a risk of moisture exposure.

Pregnancy and Breastfeeding

Both PTU and methimazole are in the FDA pregnancy category D, which means these drugs are known to be harmful to unborn babies. Babies of mothers taking antithyroid drugs have a higher risk of goiter, hypothyroidism, or even cretinism. The risk of hyperthyroidism is, however, greater than the risk of taking a low dose of the medication, so antithyroid drugs are used in pregnancy. Typically, your doctor will recommend the smallest possible dose that will control your condition. Methimazole more easily crosses the placental membranes, meaning there is a slightly greater risk to an unborn baby of side effects. In addition, rare instances of a condition called aplasia cutis, which causes scalp defects, have been seen in babies born to mothers who took methimazole during pregnancy. These scalp defects have not been seen in babies of mothers who took PTU, so PTU is the recommended drug during pregnancy.

Breastfeeding while on antithyroid drugs is controversial. Some physicians say it is safe, but they prefer PTU over methimazole, since methimazole crosses into breast milk more easily. Doctors also recommend using the lowest possible dose of PTU and taking it right after nursing. Other practitioners have concerns about use of any of these drugs during breastfeeding. More details on the issues surrounding antithyroid drugs during pregnancy and breastfeeding are discussed in chapter 8.

More Common Side Effects

Minor side effects occur in some 5 to 10 percent of patients taking antithyroid drugs. You should discuss these symptoms and side effects with your doctor right away, but many of them may not require medical attention, and you may find they go away as you become more used to the medication. These side effects include:

- Mild temporary fever
- Skin rash
- Itching
- Hives
- Abnormal hair loss
- Upset stomach or nausea
- Loss of taste, or metallic taste
- Abnormal sensations (tingling, prickling, burning, tightness, and pulling)
- Joint and muscle aches
- Drowsiness
- Dizziness

Some people have found that taking an antihistamine eliminates itching and hives. Occasionally, patients are allergic to one or both antithyroid drugs and will have itching, hives, and other allergic reactions that are not resolved by antihistamines. In this case, other options need to be discussed with your physician.

Serious Side Effects

More serious side effects are quite rare, affecting 0.2 to 0.5 percent of patients. Liver problems, although uncommon, can be a serious side effect of antithyroid drugs. While taking antithyroid drugs, you should notify your doctor if you have any of the signs and symptoms of liver problems, including abdominal pain, nausea, loss of appetite, a yellowing of the skin or eyes, light-colored stools, or dark urine. Most liver problems will resolve after you're taken off the antithyroid drug, but PTU-related liver hepatitis may be fatal even after medication is discontinued, especially if you are thyrotoxic. Your doctor should test liver function regularly while you are taking antithyroid drugs.

Agranulocytosis is a condition where the bone marrow suddenly stops making white blood cells, which greatly increases your risk of serious, even life-threatening infection, bleeding, anemia, and other serious conditions. Any of the following symptoms should be reported immediately to your physician: fever, chills, sore throat, hoarseness, sore mouth, sores in the mouth, coughing, painful urination, shortness of breath, swelling of feet or lower legs, swollen lymph nodes, swollen salivary glands, difficult urination, blood in your urine, unusual bleeding, unusual bruising, red spots on the skin, severe skin rash, nosebleeds, black stools, bloody stools, unusual tiredness, unusual weakness, or any feeling of significant discomfort, illness, or weakness. Your doctor will test your white blood cell (WBC) count. If there are signs of potential agranulocytosis, your doctor will have you stop the antithyroid drug right away because you are at risk of a blood infection. Most patients recover from agranulocytosis if the antithyroid drug is stopped and antibiotic therapy is started. (Your doctor will then decide if it's safe for you to go back on antithyroid drugs.)

While rare, you are considered at higher risk for agranulocytosis if:

- You are in your first 3 months of treatment
- You are over 40
- You are taking PTU, versus methimazole
- You are on a daily dose of methimazole of 40 mg or more
- You have been exposed to infections or live viruses

To reduce your risk of agranulocytosis, you may want to avoid contact with people who have colds, flu, or contagious illnesses. Don't get any "live" vaccines while you're taking antithyroid drugs. You should also avoid contact with others who have recently been vaccinated with a live vaccine—for example, the oral polio vaccine—because they may be infectious.

Many doctors don't perform regular white blood cell counts to monitor patients on an antithyroid drug because it's generally thought by practitioners that agranulocytosis is not predictable; it can come on without any warning in just several hours. A 12-year study of over 15,000 Graves' disease patients showed that 55 (0.4 percent) developed agranulocytosis, and only 12 of the 55 were symptomatic. The other cases were discovered during routine screening. To protect yourself, insist on a baseline WBC before you start treatment, and you may want to push for the doctor to run a WBC every time your blood is taken to check thyroid function, particularly early on in your treatment.

Several animal studies have shown a slightly increased cancer risk associated with antithyroid drugs, but their applicability to humans is not known. More studies on the potential cancer risks of antithyroid drugs are needed.

Monitoring
Typically, your thyroid hormone levels (TSH, T4, free T4, and T3) should be reassessed 4 weeks after you begin antithyroid treatment. If your thyroid hormone levels have not decreased signifi-

cantly, your antithyroid dosage may need to be increased. If your thyroid hormone levels have decreased significantly, your dosage of antithyroid medication may be reduced in order to prevent hypothyroidism from developing.

Most physicians recommend retesting every 2 to 4 months until you are euthyroid. Once you are euthyroid, you should be monitored at least every 4 to 6 months.

Withdrawing the Drug

Some doctors suggest withdrawal of antithyroid drugs after a year to see if you are in a remission. You may be instructed to simply stop taking your antithyroid drugs, but in his book *The Thyroid Solution*, thyroid expert Dr. Ridha Arem recommends tapering your dose:

> *With methimazole, I usually decrease the dose first by 5 milligrams daily until the patient has reached a dose of 5 milligrams per day; then the dose is dropped to 5 milligrams every other day, then to 5 milligrams twice a week (on Sunday and Wednesday) before stopping the medication. Only if the TSH remains normal while you are taking 5 milligrams twice a week for at least two months should you stop taking the medication. If the TSH is not normal, you may become hyperthyroid again, and the vicious cycle will resume.*

Remission on Antithyroid Drugs

The possibility of remission with antithyroid drugs is not typically discussed in the United States, because radioactive iodine (RAI) treatment to permanently kill off the thyroid is almost always recommended after diagnosis. But remission from Graves' disease and hyperthyroidism is a very real possibility using antithyroid drugs and is considered the objective for treatment everywhere except the United States.

Experts don't really know how or why remission—that is, normal, or euthyroid, thyroid levels—happens. Whether the remission is spontaneous or due to the reduction of the hyperthyroid state, or whether the drugs have an effect on the immune system, is not known. An estimated 30 to 50 percent of patients achieve a remission when taking an antithyroid drug for at least 6 months to a year. Remission on antithyroid drugs is most likely if:

- You have mild or subclinical hyperthyroidism
- You have a small goiter
- You are not a smoker
- You do not have high levels of blocking antibodies
- You are not a child, teen, or young adult
- You do not have ophthalmopathy

People who have more serious hyperthyroidism, have a large goiter, smoke, have high levels of blocking antibodies, have ophthalmopathy, and/or are a child, teenager, or young adult have less of a chance of permanent remission on antithyroid drug therapy.

Some studies have shown that remission rates are higher when you take antithyroid drugs for more than 18 months to 24 months, versus shorter periods of 6 to 12 months, but the findings are still controversial. One Norwegian study found that some 62% of patients were in remission at the 1-year point and 52% were still in remission at 2 years for 18 to 24 months, after taking either methimazole or PTU.

It's been shown that as many as 30 to 40 percent of patients treated with antithyroid drugs remain in remission 10 years after they stop their drug treatment. Half of the patients who have a remission will, however, have a recurrence. If hyperthyroidism returns after treatment with an antithyroid drug, many physicians recommend destructive treatment such as RAI or surgery.

Following remission, only 20 percent of patients treated with antithyroid drugs become hypothyroid after 20 years.

Long-Term Use

Generally, many physicians believe that treating for periods longer than approximately 18 months is not likely to help you achieve remission compared to longer treatment periods. Many patients, however, report that they are stabilized on long-term use of low-dose antithyroid drugs, with no side effects.

Doreen, a patient in her late twenties, was given a low dose of RAI that didn't work. When her doctor suggested a second round, she refused, explaining:

> I continue to see my endocrinologist for regular blood work and I am now only taking 2.5 mg of methimazole every 2 out of 3 days. My endo has referred to me as "misguided" for not taking his advice to do RAI, but after everything I've read about it, I'm just not comfortable with the idea. My TSH has been normal more often than not in the past couple of years. I think I've finally found a dosage that works for me. My endo would still like to wean me off of the methimazole completely, but every time he lowers my dose, I go back to being hyper. I'm trying to convince him that I'm fine taking such a low dose!

Methimazole or PTU: Which Should You Take?

As noted, PTU is the drug of choice in the United States. Methimazole and carbimazole are primarily used outside the United States, and PTU may not even be available in some parts of the world. But when you have a choice, which drug should you take: methimazole or PTU?

Generally, the research shows that while both drugs are effective, methimazole may be slightly more effective. Methimazole at lower doses—for example, 5–10 mg/day—is considered to be less of a risk than PTU for the more serious side effects such as agranulocytosis or liver problems. Overall, the rate of agranulocytosis for both drugs ranges from 0.2 to 0.5 percent, but the number of cases in methimazole patients on low doses is very small. Rare but serious side effects, including drug-induced hepatitis and antineutrophil cytoplasmic antibody-positive vasculitis (an inflammation of the blood vessels) are more typical of PTU and are rarely seen in patients taking methimazole. Because methimazole only has to be taken once a day and PTU must be taken three to four times throughout the day to be effective, some patients prefer methimazole.

If you are taking antithyroid drugs in preparation for RAI, you should be taking methimazole or switch to it in the month prior to RAI. PTU has been shown in numerous research studies to substantially reduce the effectiveness of RAI. If remaining on PTU prior to RAI, the dose of radioactive iodine may need to be increased by as much as 25 percent to overcome the radioresistant side effect of taking PTU.

If you have severe thyrotoxicosis, your doctor may recommend PTU because of its fast-acting nature. PTU is not a long-lasting drug, so you have to take it several times throughout the day to maintain control over symptoms. But some patients find that by carefully timing when they take their PTU throughout the day, they can achieve better symptom control on lower doses of medication.

Methimazole is considered ten times more potent than PTU, which means it presents a slightly higher risk for liver damage. At lower doses the cost of methimazole and PTU are similar, but at higher doses PTU is less expensive than methimazole. If you are pregnant or breastfeeding, PTU does not cross over the placenta or into breast milk as readily as methimazole, so it is the preferred drug in these cases.

▮ Block-Replace Therapy

Block-replace therapy (BRT) is a controversial form of hyperthyroidism treatment. The theory behind it is that you are given enough antithyroid drug to shut down your thyroid completely, suppressing TSH and inhibiting the autoimmune process. You are then given replacement doses of thyroid hormone to restore you to normal thyroid function.

BRT garnered international interest after the results of a study were published in 1991 in the *New England Journal of Medicine*. Japanese researchers found that patients who were given methimazole plus levothyroxine, one combination of drugs commonly used in BRT, for 12 months, then levothyroxine alone for 36 months, had a 98.3 percent remission rate. The remission rate for methimazole alone was 65 percent. BRT also lowered antibody levels, whereas antithyroid drugs alone did not. Subsequent researchers, however, have been unable to reproduce these high remission rates. Because the results have not been reproducible, some doctors believe there is no benefit to BRT.

Other practitioners have continued to recommend BRT over antithyroid drugs alone, believing that it does result in high remission rates. They claim that the reason the Japanese study results have not been repeated was that the study itself used tangible guidelines, including T3 suppression tests, to determine when the patient entered remission. Specific guidelines to actually document remission were rarely used in the follow-up studies, however. These practitioners believe that the response of their patients justifies continued use of the BRT regimen.

More common, however, are doctors who believe that although studies weren't able to reproduce the high remission rates seen in the Japanese research, BRT is still preferable for most patients because it is easier to maintain normal thyroid levels, which ultimately means patients on BRT make fewer visits to the doctor than those on antithyroid drugs alone. BRT also appears to achieve remission more quickly than antithyroid drugs alone. In one study, the remission rate 6 months after stopping BRT was 59 percent and after 12 months on BRT it was 65 percent.

Dr. Richard Shames, *thyroid power* author and expert, advocates block-replace therapy:

> *Some patients simply do better with block-replace. I've had people that really love it. They seem to be holding down their own thyroid production with the supplements and 5 mg of Tapazole, and then taking 12.5 or 25 mcg of thyroxine, or a compounded thyroxine cream. They can block the gland further if they also have a little T3 added.*

Some patients are not good candidates for BRT. For example, while BRT can be used with children, the higher dose of antithyroid drugs needed as part of BRT outweighs the potential benefits. Patients who are particularly sensitive to thyroid hormone drugs or who have heart problems may experience added symptoms on BRT. Because higher doses of antithyroid drugs are needed, there is also a slightly greater risk of side effects from those drugs.

▮ Beta-Blockers

Beta-adrenergic receptor antagonists (known as beta blockers) are often used as part of hyperthyroidism treatment because they help alleviate the effects of excess thyroid hormone on the heart and circulation, especially rapid heart rate (tachycardia), blood pressure, palpitations, tremor, and irregular rhythms (arrhythmias). Beta blockers also reduce breathing rate, excessive sweating and heat intolerance, and feelings of nervousness and anxiety. Some beta blockers can help prevent T4 to T3 conversion. They don't, however, slow the metabolic rate itself.

Propranolol (pronounced pro-PRAH-no-lall) is the most recommended and studied beta blocker for hyperthyroidism. The most common brand name for propranolol is Inderal; another brand is InnoPran.

While propranolol is considered the first beta blocker to try for Graves' and hyperthyroidism patients, others that are sometimes given include atenolol (Tenormin) and metoprolol (Lopressor, Toprol XL). The effects of most beta blockers are usually fairly rapid, sometimes even within 10 to 15 minutes.

Talk to Your Doctor

If you have asthma, severe allergies, emphysema, or any lung disease or bronchial condition, beta blockers will probably not be recommended for you, since they may aggravate these conditions significantly. Be sure you make your doctor aware of these or any other health conditions. In particular, the following disorders may be adversely affected by beta blockers, so be sure to discuss them with your practitioner:

- Heart problems such as low blood pressure, a slow heart rate, heart block, sick sinus syndrome, a pacemaker, heart failure
- Diabetes
- Depression
- Kidney disease
- Liver disease
- Circulation problems
- Gout
- Lupus erythematosus
- Pancreatic disease

- Kidney disease
- Liver disease
- Depression
- Myasthenia gravis
- Pheochromocytoma
- Psoriasis
- Raynaud's syndrome

Talk to your doctor or pharmacist before taking over-the-counter allergy or cold remedies. Be sure to let your doctor know that you are taking this drug before you have any medical tests (particularly allergy skin tests) or emergency treatment or surgery, including dental surgery.

If you can't use a beta blocker, your doctor may be able to give you another medicine that has a similar effect such as reserpine or guanethidine.

Interactions

There are various interaction possibilities between beta blockers and other drugs. Be sure you discuss these with your doctor before taking beta blockers. You should especially mention the following:

- Acid blockers such as cimetidine (Tagamet)
- Allergy shots
- Aluminum-containing drugs such as Mylanta
- Aminophylline (e.g., Somophyllin)
- Birth-control pills
- Blood thinners such as warfarin (Coumadin)
- Caffeine (e.g., NoDoz)
- Calcium
- Calcium channel blockers such as amlodipine (Norvasc), diltiazem (Cardizem), nifedipine (Procardia), and others

- Cocaine
- Diabetes medications such as insulin, glyburide (Diabeta, Micronase, Glynase), glipizide (Glucotrol), chlorpropamide (Diabinese), and metformin (Glucophage/Glucotrol)
- Diuretics
- Dyphylline (e.g., Lufylline)
- Guanabenz (e.g., Wytensin)
- Haloperidol (Haldol)
- Heart medicines such as nifedipine (Procardia, Adalat), reserpine (Serpasil), verapamil (Calan, Verelan, Isoptin), diltiazem (Cardizem, Dilacor XR), clonidine (Catapres), digoxin (Lanoxin), and digitalis
- Lithium
- Monoamine oxidase (MAO) inhibitors such as phenelzine (Nardil), selegiline (Eldepryl), and others
- Nonsteroidal antiinflammatory drugs (NSAIDs) such as ibuprofen (Motrin, Advil, others), naproxen (Aleve, Anaprox, Naprosyn, others), ketoprofen (Orudis, Orudis KT, Oruvail), and aspirin
- Oxtriphylline (e.g., Choledyl)
- Penicillins
- Prescription or over-the-counter cough and cold medications
- Prescription or over-the-counter diet pills
- Respiratory drugs such as albuterol (Ventolin, Proventil, Volmax, others), bitolterol (Tornalate), metaproterenol (Alupent, Metaprel), pirbuterol (Maxair), terbutaline (Brethaire, Brethine, Bricanyl), and theophylline (Theo-Dur, Theochron, Theolair)
- Various antibiotics

Dosing

Try to take your beta blockers at the same time(s) every day. Remember if you are taking any long-acting or time-released versions that you should not crush or break open the pills. If you miss a dose, try to take it as soon as you remember. But if you are close to the time to take your next dose, skip the missed dose and just take your next dose—don't double your dose.

Always follow your doctor's instructions regarding dosage. But for general information, the typical doses for hyperthyroidism would be 20 to 40 mg of propranolol up to five times a day or 50 to 100 mg of atenolol or metroprolol, which can be taken once a day.

Storage

You should keep these medications in their original container with the lid or cap tightly closed, and always out of reach of children. You should store it at room temperature, away from heat and moisture, ideally not in the bathroom. Properly dispose of any outdated medication.

Pregnancy and Breastfeeding

Beta blockers fall into FDA category C, so their use is typically not recommended during pregnancy. It is not known whether propranolol is dangerous to unborns, but some beta blockers during pregnancy have been linked to breathing problems, a slowed heart rate, and lowered blood pressure in newborns. If you become pregnant while taking these drugs, you should advise your physician immediately. Since beta blockers, especially propranolol, atenolol, and metoprolol, pass into breast milk, they may affect your baby and are not recommended during breastfeeding. Consult your doctor before breastfeeding if you are taking these drugs.

More Common Side Effects

Some of the more common but less serious side effects of beta blockers include:

- Fatigue
- Confusion
- Headache
- Dizziness
- Weak pulse
- Slowed heart rate
- Diarrhea or constipation
- Nausea and vomiting
- Depression
- Nightmares
- Impotence in men

Serious Side Effects

Rare but serious side effects of beta blockers are wheezing, shortness of breath, hives, difficulty breathing, closing of the throat, swelling of the lips, tongue, or face. These symptoms are evidence of a potentially life-threatening allergic reaction. Call your doctor or go to the emergency room immediately if you experience any of them.

Other serious symptoms that you should discuss with your doctor immediately include:

- Irregular heartbeat
- Pain or cramping in your legs
- Rapid, sudden-onset weight gain such as more than 2 pounds a day or 5 pounds a week
- Chest pain or heart pain
- Unusually cold, blue, or painful feet and hands
- Significant skin rash

Withdrawing the Drug

Suddenly stopping beta blockers is not typically recommended, since this can be risky to your heart. Your doctor will discuss a plan to taper your dose to a point where you can safely stop taking the drug.

■ Blockades

Some drugs fall into the category of blockades—that is, they block the release of thyroid hormone from the gland. Blockades should not be used for long-term therapies. They must be given carefully, but there are situations where they may help.

Blockades can include iodine preparations and lithium. Some of the iodine preparations given for rapid blocking of thyroid hormone release include:

- Sodium iodide
- Saturated solution of potassium iodide (SSKI)
- Lugol's solution
- Iopanoic acid (Telepaque)
- Dexamethasone (Decadron)

Iodine preparations should only be taken on the advice of a knowledgeable physician, since excess iodine may worsen symptoms. Iodines should not be used along with lithium, however, as they can rapidly cause hypothyroidism.

Lithium can block the release of iodine and thyroid hormone from the thyroid. It is sometimes used as a blockade drug before RAI to prevent thyroid storm or to treat thyroid storm. While thyroid storm is considered rare, it is more of a risk for older patients and those who have underlying heart disease. Some researchers have theorized that giving patients methimazole up to the point of RAI may help reduce the risk of thyroid storm after RAI, but this has not shown to be effective. Instead, research has shown that a 2- to 3-week course of lithium carbonate begun the day after methimazole is stopped can prevent the post-RAI increases in circulating thyroid hormone that lead to thyroid storm. Lithium therapy is considered a safe and effective way to quickly control hyperthyroidism.

Lithium has been used as an option for patients who have recurrent thyrotoxicosis that is not sufficiently responsive to antithyroid drugs. Some research has also shown that lithium may be helpful when given to patients who go off antithyroid drugs prior to RAI therapy. A short course (6 to 7 days) of lithium can be a useful adjunct to RAI treatment because it has been shown to more quickly reduce thyrotoxicosis and helps prevent worsening hyperthyroidism due to the stoppage of antithyroid drugs prior to RAI.

▌ Corticosteroids/Glucocorticoids

Corticosteroids (pronounced kor-ti-koe-STER-oyds), which are cortisone-like medicines, help to reduce inflammation and can calm down the body's immune response. In addition to the antiinflammatory effects, steroids are thought to lessen T4 to T3 conversion and reduce formation of antibodies. Steroid drugs are primarily reserved for use during thyroid storm and when thyroid eye disease/ophthalmopathy is severe, is rapidly progressing, or a compressed optic nerve is threatening eyesight.

Various steroids that can be given orally include:

- Hydrocortisone (Hydrocortone, Cortef, Hydrocort, Hydro-Tex, Solu-Cortef)
- Prednisone (Deltasone, Meticorten, Orasone, Sterapred)
- Methylprednisolone (Medrol, Solu-Medrol, Depo-Medrol)

When eyesight is endangered, intravenous pulse therapy is sometimes recommended. This usually involves intravenous methylprednisolone given daily for 2 to 3 days a total of three to five times over a 3- to 5-week period.

Talk to Your Doctor

Before starting corticosteroid therapy, be particularly careful to inform your doctor of your full medical history, including other conditions you have and medications you are taking. These drugs can affect many other medical conditions, so your doctor will need complete information in order to properly treat you. Some conditions that you need to be particularly sure your doctor is aware of include:

- Viral infections, including acquired immunodeficiency syndrome (AIDS) and herpes
- Bacterial or fungal infections
- Diabetes
- Kidney disease, dialysis, or stones
- Liver disease
- High blood pressure or heart disease
- Ulcerative colitis, diverticulitis, or stomach ulcers
- Myasthenia gravis
- Human immunodeficiency virus (HIV) infection
- Recent surgery or injury
- Tuberculosis (active, inactive, or a past history)
- Chickenpox (including a recent exposure)
- Measles (including a recent exposure)
- Glaucoma
- High cholesterol
- Osteoporosis
- Lupus

Be sure to talk to your doctor and get approval before you have any vaccinations or immunizations while you are taking these drugs. You should also discuss with your doctor in advance if someone living in your home is planning to get the live oral polio vaccine because there is a risk that you can contract polio if exposed while on corticosteroids. In addition, you should avoid close contact with others who have recently taken the oral polio vaccine.

You should avoid contact with anyone who has chickenpox or measles. This is particularly important for children taking corticosteroid drugs. If you think you've been exposed to the chickenpox or measles virus, contact your doctor immediately.

If you are on corticosteroids for any length of time, ask your doctor whether you should carry some form of medical identification listing the drugs that you are taking, including the corticosteroid. Let the doctor know before you have any skin tests, since corticosteroids can cause incorrect results. And notify your doctor that you are taking corticosteroid drugs before having surgery, including dental surgery, or emergency treatment of any kind.

Interactions

Tell your physician about all drugs you are taking. Only your practitioner can decide if you can take various drugs at the same time, but you should be careful to note use of the following:

- Aminoglutethimide (e.g., Cytadren)
- Amphotericin B (e.g., Fungizone)
- Antacids (in large amounts)
- Barbiturates
- Carbamazepine (e.g., Tegretol)
- Cyclosporine (e.g., Sandimmune)
- Diabetes drugs, insulin
- Digitalis glycosides

- Diuretics (water pills), especially those containing potassium
- Estrogens
- Griseofulvin (e.g., Fulvicin)
- Mitotane (e.g., Lysodren)
- Phenylbutazone (e.g., Butazolidin)
- Phenytoin (e.g., Dilantin)
- Potassium supplements
- Primidone (e.g., Mysoline)
- Rifampin (e.g., Rifadin)
- Ritodrine (e.g., Yutopar)
- Sodium-containing medicine
- Somatrem (e.g., Protropin)
- Somatropin (e.g., Humatrope)

Dosing

Take these drugs exactly as directed by your physician. Some people find that taking corticosteroids with food and milk or water can help prevent stomach upset. Alcohol tends to aggravate stomach problems in people taking corticosteroids, so you should avoid drinking unless you have discussed it first with your doctor.

Storage

You should keep these medications in their original container with the lid or cap tightly closed, and always out of reach of children. You should store it at room temperature, away from heat and moisture, ideally not in the bathroom. Properly dispose of any outdated medication.

Pregnancy and Breastfeeding

Corticosteroid drugs are in the FDA pregnancy category C, meaning that it is not known if these drugs will harm your unborn baby. Studies have not been done to determine if using these drugs during pregnancy is dangerous. Animal studies have shown that corticosteroids can cause birth defects, however, and these drugs are typically not recommended by doctors during pregnancy. Be sure to contact your doctor immediately if you become pregnant while taking these drugs.

Corticosteroids can pass into breast milk. They can have a negative effect on your baby's growth, and are not typically recommended while breastfeeding. Talk to your doctor about whether you are on a dose that permits breastfeeding, or if you need to take another drug or stop breastfeeding during corticosteroid treatment.

More Common Side Effects

You should contact your doctor if you have any of the less serious and more common side effects of corticosteroids, which include:

- Insomnia
- Nausea, vomiting, indigestion, or stomach upset
- Fatigue or dizziness
- Muscle weakness or joint pain
- Problems with diabetes control
- Increased hunger or thirst
- Nervousness or restlessness

Side effects that are less common and are usually only seen with high doses should always be reported to your doctor right away, including:

- Acne
- Increased hair growth
- Thinning of skin
- Roundness or puffiness in the face
- Menstrual problems
- Wounds that will not heal
- Frequent urination

Corticosteroids may lower your ability to fight off infection, so contact your doctor if you notice any signs of infection such as fever, sore throat, or a cough.

Serious Side Effects

You should contact your doctor immediately or go to the emergency room if you have any of the most serious side effects, which include:

- Allergic reaction (i.e., difficulty breathing; throat closing; swelling of lips, tongue, throat, or face; hives)
- Rapid weight gain (i.e., more than 5 pounds in a day or two)
- Increased blood pressure
- Severe headache
- Blurred vision
- Swelling in feet, legs, or hands
- Confusion
- Sudden blindness
- Irregular heartbeat

Withdrawing the Drug

Be sure to ask your doctor for specific advice on how best to stop taking your corticosteroid drug. Generally, if you've been taking corticosteroids for several weeks, it's not recommended to stop taking these drugs abruptly, since this can cause a variety of dangerous side effects. Usually, doctors recommend a gradual tapering of your dosage.

■ Stimulants

Never take stimulants such as ephedrine or pseudoephedrine (Sudafed) without consulting your doctor. Also be careful about procaine (Novocain) at the dentist's office. These drugs can trigger a racing heartbeat in people who are hyperthyroid.

Tammy talks about the complications that she experienced with a bad throat infection. Her doctor prescribed an antibiotic and told her to take Sudafed:

> *Later that night, I said to my husband, "John, help me. . . . I don't feel so good." My heart was pounding out of my chest, 170 plus beats per minute. The ambulance came. . . . They couldn't understand—was I having a heart attack? What was going on? At the emergency room, my heart went up and down, continuing this erratic rhythm and escalating. They ran tests. They took blood work, and at the end of the time, told me it's anxiety! Never looking into the Sudafed 12-hour time-released tablet I had taken. Now I know that was the culprit, mixed with my overactive thyroid condition. It was a risky situation.*

6

Radioactive Iodine (RAI) Treatment and Surgery

■ Radioactive Iodine (RAI) Treatment

In the United States, radioactive iodine (RAI) is the preferred treatment for most people with Graves' disease and hyperthyroidism. Some people refer to RAI as the radioactive cocktail, a chemical thyroidectomy, chemical surgery, or ablation.

One survey of North American endocrinologists found that 69 percent of them prefer RAI over antithyroid drugs for initial treatment of adults with Graves' disease and hyperthyroidism. There are definitely some shades of gray, however. Some specialists recommend that the first episode of Graves' disease treated should always be with antithyroid drugs, except in the case of patients 50 and older, who should have RAI to reduce the possibility of hyperthyroidism-induced atrial fibrillation. There is a subset of practitioners who are more comfortable using RAI but are judicious in using it with women of childbearing age and don't typically use it with children. Finally, at the other end of the spectrum, some doctors advocate RAI for all patients, including children, as the first-line treatment.

RAI is infrequently used in Europe and other parts of the world, where medications are almost always tried as a first-line treatment. Outside the United States, RAI is also rarely used on women under 40 and almost never on children.

RAI was first studied in the United States in the mid- to late 1940s, when doctors examined people who had been exposed to high levels of radiation during atomic bomb tests. It was discovered that the radioactive exposure had caused thyroid dysfunction. RAI was later systematized for use as a hyperthyroidism treatment. It is based on the fact that the thyroid absorbs and concentrates iodine. RAI is like regular iodine we get in foods and supplements, except it carries the radioactivity with it to the thyroid.

Among doctors in the United States, RAI is viewed as a simple treatment. In their view, you take the radioactive iodine as a pill or drink, and it ablates all or part of the thyroid tissue, reversing the hyperthyroidism in many cases after a single dose.

Risks over the Next Few Months

Some studies have found no increased risk of cancer, leukemia, infertility, or birth defects associated with RAI. There are other studies that have shown that although the overall risk is low, there is actually a slightly increased risk of thyroid and bowel cancer after RAI.

RAI is considered by mainstream endocrinologists to have no other specific risks or long-lasting side effects, although one of the primary results in many patients is hypothyroidism—an underactive thyroid. Approximately 90 percent of RAI patients, in fact, are hypothyroid within 10 years of their treatment.

The American view of RAI is summed up clearly by a leading endocrinologist, Dr. Hossein Gharib, professor of medicine at the Mayo Clinic College of Medicine and a past president of the American Association of Clinical Endocrinologists. Dr. Gharib told me:

RAI is the preferred treatment for Graves' disease. I do not consider hypothyroidism after therapy a complication. It is effective, cost-effective, and safe. We have used it at Mayo for 55 years with great success.

Before You Have RAI

If you are a woman of childbearing age, you should always have a pregnancy test. RAI can be extremely damaging to the fetal thyroid and is never given to pregnant women.

You should avoid taking any iodine or iodine-containing drugs for at least 2 weeks before RAI. Talk to your physician before taking anything that may contain iodine.

Be particularly careful about medical tests such as x-rays that may include iodine contrast dyes. Be sure to inform your doctor if you have received any x-rays using iodine contrast within the last 6 weeks.

There is disagreement as to whether you should continue taking antithyroid drugs right up to the point when you receive RAI. According to Dr. Ridha Arem, author of *The Thyroid Solution*, when choosing to use RAI, some doctors will give antithyroid drugs for several months prior to RAI to first bring thyroid levels down to normal. This may help reduce the chance that a large release of thyroid hormone post-RAI could temporarily worsen hyperthyroidism or even trigger a dangerous thyroid storm. Dr. Arem explains:

I often elect this last approach so that the patient improves— emotionally and physically—and has time to learn more about the condition and the treatment options.

There have been concerns, however, that antithyroid drugs may reduce the effectiveness of RAI. The issue appears to be which drug is taken and when it is stopped prior to RAI. According to research, the antithyroid drugs methimazole and carbimazole can be taken up to 3 to 5 days before RAI without reducing the effectiveness of RAI.

PTU, however, appears to take longer to clear out of your system and can make you more resistant to RAI. It should be stopped at least 2 weeks before RAI. You can be switched from PTU to methimazole so that you can take your antithyroid drug longer. Dr. Arem recommends:

> *If the medication you have been taking is PTU, make sure that you are switched to Tapazole three to four weeks prior to the radioiodine treatment. Recent research has concluded that PTU treatment causes the gland to become more resistant to radioiodine treatment.*

If you can't stop PTU, then your doctor should consider giving a higher dose of RAI to offset the effects of PTU.

RAI and Graves' Ophthalmopathy/Eye Disease

Graves' ophthalmopathy treatment is discussed at length in chapter 7. But if you have moderate to severe eye problems, many experts recommend that you avoid RAI until your eye condition is stabilized. Research has shown that RAI carries a small risk of causing progression and worsening of Graves' ophthalmopathy. This is more of a risk if you are a smoker.

Some doctors say that RAI does not have to be avoided in people with eye problems and that the worsening effect of RAI can be prevented by administering glucocorticoids (e.g., prednisone) at the time of RAI, then slowly reducing the dose over the next 3 to 4 months.

How Is RAI Given?

RAI is typically given as a single dose of 10 to 20 millicuries in a capsule or drink. After you've ingested it, the iodine targets and enters the thyroid, where it radiates your thyroid cells, damaging and killing them. Your thyroid shrinks and thyroid function slows down.

Right After You've Had RAI

Most patients receiving RAI in Europe are quarantined for 5 days; only those receiving high levels of RAI are hospitalized or quarantined in the United States. Some experts in the United States say that doses above 30 millicuries should be given only in a hospital to prevent radioactive exposure to others.

In the first 24 hours after RAI, most practitioners recommend you avoid intimate contact, including kissing. In the first 5 days or so after RAI, you may want to limit your contact with young children and pregnant women to help protect them from radiation exposure. In particular, since the thyroid gland of infants and children is most susceptible to radiation exposure, you should avoid carrying children in a way that they will be exposed to your thyroid area and avoid any thyroid-to-thyroid contact. Some experts recommend that you simply limit contact with a baby to less than 2 hours a day the first week after treatment.

Experts recommend drinking a lot of water—some say at least four extra glasses a day—to help flush the RAI out of your system. In the days immediately after RAI, some doctors recommend following these additional guidelines to help protect those around you:

- Wash your glasses or cups and eating utensils immediately after use.
- Flush the toilet at least twice after use, and wipe the rim of the toilet bowl dry if necessary, before washing your hands thoroughly.
- Flush tissues down the toilet right away.

- Use separate towels from the rest of your family.
- Wash your hands carefully before you prepare any food for others.
- Try to stay from 2 to 3 feet—arm's length—away from others.
- Sleep alone if possible.

Some experts believe that joint activities such as sleeping in the same bed, sitting on a sofa, going to the movies, or taking long car or airplane trips should be avoided for 1 to 2 weeks after RAI. Others say that you can follow guidelines based on the amount of RAI you received. For example, follow the guidelines for 1 week if you received between 3 and 6 millicuries, 2 weeks for 6 to 12 millicuries, and 1 month for more than 12 millicuries.

Thyroid Storm Risk

Because it may take a few weeks after the treatment dose of radioactive iodine for there to be a decrease in the blood level of thyroid hormone, you are at risk for a worsening of hyperthyroidism during this period. This increased hyperthyroidism may not be a problem for many people. Patients with heart disease, such as seniors, are at greater risk during this period of overactivity, since the excess thyroid hormone may overstimulate the heart. Many practitioners prescribe antithyroid drugs for their patients who are about to undergo RAI in order to prevent thyroid storm.

Side Effects

Some people have temporary nausea and vomiting after treatment. You may want to avoid eating for several hours before and after you actually ingest the RAI. This side effect usually lasts only a day or two.

You may also have a sore throat for a few days after treatment, which is also usually treated with over-the-counter pain relievers.

Some of the RAI may be picked up by the salivary glands around the jaws and under the tongue, causing painful swelling and enlargement of these glands. This is treated by drinking plenty of fluids, by sucking on lemon drops (in order to stimulate the flow of saliva), and occasionally by taking pain medicine such as aspirin.

How Fast Does It Work?

Some people notice improvement of symptoms within 4 weeks. Meanwhile, if symptoms are especially severe, your doctor can resume antithyroid drugs and beta blockers as needed.

Some people assume that RAI works immediately—that the treatment somehow zaps the thyroid right away—but that is not the case. The RAI targets the thyroid, then destroys it over time. It usually takes 2 to 3 months, but it can take much longer.

Thyroid levels steadily reduce in some patients, eventually stabilizing in the normal range or causing hypothyroidism. In other patients, however, thyroid hormone levels may remain high after RAI, then very quickly plunge over just a few weeks, quickly causing hypothyroidism. According to Dr. Arem:

> Avoid taking high doses of antithyroid drugs after radioiodine treatment. A small amount may help bring down thyroid levels while the radioiodine is working, but high amounts can add to the radioiodine's effect and make you plunge rapidly into a severely hypothyroid state.

Some people can be unstable after RAI, fluctuating between periods of hypothyroidism and hyperthyroidism. This is seen particularly if they start on thyroid hormone replacement drugs for hypothyroidism after RAI. The thyroid hormone may reactivate remaining thyroid tissue and cause bursts of hyperthyroidism.

To decrease fluctuations, some doctors recommend block-replace treatment post-RAI using a combination of methimazole and thyroxine. Methimazole suppresses periodic bursts of hyperthyroidism while thyroxine provides the body with a predictable and steady level of thyroid hormone.

Will You Need a Second Dose?

At present, an estimated 30 percent of patients who receive RAI need to be retreated in order to resolve the overactive thyroid. You are more likely to require a second dose if:

- Your initial dose was smaller
- You are a teenager or young adult
- Your thyroid gland is particularly large, enlarged, or you have extensive goiter
- Your RAI uptake values were particularly high before RAI
- You had higher free T4 levels before RAI
- You were taking antithyroid drugs for more than 4 months—particularly PTU—before RAI

The goal in the past with RAI was to leave the patient with thyroid function in the normal range. We now know that most patients do end up hypothyroid eventually, whether after the first RAI or additional RAI treatments. Many doctors will now administer a second dose within a few months if they don't have significant results.

Research has shown that 25 to 50 percent of patients are hypothyroid a year after RAI, and 5 percent more become hypothyroid each year, until 90 percent are hypothyroid at 10 years. Some practitioners have indicated they believe that since hypothyroidism is inevitable for most patients after RAI, the failure to make a patient hypothyroid on the first treatment is actually a breakdown in the treatment process and a needless delay. This is leading to larger first doses so that the doctor can avoid having to give a second treatment and so that "success" can be achieved as quickly as possible.

The logic is that if you are going to eventually become hypothyroid anyway, it's better to have hypothyroidism identified and monitored by a practitioner right away so that it can be treated. If a patient becomes euthyroid—normal range—after RAI, she needs to be periodically evaluated in case she then becomes hypothyroid.

Some doctors feel that periodic evaluation is too complicated and it's too risky that a patient might become hypothyroid and go without treatment if she is not being regularly monitored. This is increasingly leading to a preference for higher RAI doses that will ensure hypothyroidism more quickly.

A very small percentage of people will require further treatment after a second dose fails to resolve their condition, in which case many practitioners will recommend surgery. If you have a goiter, RAI should reduce your goiter substantially within 3 months of treatment. If you have a particularly large goiter, however, researchers have determined that surgery is probably a better choice for you. When RAI is used to treat a goiter instead of surgery, it can help with symptoms such as tracheal compression and breathing. Typically, it will only reduce the size of a large goiter by 30 to 40 percent.

RAI Before Pregnancy

Many experts suggest that you should avoid becoming pregnant for 3 months to 1 year after RAI to prevent potential side effects of the radiation to the fetus. The consensus in the United States is generally that you should wait at least 6 months. In the meantime, reliable birth control should be used. It's particularly important because fertility may be increased in some women after hyperthyroidism starts to resolve.

▌ Thyroid Surgery

Thyroid surgery for Graves' disease and hyperthyroidism is controversial. It is the third treatment option typically offered in the
United States, after RAI and antithyroid drugs, while it is considered the second choice, after antithyroid drugs, in other countries.
Generally, though, there is agreement that surgery should be performed in certain situations:

- If antithyroid drugs and/or RAI have been unable to con-
  trol the condition
- If you have suspicious nodules or thyroid cancer has al-
  ready been found
- If you are experiencing an obstructed airway/difficulty
  breathing or swallowing
- If you are pregnant and are not responding to antithyroid
  drugs
- If you have a very large goiter
- If you are a child

Surgery is frequently recommended in countries outside the
United States for the following patients:

- Those who are allergic to antithyroid medications
- Children, when antithyroid drugs aren't solving the problem
- Women of childbearing age, when antithyroid drugs aren't
  solving the problem
- Those who have moderate to severe Graves' ophthalmopathy
- Those who want to get pregnant fairly soon after treatment

Surgery provides rapid relief of symptoms to most patients, especially those with a large goiter and/or severe thyrotoxicosis.

Before Surgery

Before surgery, many practitioners treat you with beta blockers for your symptoms, plus an iodine treatment such as Lugol's solution. The iodine helps to prepare the thyroid tissue for surgery, making it less vascular (which means it's less likely to bleed extensively).

Choosing a Surgeon

Thyroid surgery is not very common in the United States. Obviously, it is critical that you find a surgeon who is experienced in the type of surgery you are considering. A general surgeon or even a head/neck surgeon may not be the best choices. You should consider traveling to one of the universities or medical centers that has surgeons with extensive recent experience in thyroid surgery.

Before you select a thyroid surgeon, find out specifically how many of these surgeries the doctor performs each year. To have expertise in thyroid surgery, the surgeon should be performing at least fifty or more thyroid and parathyroid surgeries annually. A surgeon whose practice is entirely dedicated to thyroid surgery or thyroid/parathyroid surgery is almost always a better choice than a general surgeon. You also want a surgeon who has been doing this for a while, so ask how many years of experience the doctor has as well as his or her total number of operations.

Columbia-Presbyterian in New York City, one of the nation's top thyroid surgery centers, rates surgeons in terms of total number of thyroid/parathyroid surgeries performed:

- Less than 200 surgeries: inexperienced
- 200–500 surgeries: intermediate
- More than 500 surgeries: experienced
- More than 1,000 surgeries: expert

Risks

Thyroid surgery is generally quite safe with an expert surgeon. The general risk of problems related to the surgery include:

- Laryngeal nerve injury that results in permanent injury to the vocal chord and/or voice impairment occurs in 1 percent of patients. In extremely rare situations, the vocal chords may be so damaged that a tracheostomy (a tube into the throat) is needed so that the patient can breathe.
- Transient hypoparathyroidism occurs in 13 percent of patients.
- Permanent hypoparathyroidism, which usually appears the first week after surgery, occurs in 1 percent of patients.
- There is a very small risk of bleeding, which usually occurs in the first few hours after surgery, and a small risk of infection.

These complication rates are an average. The rates of an inexperienced surgeon would likely be much higher, whereas an expert thyroid surgeon typically has a negligible rate of complications.

The complication rates are also different based on whether the surgery is a partial/subtotal thyroidectomy or a total thyroidectomy:

- Risk for complications concerning recurrent laryngeal nerve paralysis after subtotal thyroidectomy: 0.6 percent
- Risk for complications concerning recurrent hypocalcemia after subtotal thyroidectomy: 0.9 percent
- Risk for complications concerning recurrent laryngeal nerve paralysis after total thyroidectomy: 1.1 percent
- Risk for complications concerning recurrent hypocalcemia after total thyroidectomy: 1.7 percent

Most patients will have a 3-inch horizontal scar from the surgery, but surgeons are usually quite adept at placing the incision in a fold in the neck, making it nearly invisible after a few months. Most surgeons use dissolvable stitches, but you may want to ask your surgeon about this ahead of time because the nonabsorbable stitches actually tend to cause less scarring. If you have any history of allergic skin reactions to stitches, you may want to ask your doctor about using hypoallergenic suture material.

Partial/Subtotal Versus Total Thyroidectomy

Some practitioners regularly perform only partial or subtotal thyroidectomies for Graves' disease and hyperthyroidism. Others believe that partial or subtotal thyroidectomy should only be done for patients with very minimal goiter and limited hyperthyroidism. Most other cases warrant total thyroidectomy.

When a subtotal or partial thyroidectomy is performed, surgeons typically do a bilateral subtotal thyroidectomy, which leaves from 1 to 5 grams on each side/lobe of the thyroid. A Harley Dunhill procedure is also popular, in which there's a total lobectomy on one side and a subtotal on the other, leaving 4 to 5 grams of thyroid tissue.

Outside the United States, total thyroidectomy—not partial thyroidectomy—is usually the standard treatment for Graves' disease. In the United States and among some other practitioners, the preference has been subtotal or partial thyroidectomy, in order to leave behind enough thyroid tissue to prevent hypothyroidism, since a total thyroidectomy has almost a 100 percent chance of causing hypothyroidism. Unfortunately, this doesn't work very often. The risk of hypothyroidism with subtotal thyroidectomy is generally very high—more than 70 percent. The risk of worsening or new Graves' ophthalmopathy is also higher with subtotal/partial thyroid surgery versus total removal.

Since one of the main reasons for partial thyroid removal is to prevent hypothyroidism, which is rarely achieved, some experts now believe there is no added benefit to subtotal thyroidectomy.

General Versus Local Anesthesia

You can have thyroid surgery done under general anesthesia, which is more common, or increasingly surgeons are able to do the surgery under local anesthesia. The benefits of local anesthesia include a shorter hospital stay, shorter actual surgery time, less vomiting, and less nausea.

If you choose local anesthesia, your doctor will typically give you numbing medication for the thyroid area, plus a mild sedative to help you stay calm. You will, however, be awake during the surgery and will be able to interact with your surgeon. Not many surgeons are trained to do thyroid surgery under local anesthesia, so if you want to proceed with this option, be sure your surgeon has done at least fifty of these surgeries.

The Surgery Itself

You will most often check into the hospital the morning of your surgery. Surgery is usually done under general anesthesia. Typically, the surgeon will cut an incision across the base of your neck in front. The incision is usually made to fall in the normal fold of the skin in your neck to make it less noticeable.

A newer technique known as endoscopic thyroid surgery involves inserting a very small magnifying camera in the neck. Carbon dioxide gas is pumped into the neck area to help make it easier to see and work on the gland. A second incision is made to insert a thin tube with a cutting edge to remove the thyroid. Because endoscopic surgery involves two small incisions of less than 1 inch, it usually leaves less visible scarring and allows a quicker return to normal activity. This type of surgery is not yet widespread, however, and you'll need to investigate to find a surgeon with experience.

Most patients remain under observation at the hospital for at least 6 hours after the surgery, at which point they may be discharged. Some people stay overnight in the hospital.

Before you are discharged, your incision will probably be covered with a clear, protective, waterproof glue called colloidium so that you can bathe or shower.

Rarely, if there is concern about bleeding or if the thyroid was very large and the surgery left a large, open space, a drain will be left in your wound to prevent fluid from accumulating. You'll need to return to the surgeon a few days later to have the drain removed.

After Surgery

It can take about a week to recover from thyroid surgery, and most people return to work and normal activities within 2 weeks. During that time, you can shower or wash your hair, but you should not swim or soak your neck. You should be able to drive again as soon as you can turn your head normally without pain or difficulty. The same rule applies to other activities, including noncontact sports. You will probably have to return to the surgeon for a follow-up visit in 3 weeks.

Some side effects you may experience after the surgery include:

- Pain when swallowing, or in the neck area: Pain can come from the breathing tube after surgery and from the surgery itself. This should subside within a few days. You should typically use an over-the-counter nonsteroidal pain reliever such as ibuprofen, ketoprofen, or aspirin to relieve discomfort if your doctor approves.
- Tension, stiffness, and tenderness in the neck: Your tendency may be to hold your head stiffly in one position after surgery, which can cause neck and muscle tension. It's good to do gentle stretching and range-of-motion exercises to prevent muscle stiffness in the neck area. Simply turning your

head to the right, then rolling your chin across the chest until your head it facing left, can help loosen tight muscles.

- Hoarse, whispery, or tired voice: Some people find that periods of hoarseness can last as long as 2 to 3 months.
- Irritation in the windpipe: If you had a breathing tube during general anesthesia, it can make you feel as if you have something stuck in your throat, or as if there's phlegm in your throat. This side effect usually goes away within 5 days.

Incision Care

While the colloidium coating over your incision makes it possible for you to bathe or shower after surgery, you should not submerge or soak your incision, and you shouldn't scrub or vigorously rub the incision. After showering, you may want to use a hair dryer on the cool setting to dry the incision.

The coating over your incision will usually turn white and peel or fall off within a week. Once the coating falls off, you can start using a scar gel such as Mederma, or aloe, vitamin E, or cocoa butter, to help with healing and minimize itching.

You might notice bruising around your incision and there may be slight swelling around the scar. If you notice significant swelling, you should contact your surgeon right away, since it could be a sign of infection.

Over time, the scar may take on a pink color and feel hard. The hardening typically peaks at about 3 weeks after surgery, then subsides over 2 to 3 months. In most cases, your scar will be minimal and may not even be noticeable within 6 months.

Postsurgical Parathyroid Damage/Hypocalcemic Syndrome

Your parathyroid glands are located near your thyroid, and their function is to control your body's calcium levels. If the parathyroids are damaged or nicked during surgery, this trauma can cause temporary or permanent shutdown, which results in a lowered calcium level called hypocalcemia. Obviously, this risk is greater if you have a less experienced surgeon. Common symptoms of hypocalcemia are:

- Numbness and tingling feeling around your lips, hands, and the bottom of your feet
- Crawly feeling on your skin
- Muscle cramps and spasms
- Bad headaches
- Anxiety
- Depression

Onset is usually within the day or two after surgery. It is rare for these symptoms to appear after 72 hours.

Treatment is temporary calcium supplementation. You may even want to have calcium—500-milligram tablets—on hand before the surgery. If you begin to feel any symptoms, take the calcium—it won't hurt you—and contact your physician. Tingling and numbness usually go away within a half hour of taking calcium. You can take calcium supplementation as often as you need it to control symptoms, but check with your doctor about your maximum calcium dosage for a day.

Hypocalcemia usually disappears in 7 to 10 days. If it does not, tell your physician. Treatment for lifelong hypocalcemia is calcium plus vitamin D.

If in a total thyroidectomy the parathyroid glands cannot be preserved, some surgeons will cut them into small pieces, then inject them into a muscle—sometimes, for example, the shoulder— where the gland parts will function to regulate the body's calcium level.

There is no agreement on how common hypocalcemia is after surgery. Some experts say that it is seen is less than 1 percent of all surgeries, but others claim it happens in 8 to 10 percent of all surgeries.

You are at higher risk for these symptoms if you have had surgery for Graves' disease rather than surgery for other causes of hyperthyroidism. Doctors are still studying why Graves' patients tend to have more of a risk.

Recurrent Laryngeal Nerve Palsy

In an estimated 1 out of every 250 thyroid surgeries, damage is done to the laryngeal nerves that control the voice. These nerves are nicked or cut during surgery. Again, the risk is far greater if your thyroid surgeon is less experienced. The primary symptoms include:

- Difficulty projecting the voice
- Hoarse voice
- Voice fatigue
- Decreased vocal range

Usually, voice changes are temporary, so the voice will return to normal within a few weeks; permanent change is rare.

7

Graves' Ophthalmopathy and Dermopathy

▍ Graves' Ophthalmopathy

In researching this chapter, I had the opportunity to talk with three trailblazers in the treatment of thyroid eye disease. The Shiley Eye Center at the University of California–San Diego has one of the nation's only dedicated thyroid eye disease clinics. Three leading ophthalmologists work as a team, seeing thyroid eye patients together as a group and focusing on an educational, patient-oriented approach to providing medical and surgical management of thyroid-related eye problems. The doctors are:

1. David B. Granet, MD, associate professor of clinical ophthalmology, who specializes in eye alignment disorders
2. Don O. Kikkawa, MD, professor of clinical ophthalmology, chief, Division of Ophthalmic Plastic and Reconstructive Surgery, who specializes in eyelid and orbital surgery
3. Leah Levi, MD, neuro-ophthalmologist and clinical professor, Department of Ophthalmology and Department of Neurosciences

Throughout this chapter, I've quoted these doctors regarding their thoughts about the treatment of thyroid eye disease–related issues.

Overview

Graves' ophthalmopathy (GO) goes by a number of other names as well, including:

- Thyroid eye disease (TED)
- Thyroid-associated ophthalmopathy (TAO)
- Dysthyroid orbitopathy
- Thyroid ophthalmopathy
- Immune exophthalmos
- Graves' eye disease
- Thyrotoxic ophthalmopathy
- Exophthalmos
- Thyrotoxic exophthalmos
- Endocrine exophthalmos

Graves' ophthalmopathy is an inflammatory condition in which the antibodies that target your thyroid also target your eyes. It typically falls into two different categories:

1. Congestive orbital eye disease: White blood cells accumulate and infiltrate your eye and muscles around the eye. This eventually causes swelling in the eye itself, the fatty tissue around the eyes, and in some cases the muscles responsible for eye movement. The areas of swelling can develop more permanent scar tissue. In general, the swelling pushes the eyeball forward, causing bulging known as proptosis or exophthalmos. The scar tissue and/or swelling can cause your muscles to become restricted, which results in double vision and retraction of your eyelids. The more serious complications tend to come from this type of eye disease.

2. Spastic eye symptoms: More common and less serious, these symptoms are the result of excess thyroid hormone and stimulation of your nervous system. Typically, this type of problem results in twitching, staring, and other irregular movements of the eye. It is worsened significantly by stimulant drugs such as ephedrine or antihistamines.

Risk factors for Graves' ophthalmopathy include:

• Having Graves' disease itself
• Having Hashimoto's disease
• Being a woman (but men are more likely to have severe Graves' ophthalmopathy)
• Being a smoker (relapse after treatment and increased severity are also more common smokers)

Stress may be a trigger factor in the development and worsening of Graves' ophthalmopathy. Many patients report that a significantly stressful event took place right before the flare-up in their eye condition.

Graves' ophthalmopathy is fairly rare. In the United States, it is seen in approximately 16 out of every 100,000 women and 2.9 out of every 100,000 men each year. Upon close examination, approximately 90 percent of people with Graves' disease show some eye involvement. But for half of these patients, the eye involvement is not particularly significant, and they may have few symptoms, if any.

Approximately 35 to 50 percent of people with Graves' disease do develop clinically significant Graves' ophthalmopathy with more noticeable symptoms. An estimated 3 to 5 percent of these patients develop a more severe form of the eye disease. Less than 5 percent of patients with Graves' eye problems experience pressure on the optic nerve, which has the potential to damage vision permanently.

About 80 percent of people with Graves' ophthalmopathy have

active Graves' disease. Among Graves' ophthalmopathy patients, their eye problems typically develop within 12 to 18 months of their initial diagnosis of thyroid disease. This does not preclude development of Graves' ophthalmopathy later, however, and there are reports of people developing Graves' ophthalmopathy as long as 20 years after the onset of Graves' disease.

Among the remaining patients, approximately 10 percent have euthyroid Graves' (no signs of active Graves') and another 10 percent are Hashimoto's patients.

Thyroid ophthalmopathy most often occurs in those aged 20 to 50. In those over 50, the condition tends to be more severe. It's rare for Graves' ophthalmopathy to affect children or adolescents.

Many people with Graves' ophthalmopathy improve, go into remission, or their eyes return to normal. Only 20 percent of patients have worsening symptoms over time, and among them, only a small percentage have serious or vision-threatening symptoms.

Spontaneous improvements can take place in Graves' ophthalmopathy. One study showed that lid retraction disappeared in 60 percent of people several years after the eye problems started. Eye muscle problems improved in 38 percent of patients. The most persistent symptom is proptosis—bulging eyes—and less than 10 percent of people have improvement in this symptom without treatment.

Symptoms

Graves' ophthalmopathy symptoms are discussed at length in chapter 2, but generally the key symptoms include:

- Eyelid retraction
- Bulging/proptosis
- Dryness, gritty feeling
- Tearing
- Puffiness

- Twitching, tics
- Staring, infrequent blinking
- Uneven motion of upper eyelid
- Lid lag
- Blurring of vision
- Reduced color brightness
- Double vision
- Light sensitivity
- Aching and soreness in the eyes

There are a variety of ways to classify eye symptoms, but one useful system is known as NOSPECS. It is a six-level classification of eye problems, as outlined in the following table:

Level	Class	Signs
0	N	No signs
1	O	Only signs are upper lid retraction and stare (may have lid lag and proptosis)
2	S	Soft tissue involvement (symptoms of excessive tearing, grittiness, pain behind the eye, light sensitivity, but no double vision)
3	P	Proptosis/exophthalmos (bulging) is significant
4	E	Extraocular muscle involvement (usually with double vision)
5	C	Corneal involvement
6	S	Sight loss (due to optic nerve involvement)

Graves' ophthalmopathy, particularly when it becomes severe, has a very negative effect on the quality of life of patients. One study found that among Graves' ophthalmopathy patients studied over a period of around 12 years, more than half had double vision and 28 percent had a reduced clarity of vision. Sixty percent had proptosis (bulging). The lifestyle implications of reduced vision and the cosmetically unacceptable appearance of being constantly wide-eyed and startled not only affect quality of life but can contribute to depression and anxiety in chronic sufferers.

Diagnosing Graves' Ophthalmopathy

It can sometimes be hard to diagnose Graves' ophthalmopathy. According to Dr. Levi:

Early on in the disease, when the change of appearance is not all that dramatic, many of the symptoms patients complain about overlap with more common conditions. Diagnosing allergies and dry eyes, for example, when there is actually underlying thyroid eye disease, is a very well-known error for many ophthalmologists. Since a regular ophthalmologist may only see two to three of these patients a year, thyroid eye disease is not at the front of the radar screen. As symptoms appear, such as when lids start retracting, or the eye bulges, then it's more obvious.

Graves' ophthalmopathy can often be diagnosed entirely by observation of a trained ophthalmologist, who will examine the eyes for signs of proptosis and can clinically identify other typical signs. A previous diagnosis of Graves' disease usually makes the diagnosis of Graves' ophthalmopathy easier.

A CT scan may be needed for evaluation of the extraocular muscles as well as the eye and the fatty tissue surrounding it. MRI is sometimes used to help get a picture of the muscles and fatty tissue around the eye as well as the state of the optic nerve.

Phases of Eye Disease

In Graves' ophthalmopathy, inflammation and infiltration typically affect the muscles, fat, and tissues that support the eye, the blood vessels and nerves that serve the eye, and the eyelids. As muscles become more inflamed and enlarged, several things can happen:

1. The eyeball gets pushed forward, causing proptosis and often a prominent stare.
2. The eye muscles may become stiff and they can't move as easily, which makes it harder for the eye itself to move, causing problems such as double vision.
3. The eye muscles may press on the optic nerve, which can interfere with vision.

Graves' ophthalmopathy is typically viewed in phases. The hot or active phase usually takes place during the first 6 to 24 months of eye disease. Symptoms typically appear and can worsen during this period.

The plateau phase is when symptoms stabilize: proptosis doesn't worsen and there aren't any new symptoms. The late phase occurs when the disease isn't active at all. Treatment is typically surgical to correct various problems and improve appearance.

Treatment of Graves' Ophthalmopathy

Most patients with Graves' ophthalmopathy will spontaneously improve, and Graves' ophthalmopathy eventually goes away in the majority of patients. Proper treatment for underlying Graves'-induced thyrotoxicosis is essential. Treating overactive thyroid can help with eye-related symptoms. One study found that eye signs improved quite a bit in 22 percent of patients on antithyroid drugs, improved slightly in 42 percent, did not change in 22 percent, and worsened in only 14 percent.

Some physicians have found that block-replace therapy, which combines antithyroid drugs with thyroid hormone replacement, maintains better stability and is more successful at preventing shifts to overt hyperthyroidism, which can help keep eye symptoms from worsening.

Smoking not only increases the risk of having Graves' ophthalmopathy for Graves' disease patients but worsens the severity of eye symptoms, makes treatments less effective, and makes Graves' ophthalmopathy relapse more likely. Graves' ophthalmopathy treatment should include a specific program to stop smoking. Talk to your doctor about some of the drugs—for example, Zyban and mild tranquilizers—that may help, and investigate the possibility of joining a support or therapy group to help you quit.

It will be helpful to have a good full-face photograph that has a close-up of your eyes taken as soon as you are diagnosed with Graves' ophthalmopathy. This will be useful down the road for comparison at various stages to help demonstrate eye changes to your doctor. Dr. Granet advises that you also bring in older pictures:

Pictures from 10 or 20 years ago to help your doctor see even subtle changes to your eyes. Your eyelids may have shifted, or you may have puffiness, but it may look normal to us, until we see pictures from before.

Treatment for Mild or Moderate Graves' Ophthalmopathy

The treatments for mild or moderate Graves' ophthalmopathy usually don't cure the problem, but they lessen discomfort until the eyes return to normal. One of the most important things you can do is focus on keeping your eyes moist, since some of the symptoms are due to excessively dry eyes:

- Use artificial tears and gels to lubricate the eyes during the day. Some good artificial tears/eyedrops you may want to use include Genteal Gel, Bion Tears, Celluvisc, Tears Naturale, and HypoTears. Avoid allergy eyedrops and those that claim they "get the red out."

- Use moisturizing ointments at night. Good lubricating ointments include LacriLube, Refresh PM, Tears Renewed, and DuoLube.
- Use a humidifier at your home and office to help put more moisture in your environment.
- Increase your intake of fluids.
- Use an essential fatty acid supplement to help with dry eyes.

Deb, a patient who is a physician herself, is a firm believer in fatty acid supplements for her Graves' ophthalmopathy:

I had read some books by Sherry Rogers, MD, and got an idea from her to try Lyprinol, which has been used for inflammatory arthritis. I figured I had an inflammatory source to my pain, so I tried it. And it made the pain go away! It kept me off steroids. Lyprinol is a concentrated omega-3 fatty acid supplement from the green-lipped mussel. I took it for a year, then figured that my eye disease had burned out and stopped it, switching to fish oil. A few months ago, I tried to switch from fish oil to flax oil; after 5 days, my eye pain returned— and went away after restarting the fish oil. So I am an absolute believer in the power of fish oil with the DHA and EPA acting as antiinflammatories.

Because it is possible to have lid retraction that prevents the eyelids from completely closing at night, some experts recommend using a lubricating ointment, then taping your eyes or using an eyeshade/blindfold/scarf/sleep mask/patch to keep eyes shut and allow the lubricant to work. Many patients report that it's helpful to sleep with your head elevated on a pillow and to even tilt up the head of your bed (by putting the head of the bed on wood blocks, for example). Elevating the head while sleeping reduces swelling in the eyes.

You may want to use cool or warm compresses or gel packs throughout the day—whatever soothes your eyes the most. Other comfort measures include:

- Avoid wind, drafts, smoke, and dust.
- Avoid bright lights.
- Use dark sunglasses (especially wraparound ones) outside and tinted glasses inside.

Specially made prisms for your glasses can help correct double-vision problems. Deb, a physician, found relief with prisms for her Graves' ophthalmopathy:

A key problem with my ophthalmopathy was the diplopia (double vision) and eyestrain. I was having a lot of neck pain as well. By the end of the day, my eyestrain was so bad that I would have to close one eye in order to see. I could not read in bed at night anymore. If I tilted my head to one side, the images would become one image; hence the neck pain. I went to two ophthalmologists who both told me that they could find no cause for my eyestrain and they did not know how much prism to give me to help this, as they could not determine a significant problem. One of these ophthalmologists was a specialist in strabismus, or lazy eyes. She ended up implying that maybe I just needed to take an antidepressant. . . . In other words, if I can't see it, you're crazy. I did not give up because it was clear to me that there was something wrong and these doctors just did not know what they were doing. But if I were a layperson, I probably would have stopped there, because I wouldn't have known enough to question them. But for the image to straighten on tilt-

ing, and for me to be fine as long as I closed one eye, made it clear to me that my eyes were not tracking together. I found an optometrist who specializes in vision therapy. She was able to do some objective testing on me that confirmed that I have a vertical phoria. . . . I now wear prism glasses that prevent the eyestrain and corrected the neck pain; I only get it if I do not wear my glasses for too long a period of time. This was yet another example of how little doctors really know!

The doctors at Shiley Eye Center use an innovative tear drainage system to keep the eyes moist. They are also leading the way in using Botox (botulinum toxin) injections to help with eye muscle imbalances and double vision. Botox temporarily paralyzes the eye muscle, which can sometimes allow the opposite muscle to tighten, thus straightening the eye. Botox may be an alternative to strabismus eye muscle surgery or eyelid surgery in some cases.

Treatment for More Severe and Rapidly Progressing Graves' Ophthalmopathy

Going beyond comfort measures into the area of medical treatment for Graves' ophthalmopathy usually means your disease is more severe and/or rapidly progressing. Typically, treatment is called for when:

- Your sight is threatened
- You are at risk of corneal perforation
- There is advanced inflammation of the soft tissues in your eye
- You have moderate to severe proptosis
- You are at risk of optic neuropathy or compression of the optic nerve
- Your appearance is of significant concern

Corticosteroids, immunosuppressants, and orbital radiation reduce symptoms in about two-thirds of patients with more severe disease. Some doctors give the corticosteroid drug prednisone to help slow the inflammation and relieve pain in Graves' ophthalmopathy. This drug rarely helps with bulging/proptosis or muscle problems, however. Typically, the drug is given orally, but occasionally doctors will give it by injection or intravenously.

A very high corticosteroid dose of up to 80 milligrams daily is typically used when the optic nerve is involved. Usually, IV therapy is done with methylprednisolone, but there is disagreement in the research about whether IV methylprednisolone is more effective than oral prednisone. Side effects of corticosteroids taken at high doses and/or over time include:

- Hypertension (high blood pressure)
- Insomnia
- Weight gain
- Bone loss
- Depression
- Psychosis
- Peptic ulcer
- Infections
- Cataracts
- Glucose intolerance
- Liver damage

There is a great deal of contradiction in the medical literature regarding the usefulness of radiation to the eyes for Graves' ophthalmopathy—a procedure known as external beam radiation, orbital radiotherapy/radiation, or irradiation of the eyes. Radiation has been used as a treatment for more than 60 years to help reduce soft-tissue inflammation and optic nerve compression. Typically, treatments are given over a 2-week period. Results have been mixed:

- One study found that external radiation to the eyes reduced swelling in two-thirds of patients, but it didn't have an effect on the eye muscle problems.
- Another study found that radiation was not as successful as corticosteroids in reducing proptosis and managing double vision.
- One research study found that radiation treatment for thyroid eye disease is not useful. Researchers found that treatment did not result in any significant improvements to the eyes in a 6-month period following the radiation.
- Another study, however, found favorable results in 50 to 60 percent of recipients, particularly when the radiation was given along with corticosteroid therapy.

There are few side effects, but in some people radiation can actually aggravate inflammation and cause hair loss at the temples for a short term. Dr. Levi has this to say about the use of orbital radiation:

We tend to reserve radiation for two sorts of desperate cases. First, the rare patient who comes in with a very rapid-onset course of thyroid eye disease, where it's not just weeks to months but progressing over a week or two. Those people we tend to put on steroids and book them for orbital radiation. The other situation is when someone comes in and they are getting an optic nerve problem because of compression of the large muscles. Most of them I start on steroids, and for most I would recommend surgery, but for those who are not good surgical candidates, radiation is an option.

Immunosuppressive therapy typically uses drugs, and in some cases chemotherapy agents, to help the course of Graves' ophthalmopathy. These therapies are considered more experimental and are not extensively used. Immunosuppressives help to change your immune system's balance to prevent the development or worsening of Graves' ophthalmopathy and to reduce antibodies against your eyes. They are often most effective when taken in conjunction with corticosteroids. Some of the treatments include:

- Methotrexate: in one study, treatment helped nearly eliminate symptoms of Graves' ophthalmopathy in some patients.
- Octreotide: patients who test positive in an octreotide III scan for somatostatin receptors in the eye may have significant improvements with this drug, but frequently with heavy side effects.
- Pentoxifylline: reduced some soft-tissue inflammation.
- Other drugs that may be of help: cyclosporine, azathioprine, and colchicine.

It's important to note that stopping smoking almost always helps increase the effectiveness of immunosuppressive treatment.

Another experimental approach is the use of intravenous immunoglobulins (IVIGs). This treatment works by blocking the production of new antibodies, helping to dissolve immune complexes that fuel autoimmune reactions. Some studies show benefits with this treatment while others don't. There are few negative side effects with IVIG.

One study found that in women who had a relapse of Graves' ophthalmopathy, eye symptoms were lessened in 75 percent, and various signs of severity were significantly decreased after treatment. If you have serious Graves' ophthalmopathy that isn't responding to other treatments, you may want to ask your doctor about IVIG.

Plasmapheresis is an experimental treatment in which blood is removed so that cells can be taken from the plasma and transfused back into you without the immunoglobulins and immune complexes in the plasma responsible for Graves' ophthalmopathy. This can be helpful in patients who have a rapidly progressing condition and is reserved for people who are not responding to other treatments.

Treatment for Optic Neuropathy

If your vision is threatened due to optic neuropathy—compression of your optic nerve—then most practitioners will prescribe intensive pulse therapy of corticosteroids, orbital radiation, and decompression surgery. This is the only time when decompression surgery will be done before your eye disease has stabilized, and it's done in order to save eyesight and prevent further permanent damage to your vision.

Treatment For Stabilized Eye Disease

According to Dr. Kikkawa, surgical treatments are not done until your eye disease has stabilized:

Usually, your eye disease must be stabilized over a period of several months—the measurements must remain the same—before you are a good candidate for surgery. Surgery is not done until the hot/active phase has stabilized, unless there is a vision threat.

The order of surgical treatment is particularly important, and all the doctors from Shiley Eye Center stress that Graves' ophthalmopathy patients should not deviate from this order:

1. Orbital decompression is done first because it can affect the movement of the eye.
2. Strabismus/muscle surgery is done next, before any eyelid repair, because the position of the eye must be stable.
3. Finally, eyelid surgery and repair is done.

Orbital decompression helps to expand the orbit area—the eye socket—to help with proptosis/exophthalmos. It allows your eye to move backward and decreases the exposure of your cornea. This surgery can also take pressure off the optic nerve. Orbital decompression is very effective in dealing with proptosis and visual acuity, but it does not tend to improve double vision. According to Dr. Kikkawa:

> The primary indications for orbital decompression are disfigurement, pain/pressure around the eye, optic neuropathy, and exposure keratopathy. There's also a compelling argument for the psychology, from the standpoint of the patient. Those who proceed—we do either a one-, two-, or three-wall decompression depending on level of proptosis. We perform surgery one eye at a time as an outpatient surgery. The patient is under general anesthesia, and the surgery typically takes 2 hours to do one side. Recovery is about a week or two, but patients can see out of the operated eye right away, although it may be blurry for a while.

Eye muscle surgery corrects double vision and misalignment of the eyes, which is sometimes referred to as strabismus. The eye muscle is cut and reattached farther back. This is most often an outpatient surgery. Dr. Granet explains:

> We do both eyes if necessary . . . and straighten the eyes by cutting the inner muscles and relieving the pressure of eyes that are being pulled down. On eyes that are asymmetric, we do asymmetric surgery; if the eyes are symmetric, then we do symmetrical surgery.

Dr. Granet has added an innovative twist to surgery:

I perform adjustable suture surgery. At the end, instead of a permanent knot, I put a slipknot, so I can later move the muscle if we haven't gotten it perfectly right. The suture can be adjusted in a nonsurgical follow-up office visit.

According to Dr. Granet, patients may have somewhat blurry vision when they return home after surgery, but they can return to reading or using the computer within a day or two. And patients can go back to work unless their job will expose them to excessive dirt or dust.

Eyelid surgery is done to repair eyelid retraction, which can cause tearing, dryness, and discomfort. This surgery helps to repair extra tissue and prolapsed fat.

RAI Treatment for Graves' Ophthalmopathy

There is controversy over whether patients who have Graves' ophthalmopathy should receive radioactive iodine (RAI) treatment. A number of studies have shown that RAI can dramatically increase thyroid-stimulating hormone (TSH) receptor antibodies after RAI, which worsens Graves' ophthalmopathy in approximately 15 percent of patients. The risk is highest for several groups of patients:

- Patients who smoke
- Patients who have severe hyperthyroidism
- Patients with higher levels of antibodies
- Patients with preexisting eye disease
- Patients who have been treated for hyperthyroidism and are now hypothyroid without sufficient thyroid hormone replacement

RAI is even thought to trigger Graves' ophthalmopathy in patients with no prior signs of eye disease. Whereas some practitioners believe that RAI should not be performed on a patient with Graves' ophthalmopathy, others feel that the risk of radioiodine-associated progression of the ophthalmopathy can be eliminated by giving the corticosteroid prednisone along with the RAI. Dr. Levi says she typically leaves the decision of whether to have RAI for Graves' ophthalmopathy to the endocrinologist:

If a patient has particularly bad eye disease and is considering RAI, then we contact the endocrinologist to review what we know and tell the patient what to expect. If there is a strong reason that the endocrinologist feels RAI is necessary, we will deal with the consequences.

But if RAI is being given to patients with Graves' ophthalmopathy, Dr. Levi does recommend corticosteroid drugs:

We actually do recommend that patients be covered with steroids before RAI, because even though it doesn't dramatically reduce the risk, there's solid evidence that steroids at least help patients who already have signs of thyroid eye disease. When people are getting RAI but they have no thyroid eye disease, no signs and no risk—for example, they're not smokers—then we don't recommend steroids.

Dr. Levi doesn't believe that a patient with Graves' ophthalmopathy should categorically choose surgery:

You have to think about the issue of surgery. You need to factor in the risk of surgery compared to the risk that RAI with steroid treatment might worsen your thyroid eye disease. You have to be working with a capable surgeon. If you're looking at the overall risk, you have to look at the individuals treating the patient, the theoretical risk of stirring up the eye disease, versus the risk of surgery with a less experienced surgeon.

Dr. Levi also cautions that if the surgeon is not experienced, you face a higher risk of nerve and parathyroid damage.

Getting the Right Practitioner for Your Eye Disease

If you suspect you have Graves' ophthalmopathy, you should see a doctor who has expertise in managing thyroid eye-related problems. You may find it difficult to get the proper diagnosis—much less treatment—from your ophthalmologist. Most doctors simply don't see many patients with thyroid-related eye problems, so many may not be familiar with the signs and symptoms. According to Dr. Granet:

The average ophthalmologist only sees a handful of patients with Graves' ophthalmopathy each year. We see [at Shiley Eye Center] in one day more than most eye doctors would see in a year.

Lynn, a Graves' disease patient who developed ophthalmopathy, describes the difficult process of getting diagnosed and treated:

My eyes were swollen and the tears were flowing constantly. Never connecting my thyroid with my eyes, I went to see an ophthalmologist. She went over my medications and history, and I did tell her that I recently had stopped Synthroid because I had turned hyperthyroid, and she never got the connection! She gave me eyedrops and that was it. Said I had dry eyes. Soon my GP called again to say that I was still hyper even when taking no meds and referred me to an endocrinologist. In the meantime, I did some research and found out that

*my eye problems were related to being hyperthyroid. A few
months later, my eyes had calmed down. I had RAI, and my
eye problems came back almost immediately. Then I found
out that RAI can bring on the eye problems—duh!*

Your local ophthalmologist may be able to treat the mildly re-
tracted eyelids and dry eyes of mild to moderate Graves' ophthalmopathy and help monitor your eyes as well as guide you on various
comfort measures. But if you have moderate to severe symptoms,
the doctors from Shiley Eye Center recommend that you head for a
nearby academic or university medical center if you can't go to a
specialty thyroid eye center. These medical centers may have more
experience in managing Graves' ophthalmopathy and the possible
surgery that might be needed.

At thyroid-specific eye clinics like Shiley, doctors stay up to date
on the latest approaches and see a larger volume of patients with the
same condition. Dr. Levi elaborates:

*It's been educational for us because we have a concentrated
period where we might see twenty to twenty-five patients—we
notice certain things I don't think we would have individually
noticed with patients scattered, one or two at a time. This
helps us to think about different approaches, understanding
what the patients are going through.*

Doctors who see a large number of Graves' ophthalmopathy patients also tend to have a better understanding of the emotional impact this disease has on patients. Dr. Levi says:

*Intellectually we knew these were unhappy patients, but it re-
ally came through to us when we saw a bunch of patients so
upset with this disease.*

Dr. Granet agrees with Dr. Levi:

> *I don't think we got it until we saw patient after patient in tears, some using the same phrases—almost word for word—about the impact the disease was having on them. It's changed the way we talk to patients. Now we are able to talk about the emotional impact of the disease, reassure patients that we know what they're going through.*

Progress is ongoing in the care of patients with thyroid eye disease, and researchers are studying radical approaches to treatment. According to Dr. Kikkawa:

> *We're continually refining the procedures and turning a guessing game into more of a science with predictability in our outcomes. But ultimately we're dealing with a disease that will best be managed on a molecular basis and surgery will eventually be obsolete, hopefully in the next decade.*

■ Graves' Dermopathy/Thyroid Dermopathy

Various skin changes occur due to Graves' disease. They primarily result from the displacement of tissue by white blood cells and chemicals—the same process that causes Graves' ophthalmopathy. Other terms for Graves' dermopathy are infiltrative dermopathy and thyroid dermopathy.

Only a small number of people with Graves' disease have significant skin involvement. In rare cases, patients who have no other symptoms develop Graves' dermopathy. These patients will typically test positive for the antibodies that establish Graves' disease, even if they are not hyperthyroid.

Most commonly, you'll develop skin-related symptoms after the thyroid condition is diagnosed—usually within 18 months of the onset of hyperthyroidism. In a small number of people, however, skin symptoms may develop before other symptoms. The two most common skin conditions associated with Graves' dermopathy are localized/pretibial myxedema (PTM) and thyroid acropachy. In addition, vitiligo, a separate autoimmune condition that is identified by colorless, unpigmented patches of skin, affects up to 7 percent of Graves' disease patients.

Localized Myxedema/Pretibial Myxedema (PTM)

Localized myxedema, or pretibial myxedema (PTM), occurs in up to 2 to 3 percent of Graves' disease patients. The condition is sometimes simply called localized edema. PTM is considered a fairly classic sign of Graves' disease. Most often it develops after the onset of hyperthyroidism itself as well as Graves' ophthalmopathy. PTM is seen in as many as 15 percent of those with severe Graves' disease.

In rare cases, PTM develops before any eye involvement or thyroid symptoms. It may actually be the factor that leads to the diagnosis of the underlying Graves' disease.

Women are three and a half times more likely to develop PTM than men. This condition is seen in children and young adults, but it's most common in older adults, particularly those in their 50s and 60s. The condition is also more common in smokers.

Waxy, red-brown lesions develop, most commonly on the front of the skin. The lesions are somewhat raised, thickened, and may even look like orange peel, or they may be leathery. PTM most commonly affects the pretibial area—the skin on the lower legs in the front. Less commonly, however, you can find the localized myxedema lesions on the tops of feet and toes, and rarely on the arms, face, shoulders, and trunk. Some studies indicate that it is more likely to develop where there has been previous scarring or skin trauma.

Occasionally, the lesions may itch, but they are rarely painful or damaging. There is a rare elephantiasic form of PTM in which lesions join together to make the entire leg appear enlarged. Usually, PTM is considered a cosmetic issue only, but corticosteroid cream or corticosteroid therapy is recommended when the condition is particularly severe. This helps reduce the inflammatory process. Treatment of the underlying hyperthyroidism can frequently help the skin complications as well.

In some cases, sunlight exposure has been reported to help. When the condition is particularly severe, steroid pulse therapy, physical therapy, manual lymphatic drainage, bandaging, surgery, or octreotide treatment may be used.

Overall, while PTM may persist for months or years, it can go into remission spontaneously. About one-fourth of all patients will have remission within 8 years. About 10 percent of patients experience eventual complete remission. A partial and sustained remission was seen in one study among as many as 38 percent of patients treated with topical corticosteriods.

Thyroid Acropachy

Thyroid acropachy is a skin condition that involves swelling and clubbing of the hands and fingers and, less commonly, the toes. Thyroid acropachy occurs in 1 percent of patients with Graves' disease.

Acropachy almost always follows pretibial myxedema, and approximately 7 percent of patients with PTM will develop acropachy. It can develop as long as 40 years after hyperthyroidism first appears.

One of the key risk factors for acropachy is cigarette smoking, and it's thought that the majority of patients who develop this complication are smokers with Graves' disease. Treatment of the underlying Graves' disease typically helps reduce acropachy.

8

Pregnancy, Breastfeeding, Infants, Children, and Teens

Graves' disease in pregnancy is not very common: only about 1 in 500 pregnant women develop Graves' disease. Another form of hyperthyroidism known as gestational transient thyrotoxicosis (GTT) is more prevalent, occurring in as many as 2 to 3 out of every 100 pregnancies. While Graves' disease can be fairly serious during pregnancy, GTT is milder. However, if left untreated or undiagnosed, hyperthyroidism can cause serious—in rare cases, even fatal—consequences for both you and your baby. It's absolutely vital to take a diagnosis of hyperthyroidism seriously and follow your doctor's recommendations.

When hyperthyroidism is not treated during pregnancy, you are at higher risk of heart problems, high blood pressure, extreme morning sickness, dramatic weight loss, anxiety, preeclampsia, congestive heart failure, placental abruption, and even thyroid storm. Thyroid storm, in fact, is a life-threatening condition that can be triggered by labor and delivery in a woman with untreated hyperthyroidism. The risk to your baby is also significant, since hyperthyroidism can cause miscarriage, intrauterine growth retardation, premature labor and delivery, hyperthyroidism, low birth weight, and even stillbirth.

The good news is that the prognosis for treated hyperthyroidism is much different, and effective treatment can almost always control hyperthyroidism in pregnancy. When the disease is treated appropriately, you will very likely have a normal, healthy pregnancy and baby.

■ Symptoms in Pregnancy

The symptoms of hyperthyroidism in pregnancy may be hard to identify because they are similar to those of pregnancy itself. Fatigue, anxiety, insomnia, hair loss—these are all symptoms many women experience in a normal pregnancy. But if you and your baby both have an abnormally rapid pulse and you have unexplained weight loss, these are red flags.

If you have GTT, you may have what seem to be more severe pregnancy symptoms. GTT develops because of the rising levels of the pregnancy hormone human chorionic gonadotropin (HCG). Elevated HCG levels stimulate your thyroid.

Some pregnant women suffer from a condition called transient hyperthyroidism of hyperemesis gravidarum (THHG). It is triggered by extreme morning sickness that involves nausea and vomiting accompanied by weight loss. Some women with Graves' disease have major heart palpitations. Morning sickness and heart flutters often happen in normal pregnancies because of the increased estrogen (which can raise antibodies) and beta HCG levels (which can stimulate the thyroid) that are typical of early pregnancy. But in women with Graves' disease, the higher level of antibodies and thyroid hormones already circulating in the bloodstream may make morning sickness and palpitations more severe.

▌Diagnosis

One of the main challenges for your practitioner is determining whether you are hyperthyroid due to GTT or Graves' disease. Doctors can't use certain diagnostic tests such as the radioactive iodine uptake test to rule out hyperthyroidism because of the harm radiation can do to your developing baby. Typically, ultrasound and blood tests for thyroid function and antibodies, as well as clinical evaluation of symptoms, will be used to make a diagnosis.

Initial testing usually includes a TSH test and free T4. Free T4 is essential, since the hormonal state of pregnancy makes total T4 less accurate. Antibody status is also frequently checked to determine if your thyroid problem is due to Graves' disease.

▌Treatment During Pregnancy

If you develop hyperthyroidism during pregnancy, it's important to have an additional consultation with an endocrinologist who can work with your obstetrician to manage your care. One survey looked at obstetrician-gynecologists' level of knowledge about thyroid disorders and their typical treatment practices. While younger practitioners were more likely to identify and treat pregnant women for thyroid conditions, some 20 percent of the ob-gyns surveyed said they don't regularly screen women for thyroid disorders. Only half of the ob-gyns felt they had received adequate training in managing thyroid disorders in pregnant patients. Few, unfortunately, felt the training was comprehensive. While more than 80 percent of the ob-gyns were confident that they could diagnose thyroid disease in a pregnant woman, fewer were confident in their ability to treat it. This points to the importance of having an endocrinologist as part of your health care team with experience in managing hyperthyroidism in pregnancy.

All of the antithyroid drugs—propylthiouracil (PTU), methimazole, and carbimazole—have been compared in pregnancy. PTU is the most water soluble and therefore doesn't transfer from mother to baby or into breast milk as efficiently as the other drugs. For this reason, as well as the fact that a slight risk of minor birth defects has been associated with methimazole and carbimazole, PTU is most likely to be recommended for pregnant women in the United States. Outside the United States, there are some areas where PTU is not available, so methimazole and carbimazole are regularly used during pregnancy. No particular problems have been associated with careful use of these drugs.

All antithyroid drugs do cross the placenta, however, and excessive doses may produce goiter and hypothyroidism in your unborn baby. The objective, therefore, is to give you the smallest dose possible that will keep your free T4 in the upper end of the normal range and prevent dangerous hyperthyroidism symptoms.

The recommended daily dose of PTU in pregnancy is typically 200 milligrams or less. If 400 milligrams or more is needed to control symptoms, your doctor may recommend a subtotal thyroidectomy during your second trimester. Doses as low as 100 milligrams of PTU can reduce T4 and increase thyroid-stimulating hormone (TSH) in your unborn baby, but PTU levels under 150 milligrams a day are rarely associated with fetal hypothyroidism.

To maintain good control of your thyroid levels, especially free T4, thyroid tests should be performed every 2 weeks at the beginning of your treatment and every 2 to 4 weeks when your thyroid levels are normal. Some doctors note that a somewhat increased heart rate is normal in pregnancy and is not necessarily a reason for your antithyroid drug dosage to be increased.

The good news is that by the second or third trimester, many of the most serious symptoms will improve, or in some cases, go away entirely. Most patients report feeling much better later in the pregnancy, since thyroid levels tend to normalize at that point. Your doctor should test your thyroid function in the third trimester. You may need to decrease your antithyroid drug dosage or even stop taking the drug entirely in the later weeks of the last trimester. Most doctors will not discontinue your antithyroid drug treatment until after your 32nd week of pregnancy because the risk of relapse is high before that time.

Beta blockers may help with significant heart-related symptoms. You cannot, however, safely take them for more than a short period of time. Longer-term use during pregnancy is associated with various dangers to your unborn baby. Typically, doctors recommend that you use a beta blocker for no more than 2 weeks, and they are most often given during the time when you are waiting for antithyroid drugs to take effect.

Treatment for THHG may be required during the first trimester. HCG levels typically fall after the first trimester, and by weeks 16 to 20, many women will feel much better. TSH may remain suppressed, however, for a time after THHG. In addition to antithyroid treatment, women with THHG may require hospitalization for intravenous fluids to replace those lost through excessive vomiting.

Iodide drugs should not be given during pregnancy because they cross the placenta and may cause goiter and/or hypothyroidism in your baby. In some cases, your doctor may recommend that you have your thyroid surgically removed during pregnancy. If surgery is recommended, it's typically performed in the second trimester (when the greatest risk of miscarriage has passed, and before the third trimester, where there's a risk of preterm labor and delivery). The reasons surgery may be recommended include:

- You are allergic to the antithyroid drugs
- You have bad side effects from antithyroid drugs
- You don't want to take the antithyroid drugs
- You need extremely high doses of antithyroid drugs to manage your condition

- You are not responding to the antithyroid drugs and still have significant symptoms
- Your baby is showing evidence of hypothyroidism due to the antithyroid drugs (typically, a slow fetal heart rate)

If you are already being treated with PTU for hyperthyroidism and become pregnant, it's likely your dosage will need adjustment, so be sure to advise your physician as soon as possible of your pregnancy so that your thyroid levels can be evaluated.

■ Postpartum Thyroid Problems

The period following childbirth can be difficult for any mother, regardless of thyroid difficulties. There's sleep deprivation, pain—especially if you've had a difficult or prolonged labor, or a C-section—worry, and simply the emotional upheaval of adding a baby to your household. Fluctuating hormones—signaling the end of pregnancy, the beginning of lactation, and so on—can make you subject to dramatic mood swings. And we've all heard about the baby blues, a period of time when you may feel unexplainably sad or depressed. But thyroid problems, which affect as many as 5 to 10 percent of all new mothers, can complicate matters, especially because they can be difficult to identify in those months after delivery.

You may go to your doctor with complaints of fatigue, anxiety, heart palpitations, irritability, or milk supply problems only to be told that these symptoms are normal for new mothers. Some women find that after they start losing weight postpartum—from the baby, from fluid loss, placental loss, breastfeeding, and so on—the weight loss doesn't stop and actually speeds up, dramatically sapping strength and energy.

If you have Graves' disease, pregnancy may worsen thyroid problems after delivery. If you are on antithyroid drugs, the dosage may be lowered in your third trimester, but after delivery you should be tested frequently, since some women find they rapidly shift back toward more acute hyperthyroidism.

Women who test positive for antithyroid antibodies early in pregnancy have a 33 to 50 percent chance of developing thyroiditis after childbirth. Postpartum thyroid problems can also appear in women who tested negative for the antibodies.

Even if you were treated successfully for Graves' disease before you became pregnant and did not require hyperthyroidism treatment during pregnancy, you are at greater risk of a thyroid problem after delivery. One study showed that 31 percent of posttreatment Graves' disease patients developed thyroid disorders after delivery. Approximately half of those patients developed postpartum thyroiditis, and the other half had a relapse of Graves' disease. Typically, the postpartum thyroiditis onset took place about 100 days after delivery, while the Graves' disease onset was far later, at around 200 days. Your risk of having a relapse of Graves' disease after delivery is higher if your thyroid-stimulating immunoglobulin (TSI) antibodies are higher in late pregnancy.

A woman with postpartum thyroid problems usually starts out by entering a hyperthyroid phase. More noticeable symptoms may include:

- Feeling particularly warm or hot when others feel cool
- Muscle weakness
- Tremulousness, anxiousness, nervousness, or irritability
- Rapid heart rate
- Overall weakness
- Rapid weight loss
- Diarrhea
- Tiredness
- Insomnia
- Low milk supply for breastfeeding

All of these symptoms can be easily mistaken as normal symptoms after pregnancy. In order to correctly diagnose postpartum thyroiditis, your health care provider first needs to distinguish it from Graves' disease. To diagnose Graves', radioactive iodine uptake, TSH, and T4 tests must be performed. A diagnosis of Graves' disease would show high uptake, whereas postpartum thyroiditis would show low uptake. (If you are breastfeeding, there is controversy over use of the uptake test. See the section on breastfeeding for more information.)

If you have thyroiditis and not Graves' disease, your hyperthyroidism symptoms may shift into hypothyroidism symptoms, including fatigue, exhaustion, constipation, weight gain, memory and concentration problems, feeling cold, muscle and joint pains. Then you may bounce between the two before things settle down.

No treatment is necessary for some women with postpartum thyroiditis because their condition resolves on its own. Most women will return to normal several months to a year after postpartum thyroid diagnosis and will never have another problem. Other women have postpartum thyroid problems after every pregnancy, but otherwise things return to normal until menopause, when thyroid problems reappear. Possibly up to 30 percent of women end up hypothyroid because their thyroid glands were too heavily damaged by the imbalance or because the pregnancy activated an inherent case of autoimmune thyroid disease.

If you gradually return to normal, your doctor will prescribe frequent thyroid function tests in order to monitor your condition. For those whose hyperthyroidism symptoms require treatment, beta blockers are typically given for symptom relief. More radical treatments—antithyroid medications, radioactive iodine (RAI), and so on—are not done as often for postpartum thyroiditis because it's not always known if the situation will be permanent.

For women in the hypothyroid phase, doctors can prescribe thyroid replacement hormones, such as Synthroid or Armour, until

TSH levels stabilize. Keep in mind, however, that once you've had an episode of postpartum thyroid problems, you are much more likely to develop a thyroid problem later during a period of stress, a subsequent pregnancy, or menopause.

■ Pregnancy After Hyperthyroidism Treatment

If you aren't pregnant yet and you have a severe or advanced case of hyperthyroidism that is difficult to control with antithyroid drugs, many doctors recommend that you permanently deal with the hyperthyroidism before you become pregnant, either by surgical removal of your thyroid gland or ablation of the thyroid with RAI. Both options will typically shift you from being hyperthyroid to being hypothyroid. If you have thyroid surgery, you should get stabilized on thyroid hormone replacement become you become pregnant. If you've had RAI, most doctors recommend waiting 4 to 6 months and getting your thyroid hormone replacement regimen stabilized before getting pregnant to reduce even the slightest risk of radioactivity to your baby. If you want to get pregnant quickly, surgery may be your best option. Getting pregnant while hypothyroid can sometimes be tricky, and carefully managing hypothyroidism during pregnancy is essential for the health of both mother and baby. Comprehensive information on hypothyroidism and pregnancy is featured in my book *Living Well with Hypothyroidism*.

If you have been treated for Graves' disease with either RAI or surgery and you are planning to become pregnant, you should know that you may still have a high reading of thyroid antibodies in your bloodstream. Some doctors now recommend a course of antithyroid drugs to bring your level of antibodies to a normal, manageable level before pregnancy.

▌Breastfeeding While You Are Hyperthyroid

No doubt, you are well aware of the benefits of breastfeeding your child. Breastfed infants reportedly score better on IQ tests, are sick less often, and enjoy better overall health. When you breastfeed, it's thought to lower your risk of breast cancer and other types of cancer. You also use up more calories and may return to your prepregnancy weight more quickly.

Hyperthyroidism shouldn't prevent most people from breastfeeding. There are, however, some key issues to keep in mind.

Milk Supply Issues

Milk supply issues are more common in women with postpartum thyroid problems. The hormone prolactin is responsible for the production of breast milk. It is stimulated by thyrotropin-releasing hormone (TRH), which in turn stimulates TSH. When your levels of TRH are low, prolactin is insufficient, so you may have difficulty producing enough breast milk to nourish your baby.

If you are having milk supply problems, be sure to have your thyroid evaluated as soon as possible, and ask your doctor for recommendations to increase milk supply. Consult with a lactation specialist or the La Leche League for additional suggestions on herbs, nutritional changes, breast pumping techniques, and lifestyle issues that can help you increase milk supply.

Antithyroid Drugs While Breastfeeding

Whether a nursing mother with Graves' disease or hyperthyroidism should take antithyroid drugs while breastfeeding is controversial. Some experts believe that it is safe for a woman to use either propylthiouracil (PTU) or methimazole while breastfeeding as long as the dosage is low.

Some breastfeeding advocates and some doctors believe that mothers on low doses of PTU can continue to breastfeed. PTU is considered the preferred drug, since methimazole concentrates in breast milk more easily. The argument is that the benefits of breastfeeding outweigh breast milk consumption with a little PTU, as long as you can monitor the baby's levels. To avoid transmission of excessive PTU to the baby, doctors may suggest taking PTU in divided doses after each feeding. In addition, doctors caution that careful monitoring of the breastfeeding infant's thyroid function at least every 3 months is essential while you are on antithyroid drugs.

Some studies have found no ill effects in the infants when mothers were being treated with relatively low doses of PTU (50–300 mg/day). One study looked at hyperthyroid mothers who were breastfeeding and continued taking PTU after delivery despite elevated TSH levels (indicative of PTU-induced hypothyroidism) in their newborns. The TSH levels of the newborns normalized even though the mothers continued on PTU therapy, which indicates that PTU treatment of breastfeeding mothers may not be harmful to their babies. Another study looked at children of thyrotoxic mothers who breastfed while taking methimazole at maximum doses of 20 to 30 milligrams per day. These children, who were evaluated for more than 2 years, had normal thyroid function throughout that time, and subsequent evaluation showed normal thyroid function, along with normal physical and intellectual development

However, there was a study that found infants exposed to PTU in utero tended to be more hyperactive and reactive to stimuli, which suggests an attention disorder, but no evidence of reduced intelligence was found. According to some endocrinologists and drug warnings, postpartum patients receiving methimazole (Tapazole) should not nurse their babies.

Despite the fact that some studies show it to be safe, some doctors are not convinced that breastfeeding should be encouraged in women taking antithyroid drugs. A July 2000 study in the journal

Pediatrics found that more than one-third of pediatricians and endocrinologists still advise against breastfeeding for those mothers taking PTU. They cite concerns over potential nonthyroid side effects of antithyroid drugs. For example, autoimmune disorders such as lupus and arthritis might be rare but serious complications of antithyroid drugs. Ultimately, whether you breastfeed will be a decision that you need to make with your doctor based on your health situation and the needs of your baby.

Thyroid Uptake Scans While Breastfeeding

A radioactive iodine uptake (RAI-U) thyroid scan is typically not recommended while breastfeeding. A thyroid scan involves an injection of radioactive iodine. RAI will pass into the milk for weeks and can concentrate in the baby's thyroid. If a doctor suggests a thyroid scan, you can ask whether an alternative diagnostic procedure—for example, blood testing or fine-needle aspiration—can be performed instead of the scan or if the test is necessary in the first place. The primary reason for a scan in a nursing mother is to determine whether she has postpartum thyroiditis (frequently a temporary condition) or Graves' disease.

If a scan must be done, it is possible to use technetium rather than radioactive iodine, according to breastfeeding expert Dr. Jack Newman:

> *Technetium has a half-life [the length of time it takes for half of the drug to leave the body] of 6 hours, which means that after 5 half-lives it will be gone from the mother's body. Thus, 30 hours after injection all of it will be gone and the mother can nurse her baby without concern about his getting radiation.*

If you do get an uptake test, you should pump and store as much milk as possible to cover the time when you can't breastfeed. After the scan, to keep your supply up, "pump and dump"—that is, use a breast pump and discard the milk until you've been given the okay from your doctor to resume breastfeeding.

Radioactive Iodine (RAI) Treatment While Breastfeeding

While the most popular treatment for Graves' disease and hyperthyroidism in the United States is RAI, this treatment should be deferred in women who are breastfeeding. The radioactive iodine appears in the breast milk and can pose a definite danger to the infant's thyroid. If RAI must be done, you'll have to stop breastfeeding beforehand.

When You Use Formula: An Important Note

If you need or choose to use formula for your baby, how can you choose which one to use? Some studies suggest that staying away from soy formulas for infants is a good idea, particularly when you have a thyroid condition. According to environmental scientist Dr. Mike Fitzpatrick, infants fed a steady diet of soy formula are more at risk for developing thyroid disease. Soy baby milks—and other soy products for children and adults alike, he attests—have high levels of isoflavones, which are strong antithyroid agents.

Dr. Fitzpatrick has spoken on behalf of the New Zealand Ministry of Health regarding its position on the issue:

> The Ministry of Health has found that infants with a history of thyroid dysfunction should avoid soy formulas and soy milks. Additionally, there is potential for isoflavone exposure to cause chronic thyroid damage in all infants fed soy formulas.

Dr. Fitzpatrick says that exposing infants to isoflavones is unnecessary and that the risk of harm could be avoided if manufacturers removed isoflavones from soy formulas. "In the interim," he states, "it is appropriate for medical practitioners to monitor the thyroid status of infants fed soy formulas."

In the 1950s and 1960s, there were several studies involving a higher increase in goiters among children who were fed soy formulas. Since then, iodine has been added to most soy formulas, but the goitrogenic (goiter-producing) isoflavones are still present. If you choose a formula, make sure you choose one of the newer formulas rich in docosahexgenoic acid (DHA) and arachidonic acid (ARA).

▮ Hyperthyroidism in Your Baby

If you have Graves' disease now or had it in the past, and particularly if your Graves' disease is not sufficiently treated and controlled during pregnancy, your baby is at greater risk of developing thyroid problems during the pregnancy. Your TRAb/TSI antibodies can cross the placenta and stimulate your baby's thyroid gland either during your pregnancy or right before the baby is born. These conditions are known as fetal thyrotoxicosis and neonatal thyrotoxicosis—hyperthyroidism before or after birth.

If left untreated, the mortality rate for thyrotoxicosis in a fetus or newborn can be as high as 30 percent, so it is essential that your antibodies be evaluated during pregnancy. Your TRAb/TSI levels should be evaluated early in your pregnancy, since high levels pose a first-trimester risk of miscarriage. And they should be evaluated again in the third trimester, when there's a risk that they will rise before delivery, making the baby hyperthyroid. (Note, however, that not all infants whose mothers test high for these antibodies will develop an overactive thyroid gland.) After birth, your newborn's thyroid function should be monitored regularly in the early weeks.

Fetal Thyrotoxicosis
In fetal thyrotoxicosis, antibodies stimulate your unborn baby's thyroid, making your baby hyperthyroid in utero. Signs your doctor should look for include:

- Fetal goiter, visible on ultrasound
- Rapid fetal heart rate, over 160 beats per minute
- Increased movement of the baby
- Accelerated bone maturity
- Fetal growth retardation

While you are pregnant, your obstetrician should conduct periodic fetal monitoring. The doctor should regularly evaluate your baby's heart rate as well as conduct periodic ultrasounds to monitor your baby's thyroid size, growth, bone development, and signs for for craniosynostosis, a skull irregularity that can develop in unborn babies with hyperthyroidism.

To treat hyperthyroidism in your unborn baby, you'll typically be given antithyroid drugs if you are not already on them, or the dosage will be increased. The drug most often given is methimazole because it can cross the placental membrane. If you are not already on methimazole drugs and your thyroid function is normal, you may need to take thyroid hormone replacement medication to help offset the antithyroid effects of the drug on your own thyroid function. These drugs do not cross the placenta as readily, so they aren't as likely to cancel out the helpful effects of the antithyroid drugs for your baby.

Neonatal Thyrotoxicosis

Newborns who have neonatal thyrotoxicosis are often low birth weight, have a high heart rate, fail to gain weight and may even lose weight, are often irritable and not easily soothed, and may have a yellowish cast to their skin. Your baby should have a blood test right after birth to evaluate thyroid function. Neonatal thyrotoxicosis can cause stunted growth, an irregular heart rate, bone and growth problems, skull abnormalities, and other potentially dangerous problems. Once diagnosed, however, sick newborns can be treated with antithyroid drugs.

Your newborn may test completely normal and be sent home with a clean bill of health. However, 7 to 10 days later, he or she may come down with hyperthyroid symptoms. The antithyroid drug you took may have passed through the placenta and bloodstream to your baby, hiding his or her hyperthyroid condition until the medications wear off. Treatment of hyperthyroidism in babies is usually a combination of PTU and the beta blocker propranolol. Your doctor will monitor your baby carefully, and typically, your doctor will be able to discontinue treatment after several months.

Your doctor and your endocrinologist know that you're hyperthyroid. But the attending physicians, obstetricians, pediatricians, and nurses at the hospital where you deliver your baby may not. Or the information may get lost or forgotten in the excitement of childbirth. So with rare but possible scenarios such as neonatal thyrotoxicosis, it's absolutely essential that you let every health care provider who comes in contact with you know of your condition. You may want to appoint a patient advocate—your spouse, a friend, or another health care professional—to act on your behalf.

■ Hyperthyroidism in Children and Teenagers

While thyroid conditions in children and teenagers are not common, they can still appear. The symptoms of hyperthyroidism in children and teens are outlined in chapters 2 and 3. Children and teenagers who are hyperthyroid almost always have Graves' disease. Severe Graves' disease and significant ophthalmopathy are fairly rare in this group.

Until recently, antithyroid drugs have generally been the preferred treatment in children and teenagers. A 2- to 4-year course typically controls the disease in 85 percent of children. Spontaneous remissions also tend to occur in as many as 25 percent of children and teens.

When the hyperthyroidism is severe and is not successfully controlled by antithyroid drugs, the next step is surgery or RAI. Some thyroid experts, in particular those outside the United States, consider surgery preferable to RAI because there are concerns that a child's thyroid should not be exposed to radiation. In the past, RAI has been associated with an increased risk of benign thyroid tumors in children as well as an increased risk of thyroid cancer. It's known that there is a huge increase in the risk of thyroid cancer in young children exposed to external radiation. The theory that there may be a small increase in the risk of thyroid cancer in younger children treated with RAI is based on this knowledge. There is no specific long-term data showing an increase in thyroid cancer or abnormalities in offspring of older children and adults who have received RAI.

One European study found that many children achieved long-term remission with antithyroid drugs after taking the drugs for approximately 3 years. Because surgery and RAI resulted in high rates of hypothyroidism among the children, the researchers recommended that antithyroid drugs remain the first-line therapy in children, followed by surgery, with caution exercised in the use of RAI.

The push to use RAI for children has become stronger only in the United States, however, where studies have found that children and adolescents had high remission rates on RAI with few complications. Research has shown that RAI does not typically worsen eye disease in children, who usually do not have a severe form of ophthalmopathy. So the debate continues, with doctors in the United States increasingly pushing for RAI as a treatment for children and doctors elsewhere turning to antithyroid drugs, then surgery, using RAI only as a last resort.

PART THREE

Integrative/Holistic Treatment Options

9

Alternative Approaches for Graves' Disease and Hyperthyroidism

If you are suffering hyperthyroidism symptoms, your practitioner will probably be anxious to treat you quickly to resolve your condition. You may have acute symptoms that should not be left untreated such as rapid heart rate, palpitations, and high blood pressure. If untreated, your practitioner knows that hyperthyroidism may progress to life-threatening thyroid storm.

Unfortunately, in the United States, the standard of care is to push from the beginning for a permanent, irreversible treatment—usually radioactive iodine (RAI), and less often, surgery—and to push for you to have this treatment as quickly as possible. This aggressive approach means that you may have little time to consider your options, and in particular, to pursue alternative approaches that might help your Graves' disease and hyperthyroidism go into remission, which happens in up to one-third of all cases.

Unfortunately, RAI and surgery both carry the possibility of significant side effects—the main one being lifelong hypothyroidism. However, most experts consider the side effects of treatment to be preferable to the complications or dangers of long-term, worsening hyperthyroidism.

If you do not have severe or life-threatening hyperthyroidism symptoms, you may want to consider a more integrative or holistic approach. The goal would be to use antithyroid drugs and alternative medicine to reduce your symptoms until you eventually go into remission on your own. Tonya is one Graves' disease patient who took this approach:

> I did not choose the treatment that most doctors suggested, which is radioactive iodine. This destroys the gland, and then many times you must go on hormone replacement therapy because your thyroid can no longer produce thyroid hormone. My thinking was that perhaps stressors in my life and not taking care of myself had led to this imbalance, so perhaps changing all those things would lead me to better health. I did take the prescription medication that was prescribed, and in addition I started to eat better, exercise more, and practice skilled relaxation. I got a lot of information from Dr. Weil's books. I am proud to say that I still have a functioning thyroid gland and it is very close to functioning normally all by itself.

Ultimately, the end result of a rush toward permanent treatment is almost always lifelong hypothyroidism, which requires regular monitoring, care, and prescription medication for life. It brings along a whole new host of symptoms and chronic health concerns. The end result of a more alternative approach? Possible remission and normalization of your thyroid function.

This chapter reviews some of the more effective holistic and integrative approaches for dealing with Graves' disease, hyperthyroidism, and their associated symptoms. A comprehensive nutritional approach developed over years of trial and error by patient advocate John Johnson and refined by an online support group that meets at his site is featured in the following chapter.

▌Dietary Changes

Some of the dietary changes you can make include:

- Limiting dietary and supplemental iodine to less than 150 micrograms daily: This means avoiding iodine supplements, kelp supplements, seaweed, fucus, bladder wrack, and iodized salt. (Sea salt is not a problem, however.)
- Adding more goitrogens, which can help block iodine absorption: Some of the more common goitrogenic foods are brussels sprouts, rutabaga, turnips, kohlrabi, radishes, cauliflower, millet, cabbage, kale, soy products, horseradish, mustard, corn, broccoli, turnips, carrots, peaches, strawberries, peanuts, spinach, watercress, mustard greens, and walnuts.
- Eating more foods with essential fatty acids: These nutrients help calm inflammation. Foods include fatty fish, olive oil, avocados, and olives.
- Eliminating aspartame and other artificial sweeteners because of suspected linkages to autoimmune disease, especially Graves' disease.

Deb, a physician coping with her own Graves' disease, turned to alternatives after long-term antithyroid drug therapy wasn't completely relieving her condition:

My grandmother had had Graves' disease and had gone into remission, so I was hoping that I would if I could just figure out what had triggered me and remove the inciting factor. I found out I had leaky gut and yeast overgrowth, went on a wheat-free, dairy-free diet, took enzymes and acidophilus and glutamine. (The question remains: Which came first—leaky gut from yeast overgrowth from the antibiotics I took for my skin, leading to production of the thyroid-stimulating antibody, or did the chronic diarrhea from the Graves' cause the leaky gut?) I had all the mercury removed from my teeth and had all biocompatible restorations done in place of the prior fillings. I developed multiple chemical sensitivity and figured out that my liver was not properly detoxifying things in my environment, and developed a nutritional protocol for myself.

▮ Chinese Medicine

Chinese medicine originated from Taoism about 4,000 years ago. It is designed to balance the health of an individual with his or her surroundings. Central to that balance is *qi* (pronounced "chee"), which translates as "vital energy" or "life force." Qi flows through the body via pathways known as meridians and is exchanged with the body's surroundings. A body is in optimal health when qi is free and balanced. In addition to qi, Chinese medicine relies on the concept of yin and yang, the interdependent opposites that represent different organs and health. Chinese medicine diagnostic techniques include observation, listening, questioning, and palpation, including feeling special pulse qualities and sensitivity of body parts. Chinese medicine treatments include diet, exercises such as tai chi and qi gong breathing, herbal preparations, acupuncture, acupressure massage, physical therapy, and moxibustion, which is the use of heat at specific energy points on the body applied either directly or with acupuncture needles as a way to add energy.

Acupuncture is now an established practice in the United States as part of Chinese medicine and even more so on its own. Americans make an estimated 9 million to 12 million visits to acupuncturists annually, and more than 3,000 conventionally trained U.S. physicians also practice acupuncture.

Acupuncture requires inserting very thin, fine needles at different key energy points to regulate or correct the flow of qi and restore health. Acupuncture treatment taps into points along meridians, each having different therapeutic functions within the body. Most of the time, patients don't feel the acupuncture needles at all; occasionally, the worst they might feel is a slight pinch for a second. As a regular recipient of acupuncture treatment and someone who really doesn't like shots, I can tell you that despite how it looks, acupuncture does not hurt when done properly. It's also safe. Most practitioners use disposable needles, and it's a good idea to ask your acupuncturist to use them.

There are many verified studies from Asia that show successful application of Chinese medicine for immunologically based diseases, including thyroid problems. One 2003 study, for example, found that a Chinese herbal remedy known as Xiehuo Yangyin powder (XHYY) was able to achieve faster improvement in hyperthyroidism symptoms and reduction of thyroid hormone levels when taken with methimazole than the methimazole alone. Patients had more rapid improvement and could take less antithyroid drug (which also makes it safer and less likely to cause any side effects).

Early in her illness, Deb, had muscle weakness, even finding herself so weak that at times she could barely stand. She verifies her successful treatment with acupuncture:

One thing that helped me incredibly with this symptom was acupuncture. I would drag myself into the acupuncturist's office, walking weakly and haltingly, and I would get up off the table and be able to walk purposefully and with normal strength.

Chinese medicine specialist and acupuncturist Shasta Tierra-Tayam believes you should always try to work with a person's whole environment, lifestyle, foods, medications, herbs, treatments, exercise, and so forth, to get the best results:

I have seen a combination of acupuncture, chi kung exercise (a type of exercise designed to improve physical and mental health), less spicy and greasy foods, and some herbal formulas with cooling, uncongesting properties help a lot within 2 months. I have seen the fast pulse rate decrease and the protruding eyes go back in, and a lot of the symptoms decrease with this more aggressive approach—three times a week of acupuncture treatments for 3 months.

When choosing a practitioner, be sure to see someone who is licensed and certified, whether a doctor or not. For physicians, top certification is from the American Academy of Medical Acupuncture (AAMA). Acupuncturists who are not doctors can be credentialed as diplomates in acupuncture (DiplAc). They may be called licensed acupuncturists (LAc or LicAc), registered acupuncturists (RAc), certified acupuncturists (CA), acupuncturists, doctors of Oriental medicine (DOM), or doctors of acupuncture (DAc). Each state has its own specific requirements for the practice of acupuncture. Either see a licensed acupuncturist or one who is nationally certified from an organization such as the National Certification Commission for Acupuncture and Oriental Medicine (NCCAOM).

■ Herbal Medicine

There are a number of herbs that are known to be useful in the treatment of hyperthyroidism:

- Lemon balm/Melissa
- Bugleweed/Lycopus

- Motherwort/leonurus
- Lemonweed/*Lithospermum ruderale*
- Creeping thyme/thymus

Most of these herbs can lower thyroid hormone secretion, inhibit thyroid-stimulating hormone (TSH), and in some cases, inhibit T4 to T3 conversion. For the best results, use in tonics prescribed by an herbalist or as a tincture—a concentrated liquid form of the herb— diluted in tea, also provided by a trained herbalist.

Some herbs should be avoided. Ashwaghanda can raise thyroid hormone levels, so it should not be used by people with hyperthyroidism. Herbs that contain iodine, such as kelp, bladder wrack, fucus, and seaweeds, should also be avoided.

Lemon Balm/Melissa

Lemon balm, also known as *Melissa officinalis,* bee balm, sweet balm, balm mint, blue balm, dropsy plant, garden balm, and common balm, is a member of the mint family and can inhibit the binding of TSH receptors. It's considered a calming herb with a relaxing, anxiety-reducing effect. It is traditionally used as a treatment for mild insomnia and for digestive problems and gas. Lemon balm is available as a dried leaf, as tea, in capsules, extracts, tinctures, and oil. Lemon balm lowers TSH levels in animals and has been used to treat Graves' disease (a condition in which the thyroid gland becomes hyperactive). You should be careful using lemon balm if you are also taking sedatives such as Ambien, benzodiazepines such as Klonopin, or barbiturates such as Fiorinal.

Bugleweed/Lycopus

Bugleweed, also known as Lycopus, Northern bugleweed, gypsywort, water bugle, sweet bugle, and Virginian water horehound, is a member of the mint family. Bugleweed has been recognized in herbal medicine as a heart tonic, and it's been shown to have the ability to slow down the heart rate and strengthen heart function. Bugleweed may decrease TSH, inhibit metabolism of iodine, and block the action of thyroid-stimulating antibodies, all of which make it a treatment for hyperthyroidism. It may help with palpitations and tremors as well.

Motherwort/Leonurus

Motherwort, also known as leonurus, lion's tail, lion's ear, throwwort, heartwort, and yi mu cao, is an herbal remedy most commonly used for relieving menstrual and labor cramps, calming nerves, lowering blood pressure, strengthening the heart, and reducing heart palpitations, arrhythmia, and rapid heartbeat. It is sometimes recommended as a treatment for overactive thyroid.

Lithospermum

Lithospermum, also known as lemonweed, koushikon, shikon, shiunko, pearl plant, Western stoneseed, stoneseed, European stoneseed, puccoon, Columbia puccoon, Columbia gromwell, common gromwell, and Western gromwell, is an herbal medicine that is used to help improve immune response and as an antiinflammatory. Lithospermum has been proven to lower thyroid hormone levels.

Thyme/Creeping Thyme

Thyme, also known as creeping thyme, wild thyme, hillwort, garden thyme, mother of thyme, penny mountain, and lemon thyme, is a member of the mint family. Thyme is a versatile herbal medicine, providing a variety of effects. In oil form, thyme can slow the heartbeat and lower body temperature, which may help with hyperthyroid symptoms.

▌Nutritional and Homeopathic Supplements

While a detailed supplement approach specific to Grave's disease and the thyroid is outlined in the Johnson protocol in the next chapter, it's important to note that a good antioxidant supplement is essential for anyone with Graves' disease and hyperthyroidism. One research study found that an antioxidant supplement that included vitamins C and E, beta-carotene, and selenium helped hyperthyroid patients taking methimazole reach normal thyroid status more quickly than patients taking methimazole alone. Two other supplements—carnitine and felvic acid—are also of interest to thyroid patients and practitioners.

Carnitine

One of the most important nutritional supplements to consider for Graves' disease and hyperthyroidism is carnitine. Carnitine, which is part of the Shames antithyroid protocol discussed in the next section, has the ability to block the action of thyroid hormone on the cells. One study looked at the effects of carnitine in women who were taking suppressive doses of thyroid hormone as a treatment for goiter. The study showed that 2 to 4 grams of carnitine daily protected against various symptoms of hyperthyroidism, including bone loss.

Another study found that 1 to 3 grams per day of carnitine resulted in an improvement in hyperthyroidism symptoms within 2 weeks, even though it did not affect blood test values. This suggests carnitine inhibits the action of the thyroid hormone rather than preventing the thyroid from actually producing hormone. Other studies have shown that carnitine can stop thyroid hormone from entering cells, which prevents its actions at the cellular level.

Fulvic Acid

Some patients have reported success with the use of supplements containing fulvic acid. Lynne was quite hyperthyroid and experiencing a range of debilitating symptoms when she was first diagnosed, explaining:

> I searched for natural remedies that would "cure" me of a hyperthyroid condition when I was diagnosed in early May 2003. My heartbeat was 100+, my T4 tested at 3.7, my T3 was 225, and TSH wasn't measurable. I was also excreting a lot of calcium in my urine, which the endocrinologist thought was as a result of the hyperthyroid condition. An iodine uptake scan revealed a score of 45 percent. In addition, my immune system was severely suppressed. I also had eczema on my legs, knees, abdomen, and elbows.

Lynne's research led her to try fulvic acid, a little-understood acid that offers minerals and trace elements formed by beneficial microbes that compost plant matter in soil. Lynne reported that a natural regimen, which included a fulvic acid mineral supplement, echinacea, burdock root infusion, omega 3s, calcium, magnesium, vitamin C, vitamin A, vitamin E, vitamin B-complex, chromium, garlic, pycnogenol, and zinc picolinate, reduced her elevated T4 levels to normal, although her T3 levels still remained above normal. After adding a probiotic super-food supplement and doing a bowel and liver detox, her T3 dropped to the high end of normal. She maintains her normal thyroid function on this natural regimen, plus healthy foods and exercise.

Homeopathic Preparations

If you've seen a cold and flu remedy called oscillococcinum on the drugstore shelf, you've seen contemporary homeopathic medicine in action. The current practice of homeopathy is based on the

200-year-old work of German doctor Samuel Hahnemann. His idea is that you can stimulate the immune system to fight illness by administering a homeopathic remedy—a microscopic, extremely diluted amount of an herb, mineral, or other substance—that would cause similar symptoms in a healthy person. The theory is "like curses like," similar to the concept behind giving a vaccine that contains some elements of the disease the vaccination is meant to prevent. Homeopathy was very popular in the U.S. in the late 1800s, but fell out of favor until recently. Currently, there are an estimated 3,000 physicians and other healthcare personnel practicing homeopathy in the United States.

I haven't heard from any patients who have been successfully treated with homeopathy for their hyperthyroidism but have heard, anecdotally, that there are some homeopathic remedies that may help with symptoms. These include kelpasan, coffea, *Natrum muriaticum*, and thyroidinum. If you are looking for a homeopath, be sure to find someone licensed with either a D.Ht. (Diplomate in Homeotherapeutics), C.C.H. (Certified in Classical Homeopathy), or D.H.A.N.P. (Diplomate of the Homeopathic Academy of Naturopathic Physicians).

■ The Shames Antithyroid Protocol

Dr. Richard Shames, who wrote the popular book *Thyroid Power* with his wife, Dr. Karilee Halo-Shames, has had success using an integrative approach for Graves' disease that combines conventional and nutritional aspects. According to Dr. Shames, he first establishes a nutritional program:

> *The therapeutic interventions for hyperthyroidism—the standard options of surgery, RAI, or antithyroid drugs—are somewhat unsavory. I have been very pleased in recent years*

to try out and be successful with a number of patients using a nutritional program.

Dr. Shames's approach includes natural antithyroid supplements and foods. His focus is on providing symptomatic relief so that you have the time to turn to a more intensive holistic program of assessing and correcting nutritional imbalances, stress-related and lifestyle issues, underlying infections, toxic exposures, and other causes and triggers of autoimmune disease.

If a person is having more difficult symptoms such as high pulse, insomnia, high blood pressure, or tremor, he will supplement the natural antithyroid approach with a low dose of a benzodiazepine drug—for example, clonazepam (Klonopin)—and a small dose of a beta blocker such as propranolol (Inderal). Dr. Shames will also include antithyroid drugs when necessary. For those patients who still need to be on an antithyroid drug while using nutritional supplements, Dr. Shames says,

Using nutritional antithyroid foods and supplements lets you use a smaller amount of PTU or Tapazole. And these drugs present a greatly reduced risk of side effects at lower doses. The risks of side effects are higher when you are taking a higher dose.

Soy

One of the first things Dr. Shames recommends is that you consider consuming more soy, which has potent thyroid-inhibiting properties:

By the time you're up to 50 mg of soy isoflavones a day, you're beginning to interfere with thyroid function. You can deliberately take advantage of this side effect. As long as the

other side effects you might encounter—too much estrogenic effect, gas/flatulence, etc.—are tolerable, you can take a fair amount of soy. Either combined with the supplements, or by itself, soy might help lower function to the extent that you can reduce or even avoid prescription antithyroid medications.

Quercetin

Quercetin is a bioflavonoid that has been very helpful for rheumatoid arthritis and chronic allergy patients. It has antiinflammatory and antihistamine qualities. At high doses, its only side effect is that it lowers thyroid hormone production. According to Dr. Shames:

By the time you get to 3 to 4 grams of quercetin—or even up to 5 grams a day—you start lowering thyroid function.

Carnitine

A key element of Dr. Shames's approach is carnitine, an amino acid that has various positive effects, and it has a significant side effect at higher doses: at levels higher than 3 to 4 grams a day (3,000–4,000 mg a day), it reduces the production of thyroid hormone. Dr. Shames says,

I make use of the side effect of this otherwise simple and very benign amino acid. I have found that a dose of two to three 500 mg carnitine tablets three times a day is in the antithyroid range. Carnitine at these doses has a similar effect to PTU or Tapazole without the side effects of these drugs.

Lipoic Acid

According to Dr. Shames, lipoic acid is an excellent antioxidant and detoxifying agent. He says this supplement also has antithyroid side effects at levels above 500 to 600 milligrams a day:

I use 600 to 800 milligrams of lipoic acid per day. Patients can take it once a day, but my preference is broken up throughout the day.

Fluoride

A final recommendation that Dr. Shames usually holds in reserve is fluoride, which was used for hyperthyroidism treatment before antithyroid drugs were developed. It can significantly reduce thyroid function, says Dr. Shames:

Most people are getting too much fluoride—and fluoridated water may be enough to lower thyroid function in sensitive people. Someone hyperthyroid might shoot for 5 to 6 mg a day of fluoride—you can get fluoride tablets, use fluoride mouthwash, etc. Fluoride can also have side effects—such as nausea, or fluorosis in children—but I don't consider them as severe as the potential side effects of Tapazole and PTU.

The Overall Approach

Dr. Shames typically recommends you start with soy, then quercetin, then carnitine, then lipoic acid. If results aren't satisfactory, fluoride can be added. Dr. Shames explains where drugs may fit in:

When things are very severe, I have them combine some of the supplements with the soy, but most people don't need to add all three supplements. If it's particularly severe, I might add 5 mg of Tapazole. I've never heard or seen—in 25 years— anybody who had side effects with that low a dose of an antithyroid drug.

Dr. Shames has found that patients can gradually cut back the number of supplements, and eventually most of his patients go into remission and become euthyroid:

Periodically, patients may flare up and have to repeat the treatment but seem to be able to control their hyperthyroidism for the most part by following my protocol.

Once the hyperthyroidism symptoms are under control, Dr. Shames provides his patients with various treatments to help "cool down" the immune system—for example, homeopathy, guided visualization, nutritional changes, heavy antioxidants, intestinal cleansing, meditation, and self-hypnosis.

▌ Mind-Body Approaches

Mind-body approaches include everything from prayer to yoga to counseling to dance to breathing. Basically, they are all practices or therapies that seek to reduce stress, establish a link between conscious thought and the body, with the goal of affecting physiological processes, and trigger the relaxation response.

Relaxation response was coined by Harvard physician Dr. Herbert Benson, the nation's foremost mind-body expert, to describe the actual physiological changes that result from relaxation and balance. In an interview with public radio host Diane Rehm, Dr. Benson articulated his thoughts:

We have found that when people regularly go into a quiet state, a large percentage of them feel the presence of a power, a force, an energy, God if you will, and they feel that presence is close to them, within them, then these people have fewer medical symptoms. Now, whether or not this is a physiological reaction independent of an external belief system, or whether or not there is indeed something out there, we cannot answer, but from the patient's point of view, they feel better.

There are many types of mind-body therapy; it's only possible to touch on a few here. But hopefully you will get ideas on approaches that are most appealing to you and where best to participate.

Meditation

One technique that is considered very effective at achieving the relaxation response is meditation. Meditation techniques are more common in Asia and are an integral part of Buddhism, Hinduism, yoga, and many Asian religions. They have been gaining popularity in other countries. Regular meditation has notable effects on blood pressure, anxiety, chronic pain, and can clinically reduce cortisol levels, a measure of the body's stress.

According to the Center for Integrative Medicine at Thomas Jefferson University Hospital in Philadelphia, meditation training can help patients with chronic illnesses reduce symptoms and improve quality of life. It helps patients cope with stress, have an improved sense of well-being, reduce body tension, and increase their clearness of thinking, all of which benefit the immune system. Researchers have also established by using magnetic resonance imaging (MRI) that meditation actually activates certain structures in the brain that control the autonomic nervous system.

Self-Hypnosis

Research reported in the *Journal of Consulting and Clinical Psychology* found that students who received hypnotic relaxation training maintained a stronger immune system compared to those who did not practice the relaxation techniques. Interestingly, the more often students practiced the relaxation techniques, the stronger their immune response system became. Dr. Leonard Holmes believes that hypnosis can be an excellent relaxation technique for almost anyone:

All hypnosis is really self-hypnosis—meaning that the person is putting him- or herself into a trance. For most of us, a trance is just a light relaxing state similar to daydreaming. Entering this state on a regular basis calms the sympathetic nervous system and reduces the levels of stress hormones in the bloodstream. Some people have even greater hypnotic ability. These are the people that you see on television acting silly with a stage hypnotist. People with high hypnotic ability can use hypnosis as a way to change things about their mind and body.

Guided Imagery

Guided imagery can be an effective technique for achieving the relaxation response and for healing. You can use your own imagery or follow a book, audiotape, or practitioner. If you are feeling very stressed, you might envision progressively relaxing each part of your body as you lie on a warm, sunny beach, or you might envision the body's healing capabilities traveling to a damaged organ.

Dr. O. Carl Simonton, author of the best-selling and highly recommended book *Getting Well Again*, talks about effective mental imagery for illness:

1. Create a mental picture of any ailment or pain that you have now, visualizing it in a form that makes sense to you.
2. Picture any treatment you are receiving and see it either eliminating the source of the ailment or pain or strengthening your body's ability to heal itself.
3. Picture your body's natural defenses and natural processes eliminating the source of the ailment or pain.
4. Imagine yourself healthy and free of the ailment or pain.
5. See yourself proceeding successfully toward meeting your goals in life.
6. Give yourself a mental pat on the back for participating in your recovery.

Chakra therapists and energy workers also recommend guided visualization to help tune and balance the energies around the thyroid. To perform a chakra-balancing visualization, sit in a comfortable upright position (in a chair or sofa, or lotus position), eyes closed. Take a few deep, cleansing breaths. The harmonic color for the thyroid is blue, so you should visualize a bright blue beam of light coming down through the top of your head and going right to your thyroid. Feel the blue energy infusing every cell of your thyroid, throat, and neck. Visualize the blue beam of energy enhancing the thyroid and curing its overactivity. Feel the blue light softly spreading all around your neck and throat. Now, say out loud, "My thyroid is energized and is working perfectly. I am safe, and loved, and filled with the energy of the Universe."

Journaling

If you've ever written a letter, e-mail, online forum post, or diary entry about something bothering you and felt better afterward, then you know about the relaxation response benefits of writing. In a 1999 study published in the *Journal of the American Medical Association,* researchers reported that some patients with chronic diseases had improvements in their health after writing about major life stresses such as car accidents or the death of a close friend or relative. The study looked at 112 patients. Each patient spent an hour per day writing. Four months after the study began, almost half of those who wrote about their stresses had experienced significant improvement in their health. "Downloading" your concerns and stresses, whether by writing in a journal or sharing your personal experiences with others who can relate via an online support group, is a natural stress-reduction activity. Expressive writing not only gives your mind a place to unload stressful concerns or worries but can be a relaxation or peaceful activity that helps to reduce stress by calming down your system and allowing you to focus better.

Yoga

When most people think of yoga, they assume it means stretching or sitting in a cross-legged lotus position. Yoga is actually an ancient science that focuses on putting the whole body, mind, and intellect in harmony with the universe. This may sound like New Age babble, but actually yoga is quite practical, with physical exercises (asanas), breathing exercises (pranayam), and meditation techniques that help achieve union and balance.

Some of the many health benefits of yoga have been conventionally tested and proven, and they are even discussed in Western medical journals. For example, certain forms of yoga have been found to have a strong antidepressant effect. Yoga has also been found to improve lung function and breathing; it can significantly reduce the amount of asthma medicines needed by asthmatic patients. Yoga is considered an effective treatment for carpal tunnel syndrome. These are just a few of the many practical applications that even mainstream medicine has found for yoga.

Yoga offers wonderful benefits in terms of generating the relaxation response and may also provide some very specific benefits for thyroid function. There is a specific asana or pose that is thought to be of great benefit to the thyroid. The half shoulder stand (viparit karani mudra) and shoulder stand (sarvangasan) positions both invert and stimulate the thyroid. According to yoga master Swami Rameshwarananda of the Yoga in Daily Life program, the shoulder stand is considered one of the most powerful positions in yoga. In addition to helping the thyroid, it is thought to prolong life through its effect on the metabolism and prana, or life energy.

In a shoulder stand, you lie flat on your back. Keeping your legs together, raise them up until they are at a right angle to your shoulders/neck, perpendicular to the floor, chin tucked into your chest, resting the weight of your body on your shoulders and elbows, arms supporting your hips. Work up to a daily session of a full 2 minutes by starting with two or three shorter sessions. Swami Ramesh-waranananda counsels that you should always stop and consult an experienced yoga instructor if doing a shoulder stand makes you feel dizzy, uncomfortable, or interferes with your breathing.

Swami Rameshwarananda also recommends the practice of pranayam (pran-a-YAM), the breathing exercises that help to cleanse and harmonize the nadi energy pathways and clear out physical, mental, and emotional obstructions. Many yoga centers and alternative health workshops offer this training.

The most basic pranayam is deep abdominal breathing. To try it yourself, lie flat on your back or stand. Put your hand on your abdomen and take a deep breath, filling your belly with air so that your hand rises, then exhale. Start basic pranayam practice by simply doing this for 10 or 15 minutes each day, and you'll be surprised at how much more relaxed yet energetic you'll feel.

There is also a specific breathing exercise designed to help the thyroid and the throat chakra. Breathe in through your nose, focusing the inhalation toward the back of your throat. Your throat should feel slightly closed or blocked while you perform this breathing exercise. Mentally, you should try to feel as if you are taking in the air *through* the front of your throat. Do this several times a day but not for long periods, since it might make you dizzy.

Energy Work/Reiki

There are many forms of energy work, where practitioners transfer healing energy to recipients, but one of the most popular and effective appears to be Reiki (ray-key). Reiki teacher, practitioner, and holistic healer Phylameana lila Desy, author of *The Everything Reiki Book,* has described Reiki as a vibrational healing modality that consists of an enormous amount of "love energy." Reiki is a form of energy work—some practitioners may touch recipients; others just pass hands over the body. The Reiki practitioner taps into a universal energy force, then passes on that energy to the recipient, who will receive it where it is most needed—mind or body. Desy explains:

> *I teach my students that Reiki is a "smart energy" because it works at the level of acceptance by each individual client. Reiki will never overwhelm someone who is not accustomed to feeling energy, as it will enter the body slowly. For someone more open to the energy, it will flow more quickly, but only at the level that is needed. Reiki is a balancing remedy. It will flow directly to whatever is in imbalance and nudge it back into a more balanced state. Reiki will address physical imbalances first before addressing the emotional, mental, and spiritual problems. For this reason alone, I think the benefits someone with a chronic illness could experience from consistent Reiki treatments are the receiving of relief from the physical and emotional suffering.*

I've had a number of Reiki treatments and personally feel that Reiki is a tremendous help, particularly when you are under stress. An hour with a good Reiki practitioner makes me feel as if I am coming away from the session with an emotional and spiritual massage. But to ensure that you get the best from this healing modality, make sure you are seeing a reputable practitioner who comes with high recommendations from others.

Spirituality and Health

Finally, it's important to mention the role of spirituality in health as part of the overall mind-body component. Holistic and mind-body medicine expert Dr. Brian Sheen believes that dealing with thyroid problems may require deep healing of the mind-body influences:

> *These mind-body influences consist of unforgiven grievances, unexpressed feelings and thoughts, and buried traumas that*

fester in the unconscious mind and interfere with the free movement of the body's natural healing systems . . . immune, endocrine, nervous, and lymphatic . . . also remodeling of daily living to learn to destress through meditation and rethink through paths such as A Course in Miracles.

In his book, *God, Faith, and Health: Exploring the Spiritual-Healing Connection,* social epidemiologist Jeff Levin acknowledges the spiritual dimension to healing:

The weight of published evidence overwhelmingly confirms that our spiritual life influences our health. This can no longer be ignored.

Some research has shown that people who are considered religious may live 7 years longer than others on average. California's Human Population Laboratory studied 5,000 people for 28 years and reported that frequent church attendance was linked to a 23 percent reduction in the chance of dying. Other studies have found that for each of the three leading causes of death in the United States—heart disease, cancer, and hypertension—people who report a religious affiliation have lower rates of illness. Researchers at Johns Hopkins University have reported that attending religious services at least once a month more than halved the risk of death due to heart disease, emphysema, suicide, and some kinds of cancers.

Other Approaches
Other mind-body approaches that may be of help include:

- Tai chi and qi gong
- Psychotherapy, cognitive therapy, or counseling
- Support group participation in person or online
- Biofeedback therapy

- Creative therapies such as art, music, and dance
- Prayer
- Massage
- Reflexology

Some other ways to reduce stress and encourage relaxation in your life include:

- Try to eat breakfast and lunch daily.
- Plan to meditate or listen to a relaxation tape for a few minutes each day.
- Instead of drinking coffee all day, switch to herbal tea or water.
- Stop multitasking. Instead, concentrate on doing one thing at a time.
- Get regular exercise.
- Avoid people who are "stress carriers" or "energy vampires."
- Take a news fast. Avoiding watching news for a day or a week.
- Don't watch the 11 P.M. news.
- Learn how to assertively turn down requests for your time.
- Learn how to properly breathe when you are feeling stressed.
- Adopt a pet.
- Drive less aggressively.
- Resist the temptation to judge or criticize others.
- Be flexible and recognize that things don't always go as you plan.
- Pray. Speak to God, your higher power, nature, or your inner guide.

10

The Johnson Nutritional Protocol

There is a precedent for the idea that nutritional imbalances may be at the root of Graves' disease and hyperthyroidism. Medical journal research has reported that supplementation with antioxidant vitamins, especially selenium, can speed up the process of becoming euthyroid when taking antithyroid drugs. But few researchers have turned their attention to identifying a comprehensive approach to managing Graves' disease and hyperthyroidism using nutritional supplementation.

This effort, however, has been undertaken by a well-known patient advocate, John Johnson, who manages a popular Web site: www.ithyroid.com. Johnson developed Graves' disease in 1997. While he suspected that hyperthyroidism was triggered by nutritional deficiency, his research could find no evidence in the medical literature of any specific connections.

Johnson had previously tackled a health problem nutritionally when he developed hypothyroidism in the mid-1980s and had to take thyroid hormone replacement medication. Although not a medical professional, he is an empowered patient and has concentrated on studying the nutritional connections to thyroid disease.

After researching various triggers, Johnson theorized that mercury toxicity from his dental fillings might be depleting certain essential nutrients, therefore causing his hypothyroidism. He had the fillings removed, his nutritional balance was restored, and his hypothyroidism resolved.

His previous success led Johnson to believe that Graves' disease and hyperthyroidism could similarly respond. He spent a number of years experimenting by informally leading a group of fellow patients. Working with foods and nutritional supplements and carefully documenting the results, Johnson set out to understand the nutritional basis of hyperthyroidism:

> Not only did I cure myself, but I also believe that I discovered that hyperthyroidism, in all its forms including Graves' disease, is a curable nutritional deficiency disease. In 1998, I began publishing the results of my research on my Web site: www.ithyroid.com. Since that time, many people have posted to the Web site or e-mailed me to tell their stories of how they recovered fully from hyperthyroidism using the information they found on my Web site.

Some of the facts we know about Graves' disease and hyperthyroidism are fascinating. Johnson says they also offer clues about the cause of the disease:

> It's a disease that women are many times more likely to develop than men. When women get the disease, it usually occurs at certain times, such as at the onset of menstruation as a teenager, during pregnancy, while breastfeeding, or at menopause. Estrogen is a factor in the disease but not the cause. People who smoke tobacco, especially female smokers, are about twice as likely to develop hyperthyroidism as nonsmokers. Some people with hyperthyroidism get Graves' oph-

thalmopathy, but high levels of thyroid hormone do not cause this disease. Thyroid disease sometimes runs in families, but it's never been shown to be a genetic disease. The theory that I developed about the cause of hyperthyroidism makes sense of all these disparate, bizarre observations about the disease.

▌ In His Own Words

John describes the development of his theory:

I knew from long experience that if what I ate or the supplements I took changed the disease symptoms, for better or worse, it had to be a nutritional disease. To find the cause of a nutritional deficiency disease it's important to observe what essential nutrients make the disease worse as well as better, because these are generally the conutrients that work with the deficient nutrient that we are trying to identify.

For example, I quickly found iodine increased my symptoms. Many people with hyperthyroidism make the same discovery and find as I did that if they avoid iodine they can control and diminish the symptoms. Many people mistakenly conclude that they are "allergic" to iodine. I believe that it's impossible to be allergic to an essential nutrient. When symptoms occur as the result of taking an essential nutrient, it means that one or more other essential nutrients are deficient. Because nutrients that work together compete with each other, when nutrient X gets sufficiently deficient and its conutrients are ingested, nutrient X gets more deficient and deficiency symptoms are manifested.

What I found was that hyperthyroidism was caused by nutritional deficiencies resulting from a complex interaction of improper nutrition, toxic metal exposure, intake of hormones including those for birth control, adaptive genes, and psychological factors like stress. However, no matter how the disease originated, the basic core mechanism of the disease was the same: a deficiency of a very important trace metal, copper.

The interesting thing about a copper deficiency is that there are so many ways to create it. Correcting the deficiency completely can take months or years when there is a heavy metal toxicity. Even when there isn't a heavy metal interfering with copper metabolism, correction can be difficult, because copper has many essential conutrients that need to be present. Also, many other essential minerals compete with copper, and taking these minerals or their conutrients can deplete copper. Moreover, once copper gets sufficiently deficient, high levels of thyroid hormone and stress hormones use up more copper, increasing the rate of depletion of the already deficient metal, thereby accelerating the development of the disease.

Many people have reported to me that upon starting a supplement program of copper, magnesium, and other conutrients, they have felt significantly better within hours. Immediate results are very gratifying, but patients need to be prepared for a long recovery. I believe that most people should recover to 90 percent within 6 months and 95 percent within a year. The process is slow because there are a lot of nutritional pieces that have to be put back together.

▌ Understanding Trace Metals

Johnson believes that understanding the nutritional mechanics of trace metals is essential for understanding the causes of hyperthyroidism and hypothyroidism, among other conditions:

Trace metals are critical because they are essential for the con-duction of electrical signals in the body. They also help the body convert one chemical or hormone into another. For ex-ample, in 1990, researchers identified the enzymes that con-vert the inactive thyroid hormone T4 into the active hormone T3. They found that these deiodinase enzymes are selenium enzymes, thus demonstrating that selenium is essential for the conversion of T4 to T3.

Trace metals that are essential to proper thyroid function in-clude iron, zinc, manganese, iodine, cobalt, selenium, and copper. All of these metals except copper seem to be involved in the pro-duction of thyroid hormones. Copper, however, appears to have a different function, limiting the amount of thyroid hormone in cir-culation.

Johnson has no doubt that hyperthyroidism is caused by a copper deficiency. There is no specific mechanism to explain the connec-tion, but he has two theories. One is that there is a copper-containing enzyme that breaks down thyroid hormone after use. The second is that copper is essential to normal immune system function and that a copper deficiency causes the overproduction of certain immune bodies that cause the disease.

Just as some nutrients need to be taken together—for example, calcium and magnesium, or B vitamins—in order to maintain nutri-tional balance, Johnson explains that trace metals also need to be balanced with other trace metals:

Zinc and copper are both very important to thyroid function. A continual intake of these metals in the wrong balance will deplete one or the other. Unlike most metals, however, the proper zinc and copper ratio depends on sex, with males needing more zinc than females and females needing more copper than males. In healthy adults an ideal ratio of zinc to copper for men is usually between 10:1 and 15:1. For menstruating women, however, the ratio needs to be lower, usually between 5:1 and 7:1. Because of the blood loss during menstruation, women need more copper and iron. Many supplement manufacturers now make separate multiples for men and women so that women get more iron and men get less. They should add in more copper for women and more zinc for men.

While many vitamins can be consumed in megavitamin doses that are thousands of times the recommended daily requirement without any particular danger, Johnson cautions that minerals, especially metals, are different:

Metals can be toxic at amounts only 4 to 10 times the daily requirement. The metals themselves are not toxic, but they have a toxic effect because they replace and deplete other essential metals, which slows down the physiological processes that depend on those metals.

Johnson believes that dietary deficiencies and excesses of trace metals occur because trace metals are unevenly distributed in our soil and food supplies. We therefore adapt to accommodate deficiencies. A good example of this adaptation process is a goiter, which is more common in iodine-deficient areas. The thyroid gland enlarges so that it can filter more blood in an attempt to gather more of the scarce mineral.

Johnson explains that specialized proteins known as metallothioneins play a role. These metallothioneins help acquire, transport, and store metals in the body, and some carry more than one metal. By this mechanism, Johnson says that metals compete with each other and deplete each other when one metal is consumed in large amounts:

One metallothionein, for example, carries copper and zinc. An excess of zinc will reduce the amount of copper that can be transported and stored, causing a functional deficiency of copper even though copper is supplied in the diet. Because the heavy metal cadmium has a chemical structure like copper and zinc, it also attaches to the same metallothionein.

■ Common Causes of Hyperthyroidism

According to Johnson, there are many things that can cause copper deficiency and hyperthyroidism. Some of these are essential nutrients that need to be avoided or reduced temporarily until copper levels return to normal.

Multiple Vitamin-Mineral Supplements

Many nutritional supplements on the market claim to contain all the nutrients you need—multiple vitamin-mineral supplements, or multiples for short. But Johnson advises caution:

Because so many essential nutrients can deplete copper, it's important to avoid these supplements. All the multiples that I've looked at have a formulation that will deplete copper and promote hyperthyroidism. When I had hyperthyroidism and was not on antithyroid drugs, taking a multiple would bring on an immediate thyroid storm.

Zinc and Vitamin B6

Johnson explains that one of the most common ways people become hyperthyroid is by getting too much zinc and not enough copper. This can occur through supplementation or by making bad food choices:

Zinc and copper work together in the body but are strong antagonists to each other. Both have strong effects on the thyroid, so I call the zinc/copper ratio the thyroid ratio. Zinc increases thyroid hormone levels and copper decreases them. Zinc deficiency is one cause of hypothyroidism. Copper deficiency will cause hyperthyroidism. Too much of either metal will deplete the other, but zinc is more effective at depleting copper than vice versa.

Some of the worst zinc supplements for hyperthyroidism are the zinc lozenges that have become popular as a cold remedy, as well as zinc/calcium combinations that women take to prevent osteoporosis. Many patients following Johnson's protocol have reported that they were taking large amounts of this kind of supplement before developing hyperthyroidism. The zinc/calcium depletes both copper and magnesium, according to Johnson, which are the two main deficiencies in hyperthyroidism:

When I had hyperthyroidism, my nutritionally oriented doctor recommended increasing my zinc intake to 100 mg per day. Many doctors recommend this because there is a study in the medical literature that shows that blood levels of zinc are low in patients with hyperthyroidism. However, zinc is probably the worst nutrient for those with hyperthyroidism. When I took 100 mg of zinc, my hyperthyroid symptoms increased significantly.

Johnson also cautions that vitamin B6 is the primary B vitamin that assists zinc metabolism, so taking B6 can have the same effect as taking zinc. Generally, he recommends avoiding vitamin B6 until you are well enough to start supplementing zinc again. Since most B-complex supplements contain B6, he recommends taking individual B vitamins because they are important to the overall nutritional approach.

Calcium and Magnesium

Johnson believes that one of the biggest deficiencies in hyperthyroidism is magnesium. Calcium and magnesium work as a pair of nutrients—taking too much of one will deplete the other. However, most nutritionists don't know that the proper utilization of both calcium and magnesium in the body is dependent on the presence of key trace metals. Johnson outlines this important issue:

In hyperthyroidism, one of the most dangerous symptoms is high, often irregular, heart rate. Taking magnesium will temporarily relieve this symptom; however, continued supplementation with magnesium will not cure the disease. The real problem is copper deficiency, because copper is essential for magnesium metabolism. When copper becomes deficient, magnesium gets functionally deficient, which means that the body's magnesium-dependent processes are reduced. While magnesium plays many important roles in the body, the one that affects people with hyperthyroidism the most is its role in muscle function. The most critically important muscles in the body that are affected by magnesium deficiency are the heart muscles.

When I was diagnosed with hyperthyroidism, I started taking 300 mg of the antithyroid drug PTU. However, after 4 days of experimenting with my calcium/magnesium supplements, I discovered that I could control the bouts of high heart rate that I was experiencing by increasing my magnesium to the point where I was taking calcium/magnesium in a 1:1 ratio rather than the normal 2:1 ratio. Although the extra calcium/magnesium slowed my heart rate, the effect was temporary. I had to retake 1,000 mg of calcium/magnesium about every 4 hours day and night.

The calcium/magnesium controlled his heart symptoms and allowed him to go off PTU, but the overall condition didn't improve until he started taking copper. Johnson adds a word of caution:

> *I now understand how dangerous it is to discontinue taking an ATD [antithyroid drug] and don't recommend that anyone do this, but that's what I did. This made my body more sensitive to nutritional effects and was probably a key factor in enabling me to determine the effects of various nutrients on hyperthyroidism.*

Cadmium, Smoking, and Salads

Smoking is a known health hazard for many diseases, including hyperthyroidism and Graves' disease. According to Johnson, eating large amounts of green leafy vegetables and salads also increases hyperthroidism risk, and interestingly the mechanism that increases the risk is the same: creating an excess amount of cadmium in the body. Tobacco smoke contains cadmium, a very toxic heavy metal that has a long life in the body. Like all plants with green leaves, tobacco naturally contains cadmium.

Johnson explains that studies with animals have shown that administration of high doses of cadmium can cause immediate hyperthyroidism. The reason is that cadmium is a copper antagonist. It is well known that cadmium toxicity interferes with zinc metabolism. It's less well known that the metallothionein protein that transports copper and zinc also transports cadmium. When cadmium is present, it occupies the binding sites on metallothionein, replacing copper and zinc and creating functional deficiencies of these metals.

Johnson cautions that in addition to avoiding smoking, other sources of cadmium such as green leafy vegetables need to be avoided until copper is replenished. Some processed foods have high levels of cadmium due to residual exposure to food processing machinery made of cadmium. Imported chocolates are known to contain high levels of cadmium. Johnson says that another food that was a problem for him was rice, including brown rice:

> *The sludge in river bottoms generally has high levels of cadmium because the heavy metal sinks. Because rice is grown submerged in water, I'm concerned that rice fields may accumulate cadmium and this winds up in the rice. My rate of recovery seemed to increase once I switched from rice to millet.*

Cadmium and Graves' Ophthalmopathy

High levels of thyroid hormone do not cause Graves' ophthalmopathy; rather, it is an antibody attack on the eye tissue. What triggers the attack and why it focuses on the eyes is not generally understood in conventional medicine. Johnson's theory is that Graves' ophthalmopathy is caused by cadmium toxicity:

> *People who smoke tobacco have a higher incidence of Graves' ophthalmopathy than nonsmokers. I met one woman who suffered from Graves' disease and severe Graves' ophthalmopathy. She had had ten sessions of radiation and two accommodation surgeries (carving out the skull bone behind the eye to make more room for the eyeball) because the radiation didn't work. I asked her if she smoked and she said no. I asked what she ate. She replied, very proud of her "good" health habits, that she ate only salads. I know it is hard to believe that eating too many salads could jeopardize your health, but when you're copper deficient, the cadmium present in green leafy vegetables may be taken up in much higher amounts than normal and cause both hyperthyroidism and Graves' ophthalmopathy.*

Johnson himself was eating what he thought was a very healthful diet, which included lots of fruit and salads, prior to developing hyperthyroidism:

As I got sicker, I increased my consumption of salads. I remember my amazement when I'd eat nothing for dinner except a fresh, all-organically grown salad and then spend all night feeling miserable with hyperthyroidism symptoms. My theory that cadmium depletes copper makes sense of this otherwise bizarre observation. At the time of my hyperthyroidism diagnosis, I had a hair analysis performed. It showed high levels of cadmium, but I never developed Graves' ophthalmopathy. One supplement that I was taking both before and while I had hyperthyroidism was 400 mcg of selenium a day. Selenium is a primary antagonist of cadmium and combines with it to escort it out of the body. Perhaps selenium protected me from developing Graves' ophthalmopathy.

Johnson theorizes that the production of free radicals during RAI may also deplete the important antioxidant glutathione peroxidase, which contains selenium, the principal nutrient responsible for moving cadmium out of the body. He believes this may be the mechanism by which RAI increases Graves' ophthalmopathy.

Immune System Stimulants

Johnson says that it's incorrect and potentially dangerous to believe that hyperthyroidism is caused by an immune system deficiency and to take products to stimulate the immune system:

Any nutritional product that is described as an immune system stimulant should be avoided. In Graves' disease the immune system is stimulating the thyroid to produce T4 by producing immune bodies that imitate the TSH molecule. Stimulating the immune system will cause your thyroid to produce more hormone and is exactly the wrong thing to do. The immune system needs control restored, and that is what copper does.

One woman who went to the health food store to get copper and other nutritional supplements that are recommended as part of Johnson's protocol asked an employee of the store where to find those products. According to Johnson:

> He told her that she shouldn't take copper since it was a toxic heavy metal. He convinced her that since hyperthyroidism is a disease of the immune system, she should take colostrum, which is the immune-stimulating substance that a baby gets from its mother's breast right after birth. When this woman took the colostrum, she went into an immediate thyroid storm. Fortunately, she lived to tell the story.

Iron

There is a higher rate of anemia in hyperthyroidism, but Johnson theorizes that it's not from iron deficiency. Rather, he says it's from copper deficiency:

> People with hyperthyroidism who develop copper deficiency anemia get symptoms known among patients as brain fog. Some people get hyperthyroidism from supplementing large amounts of iron. Because iron works so closely with copper, any amount of iron will further deplete copper in a copper-deficient body. Therefore, patients with hyperthyroidism should not only avoid iron supplements but also avoid iron-containing foods like red meat, wine, and fruits. In addition, it's important to avoid vitamins that assist iron metabolism, like vitamin B12 and folic acid. It's easy to see when you have too much iron and too little copper. Pay attention to your body temperature. Iron is warming, while copper is cooling. Hyperthyroidism makes you feel hot and sweaty. Stopping iron intake and supplementing copper will cool the body.

▌ Correcting Hyperthyroidism Nutritionally

In Johnson's opinion, the first step in dealing with hyperthyroidism nutritionally is to stop the intake of supplements, foods, hormones, immune stimulants, and toxic metals that could be causing a copper deficiency. The second step, which can be taken at the same time, is for you to begin a supplementation program that has replenishing copper as its main goal but includes getting enough of the various conutrients that help your body metabolize copper properly.

According to Johnson, it's particularly important to follow this order: identifying the most deficient nutrient and supplementing that first, then finding the next most deficient nutrient, and so on:

Starting with any nutrient, other than the most deficient, will further deplete the most deficient nutrient, making the disease worse. Taking the right supplements in the correct order is critical. It's very common for someone with hyperthyroidism to start taking only copper and see immediate and significant benefits for a few days and then have the disease symptoms come back. This is what happened to me, over and over again. What this means is that the body has run out of one or more conutrients and these deficiencies are now stopping the body from assimilating and/or using the copper. Adding the next most deficient nutrient will resume the progress.

Before starting a nutritional program for hyperthyroidism, Johnson advises getting a hair analysis to determine your mineral status:

Hair analysis is the preferred method because blood tests do not show trace mineral deficiencies well. The body has a re-markable ability to normalize the mineral levels in the blood, which masks deficiencies. I have seen several cases where the blood test showed copper to be normal but the hair analysis showed that it was very deficient.

The process of using a nutritional program to correct hyperthyroidism is not an overnight solution. Full correction of hyperthyroidism can take many months or even years. Johnson feels that it can take a long time for several reasons:

It's not only necessary to replenish copper, but when there is cadmium toxicity, a lot of stored cadmium has to be moved out of the body. Because cadmium is much heavier than copper, it takes a longer time for copper to replace the cadmium than it took the cadmium to replace the copper.

If you are presently taking an antithyroid drug (ATD) and you decide to begin a nutritional program, don't discontinue the ATD in anticipation of getting results. It's better to reduce the ATD after you get results. Always consult your physician. Keep in mind that each person will have a slightly different profile of deficiencies, so correcting the disease usually requires a fair amount of trial and error until you determine the right balance of nutrients for you.

Minerals

Copper

Johnson says that copper is usually the most deficient mineral and therefore the first one to supplement. He recommends you start with 2.5 to 3 milligrams per day and work up to a maximum of 10 milligrams per day. Most people settle on about 6 to 8 milligrams per day for 6 to 12 months. Both copper and zinc taken on an empty stomach will cause nausea and possibly vomiting, so they should always be taken on a full stomach.

Calcium and Magnesium

Johnson recommends starting with 400-milligram capsules of magnesium as needed to help slow the heart rate. You may want to add in calcium when the magnesium is as effective as you'd like. Gradually, you'll find the right ratio of calcium and magnesium. For most people, the ideal ratio will be 1:1, but in some cases there may be a need for slightly more magnesium.

Trace Elements

Johnson finds that many people need a trace mineral supplement:

There may be some ultra-trace element that is needed for copper metabolism that I haven't been able to identify. There are many of these supplements on the market with names like "colloidal minerals." Take as directed.

Boron

Johnson believes that boron is an essential conutrient for copper:

I took boron sporadically and it took me a long time to figure out that I felt better the next day after taking boron. Once I started taking 3 mg of boron a day, my rate of recovery was faster.

Silicon

Silicon is involved in collagen production, and Johnson believes it is a conutrient for copper. Many people with hyperthyroidism find that their hair breaks as well as falls out by the roots. Silicon is essential for your hair to be strong, so it's very likely to be deficient in hyperthyroidism. Take one capsule daily of a horsetail silica extract.

Lithium

Lithium is one of the alkaline minerals—along with sodium and potassium—that controls the passage of metals and other nutrients into cells. There are studies that describe a sodium-lithium counter-transport system that appears to move copper into the cells. Johnson reports that some people find taking 50 milligrams of lithium per day helps.

Selenium

Selenium is a critical element for thyroid health. Not only is it essential for the production of T4 and the conversion of T4 to T3, but it is also needed to help chelate heavy metals such as cadmium and mercury out of the bloodstream.

Other Minerals

Johnson's program focuses on adding the essential minerals back in after copper supplementation has begun. These minerals include iron, zinc, manganese, iodine, sulfur, and chromium.

Vitamins

There are some key vitamins that are essential for copper metabolism. Johnson cautions that B6, folic acid, and B12 should be limited until copper levels increase.

B-Complex Vitamins

The B-complex vitamins—B1 (thiamine), B2 (riboflavin), B3 (niacin), and B5 (pantothenic acid)—all work with copper. It's important to take equal amounts of these vitamins. Most patients find that they need between 100 and 500 milligrams of each per day. You may have to buy them separately in order to avoid B6, which pushes zinc metabolism. Also, Johnson notes that taking B3 as pure niacin seems to work better than taking it as niacinamide. (Niacin in amounts over 50 mg will produce full-body flushing, which can be a frightening side effect in some people. The flushing is considered harmless, but you should be aware of it as a potential side effect.)

Biotin

Biotin is a critical vitamin that is essential for copper metabolism. Johnson says,

> Discovering that I had to take biotin with copper was the key discovery that enabled me to recover. Most B-complex supplements don't have enough biotin. Take at least 1,200 mcg of biotin daily.

Para-Aminobenzoic Acid (PABA)

PABA is another vitamin that assists copper metabolism. Take the same milligram amount as you do of vitamins B1, B2, B3, and B5.

Choline, Inositol, and Glutathione

Johnson explains that these nutrients combine with selenium to produce glutathione peroxidase, the antioxidant that protects the thyroid gland from damage:

> Hydrogen peroxide is produced during the normal process of thyroid hormone production. Increasing these supplements will control the burning feeling in the thyroid and stop the damage being caused by too much hydrogen peroxide.

Other Recommendations

Here are some other recommendations that Johnson includes in his protocol:

- Avoid fruits until copper is replenished. According to Johnson, fruit sugars may promote copper deficiency.
- Eat sufficient protein and fat.

- Do not abuse vitamin C. Amounts of more than 5 grams (5,000 mg) per day can deplete copper. Limit vitamin C to 500 to 1,000 milligrams per day.
- Restrict iodine until you replenish copper.
- Limit manganese.
- Restrict sulfur exposure in foods (e.g., egg yolks) and in supplements, such as methylsulfonylmethane (MSM) or glucosamine and chondroitin sulfates for arthritis and joint health, since sulfur can further deplete copper.

Will It Work?

The conventional medical world has its standard treatments for Graves' disease and hyperthyroidism—treatments that focus not on any causes of the conditions or on restoring the thyroid to normal but rather on disabling the thyroid. The idea of a nutritional treatment approach is not one that most conventional physicians would espouse. But Johnson says,

> I believe that my theory offers the best explanation of what causes the disease and provides a way to correct the disease. If hyperthyroidism is a nutritional deficiency disease, following the medical establishment's advice to destroy your thyroid is only going to stop one problem, which is high levels of thyroid hormone. It doesn't correct the underlying cause of the disease. The patient is still going to suffer for years or a lifetime from other symptoms caused by the uncorrected nutritional deficiencies.

Johnson cautions about holistic practitioners who may not truly understand hyperthyroidism:

> Some practitioners aren't so cautious. These practitioners are accustomed to treating people with low vitality and low thy-

roid output. The nutritional protocols that they typically recommend for other diseases won't work with hyperthyroidism. These protocols typically contain nutrients like zinc that increase energy and thyroid production and will act as poisons to patients with hyperthyroidism.

PART FOUR

Life After Treatment

11

Hypothyroidism and Its Treatment

▮ Risks of Hypothyroidism After Treatment

Ultimately, many patients who start out with Graves' disease or hyperthyroidism will end up hypothyroid. One study found that 56 percent of patients were hypothyroid 1 year after RAI, and almost 90 percent were hypothyroid at 10 years. Hypothyroidism rates were highest in people who had Graves' disease, those who had a goiter, and those who had a high RAI dose.

Surgery usually leaves you hypothyroid as well. Total thyroidectomy always leaves you hypothyroid, and 70 percent of people who get a partial or subtotal thyroidectomy will become hypothyroid.

Drug-induced hypothyroidism is a risk if you are taking too much antithyroid drugs as a treatment for your hyperthyroidism. After starting antithyroid drugs, or having RAI or surgery, it's essential for you to watch for the potential onset of hypothyroidism.

Here are some important things to know about hypothyroidism:

- Your doctor may not tell you that hypothyroidism is a risk after RAI or surgery.

- Hypothyroidism may take years to develop after RAI, or you can have a rapid plunge in your hormone levels, leaving you quickly hypothyroid.
- Hypothyroidism typically sets in quickly after surgery.
- Untreated hypothyroidism can worsen the risk and severity of Graves' ophthalmopathy.

▌Hypothyroidism Signs and Symptoms

If you have had RAI, your doctor should periodically evaluate you for hypothyroidism. Some of the clinical signs your doctor may observe are in this checklist.

Clinical Signs of Hypothyroidism
___ Slowed Achilles reflex
___ Other slowed reflexes
___ Low body temperature
___ Slow heartbeat
___ Irregular heartbeat, palpitations
___ Blood pressure irregularities—low blood pressure, high blood pressure
___ Loss of outer edge of eyebrow hair
___ Coarse, brittle, strawlike hair
___ Loss of scalp, underarm, and/or pubic hair
___ Dry skin
___ Dry mucous membranes
___ Yellowish cast to the skin, jaundice
___ Pallor, paleness of skin, pale lips
___ Dull facial expression
___ Puffiness around the eyes
___ Slow movement
___ Slow speech

__ Hoarseness of voice
__ Edema (swelling) of the feet

You can review the following detailed checklist of hypothyroidism symptoms frequently to monitor any symptoms of concern. It is also helpful after you are being treated for hypothyroidism to determine if you are receiving sufficient treatment.

SYMPTOMS OF HYPOTHYROIDISM

Obesity/Weight Gain
__ I am obese or overweight.
__ I am gaining weight inappropriately.
__ I'm unable to lose weight with proper diet/exercise.

Weight Loss
__ I'm losing weight inappropriately.

Ascites/Fluid in the Abdomen
__ I have rapidly gained weight.
__ I am experiencing abdominal discomfort and distention.
__ I'm experiencing shortness of breath.
__ My ankles are swollen.

Digestive Problems/Constipation
__ I am constipated, sometimes severely.
__ I have frequent diarrhea.

Body Temperature
__ I have been diagnosed as having hypothermia (low body temperature).
__ My "normal" basal body temperature is lower than 97.8°F to 98.2°F.
__ I feel cold when others feel hot. I need extra sweaters when others need air conditioning.

__ I feel cold, especially in the hands and/or feet.

__ I perspire less than normal.

Tiredness/Weakness

__ I feel fatigued more than normal.

__ I feel weak.

__ I feel run-down, sluggish, lethargic.

__ I feel like I can't get enough sleep, even though I'm sleeping the amount I should need to feel well rested.

Brain Fog

__ I find it difficult to concentrate.

__ I am having trouble with my memory.

__ I find it difficult to focus.

Pulse/Blood Pressure

__ I have a slow pulse.

__ I have low blood pressure.

__ I have high blood pressure.

Cholesterol Levels

__ I have high cholesterol.

__ I have high cholesterol that is resistant to diet or drug treatment.

Skin Changes

__ My mucous membranes (i.e., mouth, eyes) are dry.

__ I have a yellowish cast to my skin.

__ My coloring is pale; my lips are pale.

__ I have a dull facial expression.

__ My eyeballs are protruding.

__ I have puffiness around my eyes.

__ My skin is rough, coarse, dry, scaly, itchy, and thick.

__ My skin is breaking out.

__ I get painful, inflamed boils in my armpits or groin.

Hair Changes

__ My hair is rough and coarse.

__ My hair is dry.

__ My hair is brittle and breaking.

__ My hair is falling out more than usual.

__ My eyebrows or eyelashes are falling out.

Nail Changes

__ My nails have been dry.

__ My nails are brittle and break more easily.

Voice Changes

__ My voice has become hoarse, husky, or gravelly.

Aches and Pains

__ I have pains, aches, and stiffness in various joints, hands, and feet.

__ I have developed carpal tunnel syndrome, or my existing carpal tunnel syndrome is getting worse.

__ I have tarsal tunnel syndrome.

__ I have plantar fasciitis (pain in the balls of the feet).

Fertility/Menstruation

__ I am having irregular menstrual cycles (longer, or heavier, or more frequent).

__ I am having trouble conceiving a baby.

__ I have started to develop ovarian cysts.

__ I have a history of one or more miscarriages.

Postpartum Symptoms
___ I have had or am having difficulty breastfeeding.
___ I am having difficulty losing weight.
___ I am losing large amounts of hair.
___ I am abnormally fatigued.
___ I'm experiencing depression and mood swings.
___ I'm having brain fog.

Breast Changes
___ My breasts are leaking milk, but I'm not lactating or breastfeeding.

Mood/Depression/Thinking
___ I feel depressed.
___ I feel restless.
___ My moods change easily.
___ I have feelings of worthlessness.
___ I have difficulty concentrating.
___ I have feelings of sadness.
___ I'm taking an antidepressant, but it doesn't seem to be working.
___ I seem to be losing interest in normal daily activities.
___ I'm more forgetful lately.
___ My mind feels like I'm in a fog.

Sex Drive
___ I have no sex drive.
___ I have a reduced sex drive.
___ I have difficulty reaching orgasm.

Eyes
___ My eyes feel gritty and dry.
___ My vision is blurry, but eyedrops help.
___ My eyes feel sensitive to light.
___ My eyes get jumpy (tics in eyes).

__ My eyes make me feel dizzy.
__ My eyes give me headaches.

Neck/Throat
__ I have strange feelings in my neck or throat—for example, a feeling of fullness, or pressure, a choking sensation, or difficulty swallowing.
__ I have a lump or what appears to be some sort of fullness or growth in my neck area.

Hearing/Tinnitus
__ I have tinnitus (ringing in the ears).
__ I have sudden hearing loss or deafness.

Infections/Resistance
__ I am getting more frequent infections or infections that last longer.
__ I get recurrent sinus infections.

Allergies
__ I have developed allergies or my allergies have become worse.

Sleeping/Snoring
__ I'm snoring more lately.
__ I have (may have) sleep apnea.

Breathing
__ I feel shortness of breath.
__ I have a tightness in my chest.
__ I feel the need to yawn to get oxygen.

Dizziness
__ I have vertigo and dizziness.
__ I feel light-headed at times.

Puffiness/Swelling

__ I have puffiness and swelling around the eyes and face.

__ I have swollen feet.

__ I have swollen hands.

__ I have swollen eyelids.

Slowness

__ My movements are slower than normal.

__ My speech is slower than normal.

Headaches

__ I have chronic headaches.

__ I get migraine headaches.

Heart Palpitations

__ I get heart palpitations, skipped beats, and heart flutters.

__ I have periods of rapid heartbeat.

Symptoms in Infants

__ My infant has a puffy face.

__ My infant has a swollen tongue.

__ My infant has a hoarse cry.

__ My infant has cold extremities.

__ My infant has mottled skin.

__ My infant has low muscle tone.

__ My infant is not eating well.

__ My infant has thick, coarse hair that grows low on the forehead.

__ My infant has a large soft spot.

__ My infant has had prolonged jaundice.

__ My infant has a herniated belly button.

__ My infant is lethargic.

__ My infant sleeps most of the time.

__ My infant appears tired even when awake.

__ My infant has persistent constipation.

__ My infant is bloated or full to the touch.

__ My infant has had little to no growth.

Symptoms in Children

__ My child is not keeping up with growth charts for height.

__ My child is having school problems.

__ My child has been diagnosed with attention deficit disorder (ADD).

__ My child is having delayed puberty.

__ My child is unusually fatigued, exhausted, or sleeping far more than usual.

__ My child is gaining weight inappropriately.

__ My child is severely constipated.

__ My child is sensitive to cold.

__ My child's hair is rough, coarse, dry, breaking, and brittle.

__ My child's hair is falling out more than usual.

__ My child's eyebrows or eyelashes are falling out.

__ My child's skin is rough, coarse, dry, scaly, itchy, and thick.

__ My child's voice has become hoarse, husky, or gravelly.

__ My child is complaining of pains, aches, and stiffness in various joints, hands, and feet.

__ My child seems depressed.

__ My child seems restless or has difficulty concentrating.

__ My child seems to be losing interest in normal daily activities.

__ My child seems more forgetful lately.

__ My child complains of strange feelings in the neck or throat, or difficulty swallowing.

__ My child seems to have some sort of fullness or growth in the neck area.

__ My child gets more frequent infections or infections that last longer.

__ My child is snoring more lately.

__ My child yawns frequently to get oxygen.

___ My child has puffiness and swelling around the eyes and face.
___ My child has swollen feet, hands, or eyelids.

Symptoms in Prepubescent or Teenage Girls

___ My child is not keeping up with growth charts for height.
___ My child is having school problems.
___ My child has been diagnosed with attention deficit disorder (ADD).
___ My child is unusually fatigued, exhausted, or sleeping far more than usual.
___ My child is gaining weight inappropriately.
___ My child is severely constipated.
___ My child is sensitive to cold.
___ My child's hair is rough, coarse, dry, breaking, and brittle.
___ My child's hair is falling out more than usual, particularly eyebrows or eyelashes.
___ My child's skin is rough, coarse, dry, scaly, itchy, and thick.
___ My child's voice has become hoarse, husky, or gravelly.
___ My child is complaining of pains, aches, and stiffness in various joints, hands, and feet.
___ My child seems depressed.
___ My child seems restless or is having difficulty concentrating.
___ My child seems to be losing interest in normal daily activities.
___ My child seems more forgetful lately.
___ My child complains of strange feelings in the neck or throat, or difficulty swallowing.
___ My child seems to have some sort of fullness or growth in the neck area.
___ My child gets more frequent infections or infections that last longer.
___ My child is snoring more lately.
___ My child yawns frequently to get oxygen.
___ My child has puffiness and swelling around the eyes and face.
___ My child has swollen feet, hands, or eyelids.
___ My child showed early appearance of breast buds.
___ My child's breasts are growing.

___ My child has had unusual vaginal bleeding before she has begun to menstruate.

___ My child has a breast discharge.

___ My child has heavy periods.

___ My child goes without menstrual periods for long periods of time.

___ My teenager has failed to get her period and is having delayed puberty.

■ Diagnosing and Treating Hypothyroidism

After treatment for Graves' disease or hyperthyroidism, your doctor should regularly test your blood for symptoms of hypothyroidism. This condition may be diagnosed if your TSH is above normal. In some cases, TSH may be high-normal, but T4/free T4 and/or T3/free T3 levels may have dropped below normal. The normal range for TSH in the United States runs from approximately 0.3 to 3.0. Individual labs can have some slight variation, but these are generally where the levels should fall, typically making someone with a TSH level above 3.0 hypothyroid.

Once you are diagnosed as hypothyroid, your doctor will put you on thyroid hormone replacement medication. The following table summarizes the various forms of thyroid hormone replacement currently available:

Generic Name	Brand Name	Description
Levothyroxine (synthetic T4)	Synthroid, Levoxyl, Unithroid, Levothroid	The most common treatment, levothyroxine provides the synthetic version of one hormone, T4. Different brands may have different fillers, dyes, and potential allergens.

(*continued*)

Generic Name	Brand Name	Description
Liothyronine (synthetic T3)	Cytomel	Drug that is often given with levothyroxine.
Liotrix (synthetic T4 + T3)	Thyrolar	A combination synthetic drug.
Time-released, compounded T3	No brands	Currently available only from compounding pharmacies.
Natural, desiccated thyroid	Armour, Biotech, Nature-throid	Derived from thyroid gland of pigs; includes T4, T3, and other thyroid hormones such as T1 and T2.

Getting hypothyroidism diagnosed and properly treated is not an easy prospect, even for someone who is already under a doctor's care for Graves' disease and/or hyperthyroidism. There is so much material that it simply can't be included here. That is why I've put together this extensive information—including guidelines, advice and support on testing, and in-depth information on the various conventional, integrative, and alternative treatment options for hypothyroidism—in my book *Living Well with Hypothyroidism*. A new edition of this bestselling book, first published in 2000 and reissued in a revised edition in 2005, has specific sections on topics of key importance, including:

- How to take your thyroid hormone
- Thyroid hormone replacement for hypothyroidism when pregnant or breastfeeding

- Interactions with other drugs and supplements
- What to do when you still don't feel well despite hypothyroidism treatment
- Food, vitamins, minerals, herbs, and other supplements for hypothyroidism

Diagnosing and treating hypothyroidism can be complicated, so you will want to understand the testing that will diagnose and monitor your condition as well as the various treatment options that help you feel your best.

12

Managing Weight Problems

One of the most troublesome problems for many Graves' and hyperthyroidism patients after radioactive iodine (RAI) or surgery, or while on long-term antithyroid therapy, is weight gain or difficulty losing weight. Your doctor may suggest that your treatment for hyperthyroidism won't cause weight gain, but that is not accurate. Typically, in most patients who are treated for hyperthyroidism, body weight, body mass index (BMI), waist circumference, and body fat are all increased after even short-term treatment of hyperthyroidism.

If you've had RAI as a treatment, you are quite likely to gain weight. One study found that among the vast majority of patients after RAI, despite being treated with levothyroxine, for their resulting hypothyroidism, the median weight gain after 6 months was 11 pounds, 20 pounds at 12 months, and 25 pounds after 2 years. Before the therapy, 27.5 percent were considered underweight by BMI calculations, and 19.3 percent were obese, with a BMI above 30. Two years after treatment, only 8.7 percent patients were underweight and 51.3 percent were obese. Overall, the researchers found that there was a 32 percent increase in obesity in previously hyperthyroid patients following RAI therapy, with the main weight gain coming in the first 2 years.

A study looking at weight gain in hyperthyroid patients concluded that the patients gained an average of 13 pounds and had a BMI increase of 8.49. Patients treated with antithyroid drugs and RAI tended to gain similar amounts of weight, but patients who had thyroidectomy gained the most weight, at 23 pounds. If a person became hypothyroid even for a short time, this was associated with more weight gain. Overall, weight increased by almost 9 pounds at 1 year and 22 pounds after 4 years, representing a mean weight gain of 8 pounds a year.

Despite restoring patients to normal thyroid-stimulating hormone (TSH) levels after hyperthyroidism, a study found that many patients had excessive weight gain, whether their treatment was RAI, surgery, or antithyroid drugs. Interestingly, thyroid cancer patients who had surgery followed by suppressive treatment to keep TSH levels very low did not typically gain weight. This study suggested that restoring hyperthyroidism patients to "normal" TSH levels using thyroid hormone replacement may be an inadequate treatment and that patients may require higher doses of medication in order to avoid weight gain.

Another study found that among people treated surgically or with RAI for toxic multinodular goiter, about 50 percent reported weight problems. The mean weight increase for women was 15.6 percent.

There are several reasons that some weight gain is common after hyperthyroidism treatment:

- After having an artificially high metabolism during hyperthyroidism, the metabolism returns to normal after hyperthyroidism treatment, but many people continue to eat at the level they were eating before, which the metabolism can no longer support.

- The high levels of circulating thyroid hormone interfere with the hormonal feedback system that controls appetite, such as leptin, insulin, and other key appetite hormones. This imbalance can go on after treatment, so your appetite remains high even as your metabolism slows down.
- Hyperthyroidism can break down muscle mass, especially in your legs and arms. As weight is added back, it tends to be fat rather than muscle. Fat does not burn calories and is less metabolically active, slowing metabolism further.

You are at greater risk of gaining weight if:

- You started out overweight
- You had Graves' disease
- You lost weight while hyperthyroid
- You are not on sufficient levels of thyroid hormone replacement

And you are at the greatest risk of weight gain if allowed to become clinically hypothyroid without thyroid hormone treatment even for a short time.

Ultimately, you shouldn't expect much in the way of sympathy from the conventional doctors and endocrinologists when it comes to weight gain or difficulty losing weight. Other patients can sympathize. I can definitely sympathize. But don't be disappointed if your doctor gives you a "get off the couch" or "eat less" response. Once your hyperthyroidism has been treated, you've become hypothyroid, and you are on thyroid hormone replacement, many doctors will simply not believe your thyroid has much to do with weight issues.

For many of us, however, being hypothyroid—no matter how we got there—is synonymous with the weight battle, and it's impossible to separate the two problems in our minds. Becoming hypothyroid is only the beginning of what becomes a lifelong battle with weight, all the while being told by doctors that weight gain or difficulty losing has nothing to do with thyroid disease. But these doctors are completely wrong.

When I became hypothyroid, I gained weight, and nothing moved the scale down an ounce. Losing weight is not easy for many people with thyroid disease. It's a slow process—a far more difficult task than it is for people without metabolic problems. It is also a problem that has caused me and millions of others far more heartache than nearly any other aftereffect of being hypothyroid.

But remember—you're not lazy or lacking willpower. Your weight problem is most likely not an emotional issue that can be shouted and bullied out of you by a television personality. You're probably not downing an entire box of donuts every night when no one else is watching. Your eating habits may not be very different than those who are at a normal weight. Your body may truly refuse to lose weight on rabbit food, Weight Watchers, or Atkins.

Your body just doesn't work the way it's supposed to, it doesn't work the way it used to, and it *does* have to do with your thyroid. Once hyperthyroidism is treated and hypothyroidism sets in, your metabolism can become so efficient at storing every calorie that even the most rigorous diet and exercise programs may not work. Your friend or spouse could go on the same diet as you, lose a pound or two a week, and you might stay the same or even gain weight. *It's not fair!*

That is the most difficult point to get past—to accept that your thyroid condition may make weight loss an unfair fight, especially in the beginning and perhaps forever. What you suspect about your body is true. You may gain weight more easily than others and you probably won't lose weight as easily or quickly as others.

The good news is that even if it's an unfair fight, you can still win! There are solutions, so let's take a look at the issue of how being hypothyroid can play a role in weight problems and what you can do to maintain a healthy weight with hypothyroidism.

∎ Weight-Loss Challenges and Solutions

Let's discuss weight-loss challenges related to hypothyroidism and talk about the solutions you can consider.

Optimize Your Thyroid Treatment

The most essential step for anyone who is hypothyroid and can't lose weight is to make sure thyroid treatment is optimized. The best diet and exercise program in the world may not allow you to lose weight if your doctor is keeping you on too low a dose of thyroid hormone replacement. Or you may be one of the many patients who can't lose weight on any dose of levothyroxine, but add in T3 or switch to natural thyroid, and your diet and exercise start working again.

How to optimize your thyroid hormone replacement treatment is discussed in great detail in my companion books, *Living Well with Hypothyroidism* and *The Thyroid Diet: Manage Your Metabolism for Lasting Weight Loss.*

Evaluate Other Drugs

Determine whether you are taking any drugs that promote weight gain and discuss your concerns with your physician. These drugs include:

- Steroid antiinflammatories (e.g., prednisone)
- Propylthiouracil (PTU)
- Lithium
- Estrogen and progesterone independently or together as the pill
- Antidiabetic drugs such as insulin
- Antidepressants, especially Prozac, Paxil, and Zoloft

- Mood-stabilizing and anticonvulsant drugs such as those given for bipolar disorder, including lithium, valproate (Depakote), and carbamazepine (Tegretol)
- Beta blockers
- Sedatives
- Tranquilizers

Check Your Blood Sugar

You should consider getting your blood sugar tested. At a minimum, you can get a glucose level from a home test kit, but preferably get a fasting glucose to evaluate whether your blood sugar is normal, high-normal, or elevated. In late 2003, the American Diabetes Association recommended that the fasting glucose range for defining prediabetes should be changed from 110 mg/dl to 100 mg/dl, meaning that a value of 100 mg/dl or higher would lead to a diagnosis of impaired fasting glucose/prediabetes/insulin resistance. If your blood sugar is high-normal or elevated, this can in part contribute to your difficulty losing weight and is a sign that you are becoming insulin resistant, are prediabetic, or are already a type 2 diabetic. If your blood sugar is elevated, you should consult with your doctor about going on an antidiabetic medication such as metformin (Glucophage). Metformin, along with diet and exercise, can actually help prevent the progression of your insulin resistance or prediabetes to full type 2 diabetes.

Consider Antidepressants or Supplements That Balance Brain Chemistry

Even if you do not suffer from depression, you might find that you have greater success fighting a stubborn weight problem if your doctor tries you on a course of antidepressants. A number of people have reported that their diet/exercise plan suddenly began to work after their doctor prescribed a short course of antidepressant medication such as Prozac, Welbutrin, Effexor, or Paxil. It's worth discussing with your doctor. Welbutrin, in particular, is thought to be helpful in curbing cravings and addictions, and it is not as likely to cause weight gain, which can be a side effect with some antidepressants.

Follow a Low-Glycemic Diet

An effective method to combat insulin resistance and the inability to properly process simple carbohydrates is eating a low-glycemic, fairly low-fat diet. Low-glycemic foods do not rank high on the glycemic index, a ranking that assigns values to foods based on their effect on blood sugar.

High-glycemic foods are sugary, starchy foods such as pasta, rice, white flour breads, cereal, desserts, and sugary drinks. You may feel frustrated that there's nothing left to eat. But you need to rethink your eating habits, shifting to a diet of low-fat protein sources (e.g., chicken, turkey, fish, leaner cuts of other meats, and low-fat dairy products) and nonstarchy, high-fiber vegetables and fruits, and certain grains.

There are numerous books and Web resources that provide information on the glycemic index of foods and beverages. But if you avoid sugar in all forms, emphasize lean sources of protein and nonstarchy vegetables, and limit fruit consumption, you are on your way toward a low-glycemic diet. And when you do eat starches, make sure they are high in fiber and eat them in small quantities.

Researchers have found that thyroid disease may actually be linked to an increased appetite for starchy/sugary carbohydrates. This increased craving appears to stem from various changes in brain chemistry and sympathetic nervous system activity due to your thyroid condition. As you eliminate the "bad" carbohydrates from your body, you'll eventually find the cravings reduced. But when they strike, you may want to try some of the products that decrease cravings, such as CraniYums serotonin-boosting supplements or homeopathic Craving Elimination Drops.

Eat Enough Calories But Not Too Many

Many thyroid patients have already switched to extremely low-calorie "starvation" diets in attempts to lose weight. This sort of diet wreaks havoc on your metabolism, making it think that you are facing starvation and turning on a whole host of appetite-increasing, fat-storing hormones. Your metabolism shifts into hoarding mode and slows down to prevent you from starving. While you may need to eat a lower-calorie diet to lose weight, diets that go lower than 1,000 to 1,200 calories per day are probably counter-productive to most people with hypothyroidism.

All the various calculators and guidelines that say the typical woman who weighs 150 pounds should eat 2,200 calories a day to maintain her weight are not likely to apply to you. At one point about a year ago, I calculated the calorie levels I'm *supposed* to be able to eat in order to maintain my weight and actually tried eating that amount every day for 2 weeks. I gained 7 pounds. That was the end of *that* experiment! I now eat about half that calorie level every day, and it's only at this level with regular exercise that I am able to lose weight or maintain weight lost over time.

Eat Enough Protein

Protein is needed to build muscle and maintain energy. Ideally, include a portion of lean protein in every meal and snack, and never eat a carbohydrate—whether vegetable, fruit, or starch—without an accompanying protein. The protein helps slow down the digestion of the carbohydrate as it converts to sugar.

Get Enough Good Fat

Essential fatty acids (EFAs) cannot be produced in the body, so you must get them through diet or supplements. The key essential fatty acids include:

- Omega-3/alpha-linolenic acid (ALA), eicosapentaenoic acid (EPA), docosahexaenoic acid (DHA): found in fresh fish from cold, deep oceans (e.g., mackerel, tuna, herring, flounder, sardines, salmon, rainbow trout, bass), linseed oil, flaxseeds and flax oil, black currant and pumpkin seeds, cod liver oil, shrimp, oysters, leafy greens, soybeans, walnuts, wheat germ, fresh sea vegetables, fish oil. Usually, your body can convert ALA into EPA and then DHA.
- Omega-6/linoleic acid/gamma-linolenic acid (GLA): found in breast milk, sesame, safflower, cotton, and sunflower seeds and oil, corn and corn oil, soybeans, raw nuts, legumes, leafy greens, black currant seeds, evening primrose oil, borage oil, spirulina, soybeans, lecithin. Linoleic acid in omega-6 can be converted into GLA.

Drink Enough Water

Hypothyroidism can cause water retention and bloating. If you feel or look bloated or swollen, you actually may not be drinking enough water. Your body will hold onto water more fiercely when you cut back on water intake. Not drinking at least 64 ounces or more of water a day is counterproductive, since it will worsen bloating and cause dehydration, which slows metabolism.

Get Enough Fiber

Fiber is essential for digestion and for optimizing your weight-loss efforts. It has minimal calories but can fill you up by adding bulk. When consumed with carbohydrates, fiber helps modulate the insulin response and normalize blood sugar. There is a fair amount of scientific support for fiber's ability to increase your feeling of fullness after you eat and reduce hunger levels. One study found that adding 14 grams of fiber per day was associated with a 10 percent decrease in calorie intake, and weight loss of 5 pounds over 4 months. Eat more raw vegetables and fruits, since they have more fiber than cooked or canned foods. Consume only high-fiber cereals and breads. Two slices of high-bran bread, for example, has 7 grams of fiber, compared to only 2 grams of fiber for white bread. Other good sources of fiber are nuts, beans, apples, oranges, broccoli, cauliflower, berries, pears, brussels sprouts, lettuce, prunes, carrots, and yams. Men up to age 50 require 38 grams of fiber a day, and women need 25 grams. Men over 50 should get at least 30 grams and women at least 21 grams. If you can't get all your fiber from food, consider a natural fiber supplement such as psyllium.

If you switch from a low-fiber to a high-fiber diet, be very careful that you are getting your thyroid medicine at least an hour before eating in the morning so that your absorption is not impaired. High-fiber diets can change your dosage requirements, so 6 to 8 weeks after starting a high-fiber diet, you may wish to have your thyroid function tested to make sure you don't need a dosage change.

Keep Track of What You Eat

Studies have shown that people who write down everything they eat lose weight even if they are not formally dieting. The act of writing everything down makes you more aware of what you eat, so you are more likely to make better choices. There are special books and journals you can buy for this purpose. One particularly good diary is the *Fat Tracker Daily Diary,* from Karen Chisholm. See www.thefattracker.com for more information. You can also use your PDA, a notepad, your computer, a calendar, or a looseleaf binder. It doesn't matter what form you select—it's the action of sitting down and thinking about your goals, what you're going to eat, and assessing what you've eaten that makes the difference.

If you want a more formalized way to keep close track of your nutritional intake and are looking for a supportive community to help you follow your chosen approach, check out tools such as Ediets, Weight Watchers Online, or Physique Transformation Program's Personal Food Analyst, all of which have detailed food-tracking programs online, as well as online support communities and forums where you can share information and encouragement with others.

▋ Tips on How to Eat

Follow Some Basic Food-Combining Rules

- Try to eat protein with nonstarchy vegetables. You don't really want to have that baked potato with the steak. You're better off with a big salad and some sautéed mushrooms on the side.
- Avoid milk and meat at the same meal. Having milk with your meat slows down digestion.
- Eat one type of protein per meal. Don't have the beef and chicken fajita combo or a surf and turf combo. Combining proteins makes them harder to digest. You can, however, add eggs to other proteins—for example, steak and eggs or ham quiche.
- Don't eat fruit with meat or heavy meals, since it becomes harder to digest and can raise blood sugar.

Eat a Big Breakfast

You should aim to eat a big breakfast that contains a substantial amount of protein. In fact, aim to eat 25 percent of your calories at breakfast. You should also eat at least 20 grams of protein at breakfast. A protein-heavy breakfast speeds up calorie burning and gets the metabolism moving. Studies have shown that people eating a certain number of calories will lose weight if they eat more calories concentrated during breakfast, whereas others on the same number of calories will stay the same or even gain if they emphasize the calorie expenditure at lunch or dinner.

Try to Eat Three Meals Instead of Multiple Mini-Meals

The controversial recommendation to eat three meals rather than grazing, or eating five or six mini-meals as is often suggested, comes from Byron Richards, a holistic nutritionist and author of the groundbreaking book *Mastering Leptin*:

> *If 5–6 small meals a day are needed to maintain energy, the metabolic situation is not in good shape. Eating very small meals may cause some weight loss, but metabolism will likely slow down before the weight goal is achieved. Even a low-calorie snack increases insulin release, thus fat-burning mode ceases or never begins. Only by increasing the amount of time between meals will proper weight loss take place.*

According to Richards, this advice to eat small, frequent meals comes from the bodybuilding and diabetic communities. Bodybuilders, says Richards, can eat more times a day because they have shortened the time that their insulin levels cycle up and down by eating consistently at high-calorie levels and burning calories intensively through their muscle development. Diabetics have a malfunctioning insulin and glucagon metabolism. They have to use calories like a drug to strictly regulate insulin levels. But these examples are not necessarily applicable for those of us who are not bodybuilders or diabetic. Richards explains that we need to condition the liver into better responsiveness and fitness by balancing our leptin. And working toward having three meals a day at 5- or 6-hour intervals is Richards's solution to optimizing leptin balance.

Eat a Lighter Dinner and Nothing Else Afterward

Dinner should be the lightest meal whenever possible. Keep in mind that few of us require large portions—if any—of the starchy carbohydrates such as pasta, bread, potatoes, and rice. If you are going to eat starches, you're better off eating them earlier in the day when your body needs the fuel and is more likely to burn it off. Richards believes that we should finish eating dinner at least 3 hours before bed and not eat after dinner. One of his key rules to balancing leptin is to allow 11 to 12 hours between dinner and breakfast.

Many experts agree with Richards that you should go to bed slightly hungry—not so hungry or starving that hunger pangs will keep you awake, but your stomach should feel nearly empty. Your body is looking for fuel to burn during the night. If you go to bed with your stomach nearly empty and your insulin levels are low, your body is much more likely to go to your fat stores.

Eat Slowly and Chew Thoroughly

Your mother always said to chew your food, and she was right! Chewing thoroughly and eating slowly is important. When you chew thoroughly, you're letting the digestive juices in your mouth and throat do their work to properly break down and begin digesting your food. At the same time, you're helping to extend the time you're actually eating, giving your brain time to receive the "I feel full" feeling that takes about 10 minutes to generate after you start eating. (How many of us are embarrassed to admit that we can eat an entire meal in *less than* 10 minutes?) When we eat too quickly, we're not giving ourselves enough time for the brain to receive the hormonal message that we've eaten and we're full.

■ Exercise and Breathing

As a confirmed couch potato with no athletic ability whatsoever, I'm the last person to talk about exercise. But there's no doubt that exercise is as potent a medicine as you can get and appears to be one of the factors that is absolutely essential to healthy weight loss or weight maintenance with hypothyroidism.

When you have a thyroid dysfunction, you may feel more fatigued than normal even with optimal treatment. This level of fatigue may mean that you exercise less and move around less, which reduces the amount of energy and calories you expend.

Thyroid disease commonly causes joint and muscle aches and pains, carpal tunnel syndrome, tarsal tunnel syndrome, and tendonitis, all of which make exercise and movement harder and may discourage you. Again, less exercise means you expend less calories.

The less you exercise and the less physically active you are, the less likely you are to burn calories from overall activity. Also, those who are inactive lose muscle mass. And reduced muscle mass means reduced metabolism because muscle burns more calories than fat even when your body is at rest.

Muscle-Building/Strength-Training Exercise

Ideally, your exercise program should include both aerobic activities and strength training. But if you have to choose just one, make sure you incorporate strength-training activities to build muscle, since it is essential to successful weight loss if you are hypothyroid.

Cynthia White, a certified aerobic instructor and personal trainer from Denton, Texas, has hypothyroidism. Cynthia highly recommends strength training, and she likes weight lifting:

Muscle is more metabolically active than fat. You don't even have to go to a gym to do this. Just buy a couple of sets of dumbbells, one set in 5 pounds and one in 10 pounds, and do the routine at home. Setting up a circuit-type routine will kill two birds with one stone. You will be working aerobically and lifting at the same time. One myth-buster: unless you are genetically blessed with a mesomorph body type (one that has a tendency to add muscle easily, which is rare for women), you will not bulk up! Trust me—I have been lifting for years and haven't bulked up yet. There are many books that can set you up with a basic weight-training program. The idea is to work the muscles, like your legs, back, chest, arms, and shoulders.

Aerobic Exercise

Regular aerobic exercise is also important. First, it's a completely natural way to help the serotonin problem. Many experts recommend 30 minutes of some vigorous aerobic activity at least five times a week as a natural mood elevator and antidepressant. Second, aerobic exercise burns calories. Third, according to Jean-Pierre Despres, PhD, professor of medicine and physical education and director of the Lipid Research Center at Laval University Hospital in Quebec:

Exercise is probably the best medication on the market to treat insulin resistance syndrome. . . . Our studies show that low-intensity, prolonged exercise—such as a daily brisk walk of 45 minutes to an hour—will substantially reduce insulin levels.

Those of us with hypothyroidism may need exercise almost as much as we need our thyroid hormone pills. Even if you're not a health spa or gym sort of person, the health experts tout the basic benefits of walking. A few minutes of brisk walking every day would be more exercise than the majority of us get and it's a terrific goal. So consider this a hypothyroidism prescription for a lifetime: Rx—take a walk and get moving!

My Approach

In the past, I regularly did yoga, and I still do it occasionally. But I've found that I like Pilates even better. While it involves stretching, breathing, and some mind-body aspects like yoga, it also focuses on the core abdominal muscles and strength building. I do an hour of mat Pilates twice a week and have done so for 2 years—the longest I've ever kept up with *any* exercise! I also joined my local gym and really enjoy doing strength-training. I also try to do the alternative nostril breathing, and abdominal breathing, at least once a day for a few minutes.

▌Other Issues

Other issues that can interfere with your ability to lose weight are discussed throughout this book and in *Living Well with Hypothyroidism,* as well as in greater depth in my book *The Thyroid Diet.* These include food allergies and sensitivities; candidiasis/yeast overgrowth; celiac disease/gluten (or wheat) sensitivity; parasites; the copper/zinc balance; adrenal imbalances; and estrogen and progesterone imbalances.

▌Supplements and Herbs for Weight Loss and Metabolism

To complement your diet and exercise program, there are hundreds of vitamins, herbs, minerals, enzymes, essential fatty acids, and combination formula supplements that promote themselves as helping to increase metabolism or make it more efficient, increase fat-burning ability, slow fat storage, balance blood sugar, and reduce appetite. I have a detailed review of these supplements in *The Thyroid Diet,* where I've listed all the supplements and provided my recommendation regarding whether they are worth trying. The most promising include alpha-lipoic acid; acetyl-l-carnitine; calcium; capsaicin/cayenne pepper; chromium picolinate; conjugated linoleic acid (CLA); CraniYums; glucosol; glutamine/L-glutamine; hoodia gordonii; pantethine; pyruvate; taurine; vitamin C; and zinc.

Other supplements that are reviewed and discussed in *The Thyroid Diet* include 5-HTP; 7-KETO; caffeine, gotu kola, guaraná, green tea extract; chitosan; coenzyme Q10; coleus; DHEA; garcinia cambogia/hydroxycitric acid (HCA); gymnema sylvestre; milk thistle; phaseolus vulgaris/starch blockers/Phase 2; and spirulina.

My Own Program

Some people ask what I take every day to aid with weight loss. In addition to a multivitamin, I take at least 1,200 milligrams of calcium, 3,500 milligrams or more of conjugated linoleic acid (CLA), approximately 800 milligrams of pure hoodia gordonii, and usually at least 1,000 milligram of vitamin C.

I also particularly like a line of weight-loss supplements called Lean for Less, from Health from the Sun/Arkopharma. When I feel that my diet needs an extra kick start, I will take all four supplements simultaneously for a few weeks, and I feel it helps get me back on track:

1. Lean for Less Thermogenic is meant to burn fat and raise metabolism. It includes green tea, coleus, and citrus aurantium, but it doesn't have other stimulants such as ma huang, ephedra, or guaraná.
2. Lean for Less Carbo Regulator is supposed to help reduce the conversion of carbohydrates into stored fat as well as reduce appetite and sweet cravings. Ingredients include

chromium picolinate, hydroxy citrate acid (garcinia cambogia fruit extract), gymnema sylvestre leaf, and holy basil leaf.

3. Lean for Less Fat Regulator is a freeze-ground preparation of nopal cactus, also known as prickly pear. Nopal cactus is reported to have a high content of gums and mucilage, giving it the unique ability to bind to fats and sugars consumed during meals and reduce their digestion and absorption into the body.

4. Lean for Less Water Regulator is a combination of vitamin C, iron, magnesium, lespedeza capitata powder, couch grass, java tea, and dandelion that decreases water retention and bloating and acts as a natural diuretic.

While Chinese medicine practitioners have been using ma huang, an herb that contains the stimulant ephedra, for centuries, the fatal abuse of ephedra-based diet pills in a few high-profile cases has ended up causing a complete FDA ban on the use of ephedra in diet formulations.

■ Especially for People with Hypothyroidism

No matter which weight-loss plan you choose, there are some particular considerations you need to keep in mind that apply specifically to you as someone with hypothyroidism:

- Don't expect to lose weight quickly. Celebrate your resounding *success* if you lose even a pound a week. Do not compare your results with those of your friends. And don't diet with a friend unless she or he is hypothyroid, too, because you're bound to feel frustrated.
- You *have* to exercise. It's not optional. Weight-bearing/muscle-building exercise is critical to raising me-

tabolism. And aerobic exercise helps burn calories. Even if you join a weight-loss center that says you can lose weight without exercise, it's not likely to be true for you.

- If you add fiber to your diet, have your thyroid function retested about 6 to 8 weeks after you stabilize at your new level of fiber intake. You may need a change in your dosage of thyroid hormone replacement.

- If you lose more than 10 percent of your body weight, it's time to get retested to see if you need a dosage adjustment.

- Many thyroid patients report that they can only lose weight when they dramatically cut down on starchy carbohydrates and sugars—bread, sugar, pasta, sodas, and desserts—and limit carbs mainly to vegetables, with some fruit. While there are thyroid patients who process carbs with no difficulty and can lose weight on a more old-fashioned food pyramid diet that emphasizes cereals, grains, and bread, they seem to be the exception rather than the rule.

- Hopping on a scale to keep track of weight loss is important—but not as important as keeping track of measurements. Particularly for thyroid patients, who may have more early results in building muscle than in losing pounds, keeping track of your measurements can provide important feedback and may even provide incentive on those days or weeks when you don't see much movement on the scale.

A comprehensive approach to losing weight with hypothyroidism, including specialized diet plans, detailed food lists, and recipes, is featured in my book *The Thyroid Diet: Managing Your Metabolism for Lasting Weight Loss*. For more information about the book, see the site http://www.GoodMetabolism.com.

13

Persistent Symptoms

There are a number of symptoms that may frequently persist after receiving treatment for hyperthyroidism.

▌ Depression

In a qualify-of-life survey I conducted among approximately 900 people with thyroid problems, 63 percent of the patients, most of whom were hypothyroid, described depression as a continuing problem despite being treated by their physicians for their thyroid condition. There is no doubt that having hypothyroidism is a key risk factor for depression. According to the Thyroid Society for Education and Research, most patients with hypothyroidism have some degree of associated depression. Ron Pies, MD, a clinical professor of psychiatry at Tufts University and a columnist for *Psychiatric Times,* estimated that as many as 40 percent of clinically hypothyroid patients experience significant depression.

Dr. Pies has speculated that there may be three reasons for the link between hypothyroidism and depression. First, a malfunctioning thyroid may actually be a marker for depression. Second, having a thyroid problem may make it easier to develop depression or worsen the symptoms of depression. Third, depression may somehow make it easier to develop autoimmune thyroid problems that may lead to hypothyroidism.

Whatever the causes, the depression associated with hypothyroidism is sometimes partially or fully relieved with sufficient thyroid hormone treatment. But the depression can continue in some cases. It may be unrelated to the hypothyroidism, it may be the body's reaction to chronic illness, or it may be an indicator that the hypothyroidism is being undertreated or not treated correctly.

If all your other hypothyroidism symptoms have been relieved by thyroid hormone replacement and depression remains, it is worthwhile to discuss treatment for depression with your doctor. However, if you still suffer depression along with continued hypothyroidism symptoms, you may want to be extra diligent to ensure that you are receiving optimal treatment for your underlying thyroid problem before accepting a diagnosis of depression. That may involve a dosage change, a change in brand, or the addition of T3 drugs.

I'm not saying not to pursue treatment for depression when it's needed. But make sure your thyroid problem is being treated as completely as possible before letting a doctor tell you that your continued symptoms are due to depression. Unlike their colleagues in endocrinology, doctors in the psychopharmacological community seem to be in tune with the concerns about undertreatment in the face of normal thyroid-stimulating hormone (TSH) values and the need for T3 drugs in some cases to help relieve depression in hypothyroid patients.

In a fascinating study that came out of Greece in 2004, researchers reported that depression can be linked to autoimmune thyroid disease. According to the lead author, Dr. K. N. Fountoulakis, "unipolar depression might be characterized by a 'low-thyroid function syndrome.'" This small study involved 60 control subjects and

30 patients experiencing major depression. Among the patients with depression, 20 female and 10 male, the age range was 21 to 60.

None of the people studied had abnormal TSH levels or abnormalities in free T3 or free T4—they would be considered to have no evidence of thyroid disease by many physicians. Yet all of the depressive patients had significantly higher levels than the control subjects of one particular measure of thyroid function—that is, thyroid-binding inhibitory immunoglobulins. And 10 out of 30 patients who had an "atypical" form of depression had significantly higher levels of thyroid microsomal antibodies—a measure of autoimmune thyroid disease—than the control subjects.

This study found a relationship between good response to the treatment for depression and the level of detectable thyroid dysfunction. Those with less thyroid dysfunction were more likely to respond to treatment for depression. Additionally, the atypical depressives—those who had significantly higher levels of thyroid microsomal antibodies—were found to be less responsive to treatment than the other people in this study.

Overall, the researchers concluded that the fact that depressed patients had increased thyroid-binding inhibitory immunoglobulins was suggestive of some sort of underlying autoimmune process independent of the type of depression. Additionally, they found that response to treatment for depression can be predicted on the basis of certain thyroid indicators, with better responses being noted when these indices were closer to normal values.

This study tells us that there appears be a relationship between the presence of thyroid antibodies and immunological dysfunction in the thyroid that predisposes some people to, or perhaps even triggers, various forms of depression. It also reinforces the fact that measuring thyroid immunological factors, including thyroid antibodies, should be part of a complete thyroid evaluation, and symptoms cannot be dismissed solely on the basis of normal TSH, T4, and T3 levels.

If your depression is a separate issue or isn't relieved by you and your doctor's best efforts at treating the underlying hypothyroidism, then the depression itself may need to be treated. This is not something to be embarrassed about; it's just an indication that your brain chemistry is interrelated with your endocrine system; without balance in one, it's hard to get balance in the other. Antidepressant treatments, such as conventional medications, herbal drugs, talk therapy, exercise, and support, can help balance brain chemistry and relieve depression.

Antidepressant Medication

The conventional treatment for depression is antidepressant medication—for example, some of the newer drugs such as mirtazapine (Remeron), venlafaxine (Effexor), nefazodone (Serzone), and bupropion (Wellbutrin); the selective serotonin reuptake inhibitors (SSRIs) such as paroxetine (Paxil), fluoxetine (Prozac), and sertraline (Zoloft); the monoamine oxidase inhibitors (MAOIs) such as phenelzine (Nardil) and tranylcypromine (Parnate); and the older tricyclic antidepressants such as sinequan (Adapin), amitriptyline (Elavil), desipramine (Norpramin), and impramine (Tofranil); and others. Your doctor should discuss the best option for you. Remember that if you take an antidepressant, it can take a few weeks or even a month or more to notice benefits. Don't give up after a week or two if you don't feel a difference. Some antidepressants can become stronger or weaker in the presence of thyroid hormone or can interfere with thyroid absorption, so discuss this with your doctor.

Alternative Antidepressant Supplements

Since there are side effects associated with many antidepressants, some people try supplements. While Saint-John's-wort (*Hypericum perforatum*) is often a popular choice, some experts believe that it can interfere with thyroid hormone replacement therapy. Other supplements used for depression include 5-HTP (5-hydroxytryptophan), an amino acid derivative and the immediate precursor to serotonin, a brain chemical responsible for feelings of well-being; and tyrosine, an amino acid that is used to create norepinephrine, a brain chemical that works as an appetite suppressant, stimulant, and antidepressant (many leading-edge researchers believe depression stems directly from a deficiency of norepinephrine). Most people need 2 to 3 weeks to notice some definite benefits. Self-treating depression with supplements isn't a good idea. If you want to experiment with Saint-John's-wort, 5-HTP, or other supplements, do it only under the guidance of a health practitioner.

Therapy

Traditional treatment for mild and moderate cases of depression can include psychotherapy. Counseling or therapy, even short term, can be useful in coping with depression, particularly in learning how to prevent and/or deal with various sources of stress. Therapy may not cure your thyroid condition, but emotional stress has a tremendous impact on disease. Learning and mastering coping skills helps to ensure that the stress has the least amount of impact on your health.

Exercise

Many doctors believe that aerobic exercise is the best antidepressant and recommend 30 minutes of vigorous aerobics at least five times a week. Others have found that brisk walking for 20 to 30 minutes daily can have a strong antidepressant effect. However you look at it, exercise stimulates a variety of positive things in the brain chemistry that can help to counteract depression. It's an essential treatment in almost every antidepressant program.

▌Fatigue

Of all the persistent symptoms in hypothyroidism, fatigue is one of the most common and most difficult to resolve. In my patient quality-of-life survey, almost 92 percent of the patients reported feeling fatigued and more exhausted than normal.

For many patients, myself included, one noticeable sign that TSH levels are getting too high and dosages may need to be adjusted is the onset of bone-numbing fatigue. It often comes on suddenly and leaves you barely able to lift your head off the pillow in the morning. You may feel like you can't get through a day without a nap, or you sleep more than usual but still feel exhausted. Frequently seen along with other symptoms you'll find on my Hypothyroidism Signs and Symptoms Checklist in chapter 11, this fatigue can be a sign that your hypothyroidism is undertreated.

Even when treatment is considered optimal, the exhaustion continues for some patients. I get many e-mails from readers who complain that they are just plain exhausted despite being treated for their thyroid disease. They want to know when they'll get their energy back.

Many doctors will tell you that the fatigue will be relieved by thyroid hormone replacement—and sometimes it is. But if you're still exhausted after you've given the medication enough time to get your levels back to normal and you've investigated whether you are receiving optimal treatment, then it's time to look into the first line of attack: Are you getting enough sleep?

According to a survey released from the National Sleep Foundation, one in three people in the United States sleeps for 6 hours or less per night—substantially less than the recommended 8 hours. The average person gets 7 hours of sleep a night, and 40 percent of adults say that they are so sleepy during the day that it interferes with their daily activities.

There is evidence that people with thyroid problems can develop some sort of dysfunction in brain chemistry that prevents them from regularly getting important stage 4 delta sleep—the deep sleep that is restorative to both energy and the immune system. During typical sleep, every 90 minutes you move from light alpha sleep (stage 1), to progressively deeper beta sleep (stage 2), to gamma (stage 3), until you reach delta sleep (stage 4), the most refreshing and restorative stage. The body recovers energy and repairs muscle tissue during stage 4. Otherwise, you can wake feeling unrefreshed and unrested. Light alpha sleep is also known as REM sleep (rapid eye movement), when you have dreams. Stages 2, 3, and 4 are non-REM sleep.

If you're not getting quality sleep, you should start by practicing good sleep hygiene. This involves not using your bed as a place for work, television watching, or reading; establishing regular bedtime routines; getting enough exercise; limiting napping; avoiding stimulants before bedtime; avoiding food later in the evening; minimizing noise and light in the bedroom; and other common-sense techniques. Ultimately, however, if you are unable to reestablish healthful sleeping patterns, you may wish to try one of these non-prescription sleep aids:

- Over-the-counter drugs, such as diphenylhydramine (Benadryl, Tylenol PM, Excedrin PM), which are not habit-forming. But some experts feel these products do not help with deep stage 4 sleep.
- Melatonin, which is particularly helpful if your body clock is off-kilter and you're unable to go to sleep until early in the morning. If you are under age 50, take 1 to 3 milligrams at bedtime; over age 50, take up to 6 milligrams at bedtime. If you wake up groggy, the dosage may be too high, so cut it back. Don't use a higher dose unless you find it to be more effective.

- Magnesium and/or calcium, 400 mg each, at night can help sleep.
- Doxylamine (Unisom for Sleep), 25 milligrams at night (an antihistamine).
- 5-HTP (5-hydroxytryptophan), 100 to 400 milligrams at night, naturally stimulates serotonin.

Some of the herbs that have been reported to help with sleep include valerian root, passionflower, and kava kava. One herbal sleep formula I particularly like was formulated by chronic fatigue syndrome/fibromyalgia practitioner Dr. Jacob Teitelbaum. His Revitalizing Sleep Formula contains the exact combination of ingredients he has found most effective in facilitating stage 4 sleep without morning grogginess. The supplement is available at most health food and vitamin stores and includes valerian (*Valeriana officinalis*) root extract; passionflower (*Passiflora incarnata*) leaf flower extract; l-theanine; hops (*Humulus lupulus*) flower extract; wild lettuce (*Lactuca virosa*) leaf extract; Jamaica dogwood (*Piscidia piscipula*) root extract; and wild lettuce (*Lactuca virosa*) leaf.

Prescription sleep aids may be appropriate for debilitating fatigue. These include:

- Tricyclic antidepressants: Antidepressants can help with relieving pain and increasing serotonin levels, which can facilitate improved sleep. Low-dose tricyclic antidepressants frequently prescribed for sleep disturbances include doxepin (Adapin, Sinequan), amitriptyline (Elavil, Etrafon, Limbitrol, Triavil), desipramine (Norpramin), and nortriptyline (Pamelor). These drugs may provide long-term benefit for improving sleep.
- Other antidepressants: Other antidepressants that may be prescribed include sertraline (Zoloft), venlafaxine (Effexor), fluvoxamine (Luvox), fluoxetine (Prozac), paroxe-

tine (Paxil), and Remeron (mirtazapine). Typically, it can take 6 weeks of using the antidepressant before it has any impact on sleep.

- Trazodone (Desyrel): It is a frequently prescribed antidepressant for sleep problems, aiding with stages 3 and 4 sleep. It's particularly helpful for those who wake up every hour, or wake up and then can't go back to sleep.
- Antianxiety/muscle relaxants/benzodiazepines: These drugs can help improve sleep, relax muscles, and modulate brain receptor sensitivity. The most frequently recommended drug is clonazepam (Klonopin), a long-acting benzodiazepine. Others include lorazepam (Ativan) and alprazolam (Xanax). These drugs may be habit-forming.
- Hypnotics: The hypnotic drugs include zolpidem (Ambien), triazolam (Halcion), temazepam (Restoril), flurazepam (Dalmane), quazepam (Doral), and estazolam (ProSom). They may be habit-forming. Zaleplon (Sonata) is considered non-habit-forming and may be a better option.

Dr. Teitelbaum believes that under the careful direction of your practitioner, you can and should mix as many prescription and herbal treatments as you need to get 7 to 8 hours of sleep without constant waking so that you feel refreshed.

Natural Energy Boosters

If you are suffering from flagging energy, you need to make sure that you are getting enough B vitamins. Vitamin B12 is essential for energy. Consider taking a B-complex, plus a separate sublingual B12. (Sublingual B12 is dissolved under your tongue and is a more effective way for the body to absorb B12.)

Another useful supplement type relates to substances that the body naturally produces for energy production. Supplements in this category include coenzyme Q10, also known as CoQ10, which supplies energy to muscles; l-carnitine; NADH (nicotinamide adenine dinucleotide), which helps cells convert food into energy; and DHEA (dehydroepiandrosterone, but be sure to be tested by your practitioner before you start this hormone).

Some people have found that the South American medicinal plant maca can help with energy. In terms of herbal remedies, while you should avoid ephedra and ma huang stimulants, you can ask your practitioner about schizandra—a Chinese herb that is used for fatigue. Ginseng, especially Siberian ginseng, as well as the supplement rhodiola, are popular for energy. Before trying any herbs, supplements, or vitamins, you should consult with your practitioner to ensure they are safe for you. Ginseng, for example, is not recommended for those with high blood pressure. Many herbs and supplements are not recommended during pregnancy.

Other Energy Tips

To help keep your metabolism stoked and your energy level high, here are some other tips:

- Make sure you eat breakfast. If you don't eat breakfast, you slow down your metabolism and send your body into hoard mode, thinking it's starving because you're going a long period of time without food.
- Don't starve. Dropping your calorie intake below 1,000 calories a day will signal to your body that you are in starvation mode. It will slow down your metabolism and reduce your energy.
- Get enough exercise. If you do it in the morning, you're likely to raise your metabolism all day.
- Water, water, water! You've heard it before, but drink those eight 8-ounce glasses of water every day. Dehydration causes fatigue.

Is It Chronic Fatigue Syndrome?

There is a higher incidence of chronic fatigue syndrome (CFS) among people with thyroid problems, and the reverse is also true. To be diagnosed with CFS, however, you must have *extreme* fatigue that is medically unexplained, lasts at least 6 months, is not the result of ongoing exertion, is not substantially relieved by rest, and causes a substantial reduction in activity levels. In addition to this extreme fatigue, there must be four or more of the following symptoms for a diagnosis of CFS:

- Substantially impaired memory/concentration
- Sore throat
- Tender neck or armpit lymph nodes
- Muscle pain
- Headaches of a new type, pattern, or severity
- Unrefreshing sleep
- Relapse of symptoms after exercise (also known as postexertional malaise) that lasts more than 24 hours
- Pain in multiple joints without joint swelling or redness

If you meet at least four of these criteria, you should pursue a diagnosis and treatment specifically for CFS. Many of the leading-edge integrative physicians know how to address the entire picture of health imbalances and symptoms represented by CFS in combination with hypothyroidism. Your first step should be to read my book *Living Well with Chronic Fatigue Syndrome and Fibromyalgia,* then visit my associated Web site, http://www.cfsfibromyalgia, for more information and help in getting diagnosed and treated.

▌ Muscle/Joint Pain

People with hypothyroidism may notice muscle or joint-related pain. Most commonly, these symptoms are due to swelling of the muscles or swelling that is pressing on nerves. Various problems include:

- General muscular weakness and pain, such as cramps and stiffness
- General joint pain, achiness, and stiffness known as arthropathy
- Tendonitis in the arms and legs
- Carpal tunnel syndrome, which involves pain, tingling, weakness, aching, or numbness in the wrist, fingers, or forearm due to swelling of membranes that compress a nerve in the forearm
- Tarsal tunnel syndrome, which is similar to carpal tunnel, with pain, tingling, burning, and other discomfort in the arch of the foot or the bottom of the foot, possibly extending into the toes
- Plantar fasciitis—that is, pain in the balls or arch of the foot, usually worse in the morning

When muscle and joint pain does not go away with proper thyroid treatment, it's time to consider several options. Is your thyroid treatment optimized in terms of TSH, T4, T3, free T4, and free T3 levels, and the addition of T3 or natural thyroid, if needed? Sometimes a change of brand, the addition of T3, or a switch to natural thyroid can relieve pain.

If you are receiving optimal thyroid treatment and are still suffering from joint and muscle problems, should you get a referral to a rheumatologist for further evaluation and possible treatment?

A trained rheumatologist can provide a more thorough evaluation for arthritis and rheumatoid arthritis. Rheumatologists are experts in joint and muscle problems, and they treat arthritis, some autoimmune conditions, various musculoskeletal pain disorders, fibromyalgia, and tendonitis. To find a rheumatologist in your area, check the American College of Rheumatology's Doctor Directory.

Antibiotic Therapy

Holistic physician David Brownstein, MD, sees many patients with thyroid disorders who complain of soreness and swelling in their joints. In his book *Overcoming Arthritis*, he describes how certain infections may be at the root of Hashimoto's thyroiditis and Graves' disease as well as various joint and muscle pains and disorders:

> *My experience has shown that many individuals suffering from autoimmune illnesses often have an underlying infectious component. I began testing my patients for bacterial infections 8 years ago, and I discovered that, in the case of thyroid patients (i.e., those with Graves', Hashimoto's or thyroiditis), the infection was located in the thyroid gland.*
>
> *In my experience, approximately 70% of those with autoimmune thyroid disorders (i.e., Graves', Hashimoto's thyroiditis) have signs of an infection. This made perfect sense to me. Perhaps these individuals had a bacterial infection (e.g., Mycoplasma) that the body was not able to clear. Mycoplasmas are a very small bacterium that can actually get inside of the cells of the body. Because of this, the immune system cells are unable to directly attack the bacteria. In order to rid the body of the bacteria, the immune system cells will often resort to attacking the body's own tissue, which has been infected with the organism.*

Dr. Brownstein uses low doses of antibiotics—often doxycycline or an antibiotic in the tetracycline family—to treat infection. The length of treatment depends on patient response. He's had some patients who have been on treatment for years because going off the antibiotic induces a flare-up in their symptoms.

I've been on low-dose antibiotics for a number of years. If I stop taking them, I start having a variety of aches and pains a few days later, including knee and elbow pain, carpal tunnel syndrome, forearm and shin pain, and flu-like total body aches. I take probiotics (supplements that contain "good" bacteria like you find in yogurt) regularly to ensure balance in my intestinal tract.

Is It Fibromyalgia?

If you are hypothyroid, you are at higher risk for developing fibromyalgia (fy-bro-my-al-ja). This common and perplexing chronic condition is characterized by widespread and often severe musculoskeletal pain, fatigue, and multiple tender points. A number of leading-edge practitioners are finding high rates of hypothyroidism in their fibromyalgia patients. Some practitioners, such as fibromyalgia researcher and expert, Dr. John Lowe, actually believe that fibromyalgia is a manifestation of hypothyroidism.

Doctors typically use the American College of Rheumatology's 1990 criteria for classifying fibromyalgia. According to these criteria, a person is considered to have fibromyalgia if he or she has widespread pain for at least 3 months in combination with tenderness in at least 11 of 18 specific tender point sites.

Pain is considered widespread when it occurs in both the left and right sides of the body above and below the waist. Cervical spine, anterior chest, thoracic spine, or low back pain must also be present. The tender points are precise areas of the body that generate pain when pressed. To be considered painful, pressure on the tender point must generate actual pain, not just tenderness. The 18 tender point sites are:

- 1, 2—Area where the neck muscles attach to the base of the skull, left and right sides (occiput)
- 3, 4—Midway between the neck and shoulder, left and right sides (trapezius)
- 5, 6—Muscles over the left and right upper inner shoulder blade, left and right sides (supraspinatus)
- 7, 8—two centimeters below the side bone at the elbow of the left and right arms (lateral epicondyle)
- 9, 10—Left and right upper outer buttocks (gluteal)
- 11, 12—Left and right hip bones (greater trochanter)
- 13, 14—Just above the left and right knees on the inside
- 15, 16—Lower neck in front, left and right sides (low cervical)
- 17, 18—Edge of upper breastbone, left and right sides (second rib)

There are a variety of other common symptoms of fibromyalgia. A detailed listing with explanations of fibromyalgia and its risks and symptoms is featured in my book *Living Well with Chronic Fatigue Syndrome and Fibromyalgia*. For more information, see the book's Web site at http://www.cfsfibromyalgia.com.

▌Hair Loss

Hair can be considered a barometer of health because hair cells are some of the fastest growing in the body. When the body is in crisis, the hair cells can shut down to redirect energy elsewhere. The types of situations that can cause hair loss include hormonal changes, poor diet and nutritional deficiencies, a variety of medications, surgery, and many medical conditions, including thyroid disease.

Many people notice rapid hair loss as a symptom of hypothyroidism. Some people actually say this is the worst symptom of their thyroid problem—this thinning hair, large amounts falling out in the shower or sink, often accompanied by changes in the hair's texture, making it dry, coarse, or easily tangled. Interestingly, some people have actually written to tell me that their thyroid problem was initially diagnosed by their hairdresser, who noticed the change!

There are three common types of hair loss. General shedding is hair lost throughout the head. You'll often notice more hair in drains and in the shower, in hair brushes, and when you brush your hair, but there are no specific patches of loss or even baldness. Typically, this is the most common form of hair loss with hypothyroidism prior to treatment. This can occasionally continue for some people after hypothyroidism treatment, particularly when taking levothyroxine drugs such as Synthroid.

A second type of hair loss is more commonly associated with fungal infection or autoimmune alopecia. It involves circular patches of hair loss and sometimes complete loss of hair in these small patches. This hair-loss problem should be evaluated by a dermatologist. Autoimmune alopecia is more common in patients who have autoimmune thyroid disease.

A third type of hair loss is male pattern hair loss: men are most susceptible, but women can have it, too. Male pattern hair loss is concentrated on the temples and top of the head. It's caused when an enzyme starts to convert the hormone testosterone on the scalp to its less useful version, dihydrotestosterone (DHT). This makes hair follicles shrink, then disappear. This condition seems to be sped up in some patients with hypothyroidism and may be the cause of continued hair loss for thyroid patients despite sufficient thyroid treatment. Normally, hair grows about a half inch a month for about 3 years, then goes into a resting period. One in ten hairs is in a resting period at any single time, and a new hair pushes the old one out after about 3 months. When more hairs go into a resting period or the conversion process speeds up, the balance becomes disrupted and hair loss occurs.

If you're experiencing hair loss and are just starting treatment for hypothyroidism, it's likely that the loss will slow down and eventually stop once hormone levels are stabilized in the normal range. This may take a few months, however. But rest assured, I've had many thousands of e-mails from people and have yet to hear from anyone who lost all his or her hair or became bald due to thyroid disease. But people, including myself, have experienced significant loss of hair volume. In my case, I'd guess at one point that I lost almost half my hair. I had long, thick hair, and it got much thinner for a while.

If you continue to lose hair, you need to make sure that it's not your particular type of thyroid hormone replacement. Prolonged or excessive hair loss is a side effect of Synthroid for some people. Many doctors do not know this even though it is a stated side effect in the Synthroid patient literature, so don't be surprised if your doctor is not aware of this possibility.

Make sure you're getting optimal treatment in terms of TSH level, other thyroid levels, and the need for additional T3. In my case, I have far fewer hair problems when I am taking a T4/T3 drug, such as Thyrolar or Armour Thyroid, than levothyroxine. When I have had major bouts of hair loss (despite low-normal TSH and being on a T4/T3 drug), I've taken the advice of several noted thyroid experts. In his book *Solved: The Riddle of Illness*, Dr. Stephen Langer points to the fact that symptoms of essential fatty acid insufficiency are very similar to hypothyroidism and recommends evening primrose oil—an excellent source of essential fatty acids—for people with hypothyroidism. The usefulness of evening primrose oil, particularly in dealing with the issues of excess hair loss with hypothyroidism, is also reinforced by endocrinologist Dr. Kenneth Blanchard:

> *For hair loss, I routinely recommend multiple vitamins, and especially evening primrose oil. If there's any sex pattern to it—*

if a woman is losing hair in partly a male pattern—then the problem is there is excessive conversion of testosterone to dihydrotestosterone at the level of the hair follicle. Evening primrose oil is an inhibitor of that conversion. So almost anybody with hair loss probably will benefit from evening primrose oil.

I can vouch for the fact that taking evening primrose oil was the only thing that calmed my hair loss down. It not only slowed, then stopped my hair loss over about 2 months, but new hair grew back. My hair was no longer straw-like, dry, and easily knotted. When I take evening primrose oil, I usually take 500 milligrams twice a day.

Look at Other Alternatives

In one study, Dr. Hugh Rushton, a professor at Portsmouth University, found that 90 percent of women with thinning hair were deficient in iron and the amino acid lysine, which is the most difficult amino acid to get via diet. Lysine helps transport iron, which is the most important element in the body and is essential for many metabolic processes. When lysine and iron levels are low, the body probably switches some hair follicles off to increase levels elsewhere. Meat, fish, and eggs are the only food sources of lysine. There are also supplements that contain lysine.

Some other natural ways to deal with hair loss include arginine, cysteine, green tea, polysorbate 80, progesterone, saw palmetto, trichosaccharide, vitamin B6, and zinc.

Prescription Treatments

A dermatologist can work with you on drug treatments, including scalp injections, drugs such as Rogaine (minoxidil) and Propecia, and other treatments that can help nonthyroid-related hair loss.

▌Low Libido/Sex Drive

According to a *Journal of the American Medical Association* (JAMA) study reported in February 1999, about 43 percent of women and 31 percent of men suffer from sexual inadequacy for various reasons, including low desire, performance anxiety, premature ejaculation, and/or pain during intercourse. Interestingly, these percentages are actually thought to be underestimates of the real level of sexual dysfunction in the United States.

While the study didn't look at the specific physical causes of sexual dysfunction, the research indicated that many of the sexual concerns are likely treatable, since they are due to physical and health issues. These health concerns can include common hormonal imbalances such as hypothyroidism.

In my quality-of-life survey, 58 percent of respondents reported having no sex drive or a reduced sex drive. Low sex drive is a common but not often talked about symptom of hypothyroidism. Unfortunately, it does not disappear despite what doctors deem is adequate treatment. Many people, especially women, still complain of a lack of sexual desire even after their doctors consider the thyroid problem sufficiently treated. If you suffer from sexual dysfunction, you need to be sure that you are getting optimal thyroid treatment, including TSH, T4/T3 levels, need for additional T3, or possible need for natural thyroid.

You also need to have your other hormones—not just thyroid—evaluated. Men should have testosterone, dehydroepiandrosterone (DHEA), and other androgen levels checked. Women should have a full hormonal profile evaluated, including estrogen levels, testosterone, and progesterone, plus DHEA. Adrenal function in women should be checked, particularly if the testosterone levels turn out to be low. Addressing imbalances in these hormones can sometimes restore sex drive to normal. Testosterone can be a tremendous aid for men in restoring libido. It is available as a pill (some brands are Android, Virilon, Testred, Oreton), as a transdermal patch (Testoderm, Androderm), by injection, and sometimes as transdermal pellets implanted under the skin.

Some women can benefit from testosterone. Doctors will frequently provide testosterone in pill form to women or as testosterone propionate cream. Supplementation with estrogen or progesterone can sometimes help. Ask your doctor about estradiol gel or patches and natural progesterone supplements rather than the conjugated estrogens that have caused so much controversy. Be careful, however, about soy-based supplements and food products that are supposed to act like estrogen to deal with menopausal symptoms. Many of these products contain levels of soy isoflavones that can worsen hypothyroidism in some women.

Low sex drive may be a result of other nonthyroid health conditions. Diabetes and hypertension/high blood pressure can cause low sex drive in both women and men. You should ask your doctor to discuss the diagnosable symptoms of depression with you so that you can assess whether you are depressed. When there are other psychological and self-esteem issues that are contributing to lower libido, therapy can sometimes help. You should also discuss other prescription drugs you are taking because some antidepressants, tranquilizers, and antihypertensives—as well as many illegal drugs such as cocaine and marijuana—can reduce sex drive.

Exercise improves blood flow to all body parts. Research has found that people who exercise regularly have higher levels of desire, greater sexual confidence and frequency, and an enhanced ability to be aroused and achieve orgasm no matter what their age. The best type of exercise is aerobics because it can trigger the release of endorphins—chemicals in the brain that create a feeling of well-being.

Drugs and Supplements

The drugs Viagra and Cialis may help with both desire and performance for men when there is sexual dysfunction. More research is needed on prescription drugs for women to help with desire.

Some herbal and natural supplements are considered effective for low sex drive. But supplements can have various and sometimes serious side effects, so you shouldn't self-treat. Talk to your practitioner regarding these products. Some supplements that may help with libido include:

- Arginine: amino acid for both men and women
- Ashwaganda: Indian ayurvedic herb, typically recommended for men
- Asian ginseng (panax): can help increase sexual energy
- Avena-sativa/oat extract (main brand is Vigorex): reportedly helps with sex drive
- Damiana: aphrodisiac herb from Mexico that is thought to stimulate testosterone production and is considered most effective in women
- DHEA: precursor hormone that your body converts to testosterone
- Ginkgo biloba: herb that can improve sexual function in men
- Horny goat weed: used by Chinese herbalists to improve sexual function in men and women
- Kava kava: herb most known for use in relaxation but can also be useful as an aphrodisiac for women
- Maca: South American herbal remedy that can help women with libido and fertility
- Yohimbe: African herb that can be a very potent sex enhancer for men
- Zinc: Low zinc levels have been associated with low sex drive in women and men

■ Perimenopause and Menopause

Perimenopause is the time frame, sometimes taking place over many years, during which the hormone levels decline and change prior to cessation of periods, causing a variety of symptoms and erratic menstrual periods. Menopause is the point when the ovaries no longer release eggs and hormones are no longer capable of producing a menstrual cycle. To be officially considered menopause, the menstrual period should have stopped for a year. Menopause typically occurs as early as the mid-40s up to the the late 50s. The menopausal history of a woman's mother is often a good gauge as to when a daughter can expect menopause. Perimenopause actually begins as early as the mid- to late 30s in some women.

Some women go through perimenopause and menopause with few symptoms. Others experience a variety of worsening symptoms, including heavy bleeding cycles, short cycles, headaches, mood swings, depression, anxiety, food cravings, weight gain, growth of fibroids, muscle and joint pain, and palpitations. Menopause educator Pat Rackowski describes it as "permanent PMS."

Does Hypothyroidism Worsen Perimenopause and Menopause?

Some experts, including Drs. Richard and Karilee Shames, say there is a significant relationship between hypothyroidism and menopause difficulties:

Low thyroid is often the ignored factor in far too many women who are simply treated with estrogen and/or progesterone. Despite increased awareness in the medical community about the issues and interventions surrounding menopause, a disturbing number of women still suffer menopause difficul-

ties. *This underlying problem is commonly coexistent hypothyroidism. Not only does low thyroid become more common as women mature, but in addition, menopause and perimenopause are transition situations which require more than the usual amount of thyroid hormone.*

According to Drs. Richard and Karilee Shames, hypothyroidism symptoms can also be confused with menopausal symptoms:

The symptoms of hot flashes, insomnia, irritability, palpitations, and the annoying "fuzzy thinking" so common in menopause can sometimes be the result of Hashimoto's thyroiditis, the most common cause of hypothyroidism. But the real complexity comes when actual symptoms of menopause are simply magnified and exaggerated because of the low thyroid situation that is now coexistent with menopause. As many thyroid sufferers are aware, low thyroid makes any illness worse. And while menopause is not an illness, it can certainly begin to feel that way when symptoms of low thyroid exacerbate the already annoying laundry list of female hormonal symptoms.

If you are hypothyroid and are also going through perimenopause or menopause, it's essential to have your thyroid function evaluated more frequently. Drs. Richard and Karilee Shames explain that many women with previously low thyroid levels will see a rise in TSH well before a rise in FSH (follicle-stimulating hormone), which is the test that usually confirms the metabolic onset of menopause. You may need adjustments in your thyroid medication in order to offset the hormonal changes taking place in your body. And optimal thyroid function is essential, as confirmed by Drs. Richard and Karilee Shames:

Frequently, the underlying hypothyroidism is such a controlling factor that simply correcting it, sometimes even with homeopathic thyroid or over-the-counter thyroid glandular, returns the whole system to fairly normal function. Menopause continues, but it is a more mild, gradual, and comfortable process. This is because thyroid is the energy throttle for the whole body, and especially the gas pedal for all of one's coping mechanisms. Once you have the energy to go through the change more gracefully, life can become more normal.

Herbs and Supplements

A variety of vitamins and herbs may help to rebalance of hormones and relieve perimenopausal and menopausal symptoms. Some of the most effective alternatives include Royal Maca (organic, provided by Whole World Botanicals), vitamin E capsules, vitamin E suppositories, Royal Jelly, folic acid with vitamin B-complex, chaste tree berry (vitex), dong quai, and black cohosh.

What about Estrogen?

While estrogen replacement therapy has been so discredited in recent years that most people are afraid of these drugs, it's important to note that all of the studies used conjugated estrogens—that is, the drug harvested from the urine of pregnant mares that was made into the formerly popular drug Premarin (*PR*egnant *MAR*e's ur*IN*e), along with progestins. Neither falls into the category of bioidentical hormones used at small physiological replacement doses that are considered to be safer, more effective alternatives by many leading-edge experts.

If a woman is truly estrogen deficient, many alternative health advocates believe that estriol may be appropriate. Estriol, a bioidentical hormone, is considered the safest of all the estrogens. It is the dominant form of estrogen made during pregnancy. It is often recommended for vaginal dryness and urinary problems. Estriol, in fact, governs the harmonious workings and the suppleness of the lower third of the urethra located in the vagina. Estriol comes in various forms, including pills, creams, and even a low-dose patch, and it's important to remember that you may only need to supplement with estrogen a few days each month.

If you do take estrogen or any hormone-balancing supplements, you should have your thyroid tested to ensure that you don't need a thyroid drug dosage adjustment. Thyroid drug effectiveness and absorption can be affected by estrogen and estrogen-like drugs.

■ Do You Have Another Autoimmune Disease?

The thyroid conditions Hashimoto's disease and Graves' disease are two of the most common autoimmune diseases, and they are the most common causes of hypothyroidism. *Autoimmune disease* refers to a category of more than eighty chronic illnesses, each very different in nature, that can affect everything from the endocrine glands (e.g., the thyroid) to organs such as the kidneys to the digestive system. Underlying all autoimmune conditions is the concept of autoimmunity.

As recently as the 1960s, medical experts believed that the immune system could only be directed against foreign invaders and could always distinguish the body's own organs and tissues from outside invaders such as bacteria and viruses. But researchers discovered that the immune system, which normally defends only against invaders, can become confused and attack the body's cells, tissues, and organs. This concept, *autoimmunity*, may be taken for granted now, but it was a groundbreaking discovery in the 1960s.

In autoimmunity, the immune system's ability to recognize what's foreign and what's part of your own body breaks down in some way. Thinking that cells or tissues or organs are foreign invaders, the immune system moves into action to be rid of the invader, starting by manufacturing antibodies known as autoantibodies and generating of T cells that have as their mission the destruction of the "invader."

In some cases, damage to tissues by the immune system may be permanent, as with the destruction of insulin-producing cells of the pancreas in type 1 diabetes. Whereas some conditions are progressive, some autoimmune diseases go into remission or even disappear. This happens, for example, in a small percentage of Graves' disease cases, or in periods of remission—sometimes months or years—in multiple sclerosis. And the hair-loss condition alopecia areata frequently resolves itself with no treatment.

Autoimmune diseases also target different parts of the body. For example, the autoimmune reaction targets the brain in multiple sclerosis, the intestinal and bowel system in Crohn's disease and irritable bowel syndrome, and the thyroid in Hashimoto's and Graves' disease. In systemic autoimmune diseases such as lupus and sarcoidosis, the affected tissues and organs may vary depending on the person. One person with lupus may have affected skin and joints, for example, whereas another may have affected skin, kidneys, and lungs.

Autoimmune diseases predominantly strike women, who suffer about 75 percent of these illnesses, according to the American Autoimmune Related Diseases Association. They are more common during childbearing years and frequently appear in women who have just had a baby, after periods of high emotional or physical stress or accidents, during periods of hormonal change such as perimenopause, and after starting birth-control pills or hormone replacement therapy. Autoimmune diseases can run in families. If a close family member has an autoimmune disease, then your risk of developing one is somewhat increased.

The most important thing you need to know is that if your hypothyroidism was triggered by Hashimoto's or Graves' disease—

which is the case for most thyroid patients—then having had one autoimmune disease puts you at risk of developing others. There are hundreds of risk factors and symptoms for autoimmune disease, and a closer look at them can help pinpoint and close in on more specific conditions. But across the board, there are very specific symptoms beyond thyroid conditions that are found in different autoimmune diseases.

Some of the most common conditions include rheumatoid arthritis, multiple sclerosis, Sjögren's syndrome, lupus, celiac disease/gluten intolerance, irritable bowel syndrome (IBS), alopecia areata, polycystic ovary syndrome (PCOS), Cushing's disease, Addison's disease, insulin-dependent type 1 diabetes, scleroderma, Raynaud's syndrome, psoriasis, and vitiligo. A detailed checklist of autoimmune symptoms, risk factors, and conditions is featured in my book *Living Well with Autoimmune Disease*. A condensed version of the checklist is online at my Web site: http://www.autoimmunebook .com. *Living Well with Autoimmune Disease* also features extensive information on conventional and alternative diagnoses and treatments for autoimmune conditions.

14

Infertility, Pregnancy, and Breastfeeding

When you are hypothyroid after treatment for Graves' disease and hyperthyroidism, your condition may make it harder to get pregnant or can make positive outcomes somewhat more difficult. Research has shown that treatment for Graves' disease doesn't necessarily improve fertility. And women who have become hypothyroid after Graves' disease and hyperthyroidism treatment may still have poor stimulation cycles, infertility, failure of the egg to implant, failures of egg donation, and miscarriage.

Untreated or undertreated hypothyroidism can cause your body to fail to release eggs. Even though you may still have periods, don't assume you're ovulating. Check with an ovulation predictor kit or talk to your doctor about testing for anovulation—that is, failure to ovulate.

Hypothyroidism can cause as a short luteal phase, which refers to the time frame between ovulation and menstruation. The luteal phase needs to be a certain length—13 to 15 days is considered normal—to nurture a fertilized egg. Doctors may diagnose you as infertile when in reality you can get pregnant but simply fail to sustain the fertilized egg. The egg miscarries right around the same time as your period would normally begin.

Some women with hypothyroidism have an excess of prolactin, the hormone responsible for the production of breast milk. While it would seem that this would be a good thing, too much prolactin during the conception period can actually impair fertility. Hypothyroidism has been linked with an increased risk of polycystic ovaries, which can also decrease fertility by causing irregularities in the menstrual cycle and sometimes no periods at all.

Dangers to mother and baby in women who are untreated or undertreated for hypothyroidism are not uncommon. One study showed that among pregnant women with either overt or subclinical (low-level) hypothyroidism:

- 21 percent of the overtly hypothyroid and 15 percent of the subclinically hypothyroid had pregnancy-induced hypertension
- 16.6 percent of the overtly hypothyroid and 8.7 percent of the subclinically hypothyroid had low-birth-weight newborns
- 6.6 percent of the overtly hypothyroid and 3.5 percent of the subclinically hypothyroid had postpartum hemorrhage
- 5 percent of the overtly hypothyroid and none of the subclinically hypothyroid had placenta abruptio
- 3.3 percent of the overtly hypothyroid and none of the subclinically hypothyroid had congenital malformations

In order for the fetal brain to develop properly, an adequate supply of thyroid hormone is vital. Lack of such hormones—as may occur in women who haven't been treated for their underactive thyroid—can cause negative effects on the baby, including lower IQ and possible learning problems. In a 1999 study in the *New En-*

gland Journal of Medicine, children born to mothers whose hypothyroidism was not being treated scored several points lower on an IQ test than children of nonthyroid patients. The study went on to note, however, that children whose mothers were undergoing treatment for an underactive thyroid scored almost the same as children born to mothers with normal thyroid function. According to thyroid expert Dr. Steven Langer:

> *Baby IQ problems result because the mother supplies all thyroid hormones for growth and development of the fetus for the first 12 weeks of pregnancy. After 12 weeks, the fetus develops its own thyroid gland; however, the mother-to-be is still the source of thyroid hormone. During those first 12 weeks, a hypothyroid mother can't always assure enough thyroid hormone for proper brain development. In some cases, miscarriage occurs at this point.*

One report in the *Journal of Medical Screening* showed that pregnant hypothyroid women who are not receiving treatment have nearly four times the risk of a late miscarriage (second trimester or later) than other women. Another study found that 6.6 percent of overtly hypothyroid mothers and 1.7 percent of subclinically hypothyroid mothers have stillbirths.

There are numerous studies indicating a relationship between thyroid autoimmunity—as determined by the presence of elevated antithyroid antibodies—and infertility and recurrent miscarriages. According to an article in the journal *Obstetrics and Gynecology,* the presence of antithyroid antibodies increases the risk of miscarriage. Several studies have indicated that women with Hashimoto's disease are two to five times more likely to have a miscarriage in the first 12 weeks of pregnancy compared with women without thyroid autoimmunity.

Elevated thyroid peroxidase antibodies (TPOAb) are also linked to an increased risk of recurrent miscarriage rate. One study found that 31 percent of women experiencing recurrent miscarriages were positive for antithyroid antibodies, thyroid peroxidase antibodies, or both. Researchers at the Pacific Fertility Center in California have shown that antithyroid antibodies can also make in vitro fertilization less successful. Fertility expert, Dr. Geoffrey Sher, says,

> The presence of antithyroid antibodies is associated with a variety of manifestations of poor reproductive performance. These range from infertility, through early miscarriage to prematurity, intrauterine growth retardation, other serious complications of late pregnancy, and even fetal death.

All this information is to underscore how important it is that you be properly monitored and treated for hypothyroidism, and that you are especially prepared before and during pregnancy. Early identification of the pregnancy, frequent testing, and proper treatment throughout pregnancy dramatically reduce the risk that hypothyroidism and thyroid autoimmunity present to both mother and baby, and can help ensure the best chance of a healthy outcome.

∎ Infertility

If you are having difficulty getting pregnant or you are experiencing miscarriages, your physician should do a complete thyroid and autoimmune workup, including TSH, total T4, free T4, total T3, free T3, antithyroid antibodies (thyroglobulin and microsomal antibodies), and antithyroid peroxidase antibodies.

Realistically, you are looking for a TSH level of 2.0 or less in a normal range of 0.3 to 3.0. Unfortunately, most laboratory tests and experts are still working off outdated lab standards that view TSH levels as high as 5.5 or 6.0 as normal. However, these levels have been shown to negatively affect fertility. If you have a TSH above 2.0, you may wish to find a sympathetic and innovative practitioner who is aware of these more recent findings as well as the optimal TSH levels for fertility and pregnancy.

Antibodies/Autoimmunity

Some of the more pioneering medical researchers and fertility specialists understand that even a high-normal TSH and/or the presence of antithyroid antibodies—even in the absence of an elevated TSH or symptoms of hypothyroidism—can be a factor in infertility or early miscarriage. A variety of immunological adjustments need to take place in a pregnant woman, and the existence of underlying autoimmune thyroid problems may set a mechanism in motion that results in a greater incidence of infertility, lower success rates with in vitro fertilization, or more frequent miscarriage.

Many doctors do not appear to know about the link between antibodies and infertility, yet it is published in conventional research journals. The respected journal *Obstetrics and Gynecology* reported that the presence of antithyroid antibodies increases the risk of miscarriage. According to research reported in the *Journal of Clinical Endocrinology and Metabolism*, the risk of miscarriage can be twice as high for women who have antithyroid antibodies.

Researchers have demonstrated that antithyroid antibodies can cause greater difficulty conceiving after in vitro fertilization, regardless of whether there are clinical symptoms of hypothyroidism. Researchers had greater success in achieving successful pregnancies when they gave low doses of heparin (an anti–blood clotting agent) and aspirin and/or intravenous immunoglobulin (IVIG) to women who had antithyroid antibodies. Dr. Geoffrey Sher and colleagues at the Pacific Fertility Center performed this research.

Keep in mind that if you are monitoring your ovulation and cycle, and if you have your thyroid and TSH levels regulated, and you still don't get pregnant after the requisite 6 months to a year, you should probably consult with a fertility specialist for additional treatment and ideas.

Some experts believe that one out of five women with thyroid antibodies will not be correctly identified when standard blood tests are used. For women who have had recurrent pregnancy loss, doctors recommend more sensitive tests such as enzyme-linked immunosorbent assays (ELISAs) or gel agglutination tests. A reproductive endocrinologist with expertise in autoimmune issues can conduct and evaluate these tests.

Low-dose heparin (an anticoagulant) with aspirin, and less commonly with prednisone (a steroid), can help ensure higher pregnancy rates. Another method for dealing with the antibodies is intravenous immunoglobulin (IVIG). A transfusion of antibodies from donors distracts your immune system, so to speak, preventing the antibodies from attacking your developing baby. According to fertility expert Dr. Geoffrey Sher, women with antithyroid antibodies have a higher success rate with in vitro fertilization when they are treated with low doses of heparin and aspirin and/or IVIG.

What You Can Do?

If you are experiencing infertility or recurrent miscarriage, you should insist on having a complete thyroid profile evaluation, including antibodies. Consider pursuing treatment if:

- Your TSH is above 2
- You have borderline low or high free T4
- You have borderline low or high free T3
- You have tested positive for thyroid antibodies

Proper thyroid treatment and optimal TSH levels can raise the likelihood of a successful pregnancy for some women. A number of women have written me to say that after extended periods of what their doctors had diagnosed as infertility, they found my information and finally insisted that their doctors test them for thyroid disease, treat high-normal TSH levels in the presence of antibodies, and/or increase their dosage of thyroid hormone to get their levels down to the TSH range of 1 to 2. And every one of those women is now a mother for the first time!

■ Preparing for Pregnancy

If you are being treated for hypothyroidism, you should take key steps to prepare for your pregnancy.

Know Your Cycles

In my own case, I needed to make sure that all the reproductive basics were covered before I planned to get pregnant, meaning I needed to answer key questions: Was I ovulating? Was my luteal phase long enough? After 20 years of periods every 28 days like clockwork, my periods came every 23 to 26 days once I became hypothyroid, so I didn't know what my cycles were actually telling me.

I started by charting my basal body temperatures in order to monitor fertility signs and ovulation as well as determine my luteal phase. My bible was a book that is absolutely essential for all women, *Taking Charge of Your Fertility,* by Toni Wechsler, MPH. With this book, I learned (for the first time I might add) the real story about the menstrual and hormonal cycles. This book is definitely a far cry from those *Now You're a Woman* pamphlets and films in grade school.

I learned how to use basal temperature and other fertility signs to chart my monthly hormonal cycle. While charting allowed me to estimate ovulation, I also used an over-the-counter ovulation predictor kit available for around $10 at the drugstore to confirm ovulation and to make sure I knew what I was doing with the charting. According to my charts and testing for 3 months, it was obvious I was ovulating and had a long enough luteal phase to sustain pregnancy. That was a good start.

Schedule a Preconception Visit to the Doctor

I had a preconception appointment with the doctor a few months earlier that had resulted in my getting an overdue measles/mumps/rubella booster vaccination and a recommendation to start taking extra folic acid, which helps prevent birth defects if taken prior to and during pregnancy. All women—not just those with a thyroid condition—who are getting ready to conceive should take a folic acid supplement for several months before attempting conception. Studies have shown that numerous birth defects, such as spina bifida, anencephaly, and other neural tube defects, have been linked to low levels of folic acid in pregnant women. Both the Centers for Disease Control and the March of Dimes recommend that women take 400 micrograms (0.4 milligrams) of synthetic folic acid every day. Neural tube defects typically appear in the growing fetus at 4 weeks of age—long before many women even know they're pregnant—which is why you need to start taking folic acid before you even try to get pregnant.

I also started taking a prenatal vitamin at that time. Many doctors prescribe prenatal vitamins with iron to their preconception patients, which is fine for thyroid patients as well as women with no thyroid problems. However, because iron interferes with the absorption of thyroid hormone, you should not take a prenatal vitamin with iron within 3 to 4 hours of your thyroid medication. This allows you to get full absorption of the thyroid hormone without interference from the iron.

Make sure your prenatal vitamin has enough iodine. It is particularly important for thyroid health, and proper iodine intake is even more essential during pregnancy. Until recently, it was assumed that iodine deficiency is not a problem in the United States, Japan, and some European countries, where iodine supplementation programs have been in place for many years. Recently, however, studies have shown that iodine intake has dropped significantly in the United States—for example, 15 percent of women of childbearing age and almost 7 percent of women during pregnancy may be iodine deficient.

Mild iodine deficiency during pregnancy can contribute to hypothyroidism, and significant iodine deficiency during pregnancy— which is seen in some countries that do not have routine iodine supplementation—can cause birth defects and even cretinism in children. The recommended dietary allowance for iodine is 200 milligrams per day during pregnancy and 75 milligrams per day while breastfeeding. A good prenatal vitamin should have enough iodine to avoid deficiency. But if you have cravings for seaweed or seafood, go ahead and indulge them (as long as you avoid the more mercury-toxic fish) because they may be a sign that your body wants more iodine.

Optimize Your TSH Level

What's the best TSH level in order to achieve a successful pregnancy? That's a tough question because different doctors have different answers. Some women may have been told that their TSH level is normal and that they shouldn't have any trouble getting pregnant, yet they suffer years of unexplained infertility or miscarriages. Others may be told not even to attempt conceiving until their thyroid level stabilizes at 1 or 2.

Part of the source of the confusion stems from the definition of normal, and much of it depends on what numbers the laboratory considers high, normal, and low. While it's a relief to get a diagnosis of normal, if you're still feeling sick or still having problems, it's no help at all to you. Insist on getting the exact number and the normal range for your lab. While the new standards indicate that the normal range is 0.3 to 3.0 (with over 3.0 being considered hypothyroid, or underactive, and under 0.3 being hyperthyroid, or overactive), many labs and practitioners are still using outdated lab guidelines, which put normal range at 0.5 to 5.5.

Even within the range of numbers set by labs, individual factors can't be overlooked. Some women might feel absolutely great with a TSH level of 3.0, and may have no difficulties getting and remaining pregnant. Other women with the exact same TSH level may feel sick, in a constant fog, and have trouble conceiving.

When I started doing my preconception workup, my TSH level was 4.1. I was feeling okay—not perfect but pretty well—and thought because I was in the normal range, this would be a good time to finally try to get pregnant. My endocrinologist (a woman with more than 20 years of experience treating women with thyroid problems and thyroid-related infertility) believed firmly that most women do not normalize unless TSH is between 1.0 and 2.0 (considered low by some doctors) and that a woman with evidence of thyroid disease can't get and/or maintain a pregnancy at a TSH higher than 1.0 or 2.0. The new Laboratory Medicine Practice Guidelines indicating a TSH target range of less than 2.0 for pregnant women had yet to be issued by the National Academy of Clinical Biochemistry.

My doctor said there weren't any specific journal papers to back up her own findings, but she'd even been treating fellow physicians suffering from infertility who'd been able to get pregnant once TSH was lowered to the 1.0 to 2.0 level. She said I might be able to get pregnant at my current level, but to sustain a pregnancy would be more difficult. So she upped my dosage of thyroid hormone replacement, targeting the TSH range of 1.0 to 2.0.

Interestingly, there was some research that backed up her opinions on normal levels during early pregnancy. There's a study reported in 1994 in the *Journal of Clinical Endocrinology and Metabolism* that looked at pregnant women with thyroid antibodies and TSH in the normal range. The study found that women with autoimmune thyroid disease had TSH values significantly higher, although still normal, in the first trimester than women with healthy pregnancies used as controls. The higher TSH level of the women with autoimmune thyroid disease was 1.6. The normal TSH level for the control group of pregnant women without autoimmune thyroid disease was 0.9. A TSH of 0.9 is a far cry from the so-called normal TSH levels of 3.0, 4.0, or 5.0 that some doctors feel are no impediment whatsoever to getting or staying pregnant. Within a month of treatment with a slightly increased dose of thyroid hormone replacement, my TSH level was down to 1.2, and I became pregnant a month after this TSH test.

▌ Managing Pregnancy

Once you are pregnant, it's not time to relax because you still need to be your own advocate, staying vigilant and knowledgeable.

Find Out as Early as Possible That You're Pregnant

Try to make sure that you find out you are pregnant as early as possible. One way is to use a home pregnancy test kit. Some kits (I like the E.P.T. kits) are sensitive as early as 10 days postconception, and you don't even have to wait for a missed period in order to get a positive result. The earlier you confirm the pregnancy, the earlier you can start taking the best possible care of yourself, setting up appointments with your practitioners, and ensuring that your hypothyroidism is properly monitored.

I tested positive on a home pregnancy test only 9 days postconception. This is fairly unusual. Some women who are pregnant don't test positive until around 14 days postconception or later. I had a blood test to confirm the pregnancy at my regular doctor's office, and I knew I was officially pregnant at only 3 weeks postconception, which is when I called to schedule my first obstetrician (ob-gyn) appointment. Experts recommend that as soon as you miss that first period, you should have a thyroid test to evaluate thyroid function.

Temporarily Increase Your Thyroid Hormone Dosage on Your Own

If you're pregnant and hypothyroid, you are likely to need an increase in your dose of thyroid hormone replacement, and that need may surface as early as a few weeks after conception, according to research reported in the *New England Journal of Medicine* in 2004. In a study conducted at Brigham and Women's Hospital and Harvard Medical School in Boston, 85 percent of pregnant women with hypothyroidism were found to require an increase in thyroid hormone replacement drug to protect the baby. Babies born to mothers with undertreated hypothyroidism are at increased risk of cognitive problems and stillbirth.

According to Dr. Erik Alexander from the Brigham and Women's Hospital and Harvard Medical School:

Hypothyroidism during pregnancy has been associated with impaired cognitive development and increased fetal mortality. During pregnancy, maternal thyroid hormone requirements increase. Although it is known that women with hypothyroidism should increase their levothyroxine dose during pregnancy, biochemical hypothyroidism occurs in many.

The study found that the increased demand for thyroid hormone was seen as early as the fifth week of gestation, leading the researchers to recommend that women themselves raise their thyroid drug intake immediately upon confirming pregnancy. According to the study authors:

We suggest that women with hypothyroidism be instructed to increase their usual levothyroxine intake by two additional doses each week immediately on confirmation of pregnancy and to contact their health care provider so that a program of test-guided dose adjustments can be instituted.

Have Your First Doctor's Visit Right Away

The first thing you should do if you suspect you're pregnant and/or have a positive pregnancy test is call your doctor's office and push to be seen as early as possible. Some doctors don't like to see pregnant patients until well into the first trimester. This is fine for some women, but as a patient with a thyroid condition it's absolutely vital that you get seen—and start the process of monitoring thyroid hormones and antibody levels—as soon as possible.

The thyroid hormone requirements of hypothyroid women increase by 25 to 50 percent soon after conception. How much of an increase in thyroid drugs you'll need may depend in part on how you became hypothyroid. Typically, women who have had radioactive iodine (RAI) for hyperthyroidism need the greatest increase—a mean increase of 46 percent, according to one study. In Hashimoto's, the mean dose increase is 26 percent. Studies have also shown that up to 25 percent of women who begin pregnancy with a normal TSH level in the first trimester and 37 percent of those with normal TSH levels in the second trimester will require a dosage increase later in the pregnancy.

My ob-gyn wanted to schedule me to come in sometime in the eighth or ninth week. I insisted on scheduling the first visit at 5 weeks postconception. At that time, I also asked for a TSH test. Interestingly, in just the 5 weeks since conception, my TSH had gone up to 3.0, from 1.2. In keeping with my endocrinologist's directions, my dosage was upped slightly, I was retested 2 weeks later, and my TSH returned to around 1.4.

In the first trimester, your baby develops arms, legs, a beating heart, a brain, and an as-yet nonworking but fully formed thyroid gland. He or she needs a steady, appropriate supply of hormones to ensure proper development, and the only place to get it is from you! Otherwise, the baby's development may suffer.

Consider Frequent Testing

In addition to being tested as soon as she confirms the pregnancy, many guidelines say that a pregnant woman with hypothyroidism should have her thyroid function checked at least once during each trimester. Normal TSH but low free T4 can be problematic during pregnancy. According to research presented at the June 2000 Endocrine Society conference, there is increasing evidence that even normal free T4 levels that fall into the lowest 10th percentile during the early stages of pregnancy can be associated with poor infant development.

Low-normal free T4 is not defined as maternal hypothyroidism when TSH is normal, but these outcomes indicate that screening and treatment for thyroid problems may be warranted in all women. The study concluded that women with a low-normal Free T4—in the lowest 10th percentile at 12 weeks gestation—are at risk for having children with developmental delay. Further, the researchers found that "TSH, during early gestation, seems to be without any value to pick up these women at risk." So you may wish to consult with a cutting-edge endocrinologist or thyroid expert who is willing to monitor not only your TSH but your free T4 levels.

After the first trimester, I had my thyroid tested every 2 months or so, and it varied no more than a few tenths of a point, requiring no adjustment in my medication throughout the entire pregnancy. It's never been so stable before or since.

Take Your Thyroid Hormone

Some women wonder if they should continue to take their thyroid hormone during pregnancy because they really don't want to take any drugs that might harm the baby. Over the last few decades, many women have become more aware of the cautions against use of prescription and nonprescription drugs during pregnancy. While these cautions are often warranted, this warning should *never* apply to hypothyroidism.

Your thyroid medication, such as Synthroid, Levoxyl, Levothroid, Armour, Thyrolar, and so on, is safe to take during pregnancy. In fact, you could be doing your baby much more harm—irreparable brain damage, for instance—if you don't take your prescribed thyroid drugs at the levels indicated by your physician. Much like an insulin-dependent diabetic cannot stop taking insulin during pregnancy, a woman who is hypothyroid should not stop taking her thyroid hormone replacement unless specifically directed to do so by her physician.

Thyroid hormone in proper doses is replacing something your body needs in order to maintain a healthy pregnancy. Insufficient thyroid hormone in early pregnancy can increase the risk of miscarriage. Later in pregnancy, it can increase the risk of stillbirth or premature delivery. And throughout the pregnancy, having an elevated TSH level can create a substantially increased risk of negatively affecting your child's psychological development, which may result in substantially lower IQ levels, reduced motor skills, and problems with attention, language, and reading throughout life.

Research reported in the *New England Journal of Medicine* in 1999 demonstrated that women with untreated underactive thyroids during pregnancy are nearly four times more likely to have children with lower IQ scores. Overall, the greatest danger for you and your unborn baby is to think that taking thyroid hormone at the proper dosage is bad for your baby. Thyroid hormone is one of the few drugs in pharmaceutical category A (low risk) for pregnant women. Studies in pregnant women show that there are no adverse effects on the fetus when thyroid medication is taken at the proper dosage.

You need to take your thyroid hormone *properly*. Here is a recap of how to ensure that you are getting maximum benefits from your thyroid medicine:

- Always check the prescription against what you receive and stick to a brand name. Don't allow generic substitutions, because generic versions may not be consistent from refill to refill.
- Most doctors feel that taking thyroid hormone on an empty stomach allows for maximum absorption. If you can, take your thyroid medicine first thing in the morning at least an hour before eating.
- If you start or stop eating high-fiber, get your thyroid rechecked because your diet may change your absorption of thyroid medicines.
- Take vitamins or supplements with iron—including pre-natal vitamins—at least 3 to 4 hours apart from your thyroid hormone. Iron can interfere with thyroid hormone absorption.
- Many pregnant women are told to add more calcium to their diet. Do not take calcium or drink calcium-fortified orange juice at the same time as thyroid hormone. Allow at least 4 hours between taking calcium and your thyroid hormone, so absorption is not affected.
- Many pregnant women take antacids due to heartburn. Don't take antacids within 3 to 4 hours of your thyroid hormone, so absorption is not affected.
- Consistency is vital to your success. If nausea prevents you from taking your pills on an empty stomach, you should take your thyroid pill every day with food rather than miss taking it. You may stabilize at a slightly higher dosage than if you were taking your pill on an empty stomach.

Enjoy the Feeling!

Most people I've talked to who have autoimmune diseases say they've actually felt *better* while pregnant. I agree. Naturally, I had the typical tiredness experienced by most pregnant women, but it was a different feeling—not the bone-numbing fatigue and brain fog I'd had with untreated hypothyroidism, but more of a sleepiness that was relieved by naps and nighttime sleep. My allergies were nearly nonexistent. I didn't get a single cold, flu, or other ailment. I've heard doctors speculate that some women with autoimmune diseases have immune systems that function almost perfectly during pregnancy, and I seemed to be one of them.

Eat Healthily and Don't Gain Too Much Weight

My main pregnancy concern was gaining more weight than I would have liked, which led to a borderline blood sugar problem late in the pregnancy that the doctor said wasn't gestational diabetes but was close to it. I thought that I ate very healthily, but looking back I realize that my diet was very heavy in carbohydrates and fruits.

I think that hypothyroidism's tendency to give some people an exaggerated insulin response and near diabetic blood sugar levels may make some pregnant women with hypothyroidism more susceptible to greater weight gain and borderline or full-blown gestational diabetes. If I had another baby, I would ask for a consult with a nutritionist to devise a low-glycemic diet that would provide sufficient nourishment for my baby and me, but it would balance blood sugar and minimize unnecessary weight gain.

Heading to the Hospital

I have one important tip for hypothyroid mothers-to-be. When you go to the hospital to have your baby, pack your thyroid hormone in your hospital overnight bag. Otherwise, it can be a major hassle to get the hospital to give you thyroid medicine, especially if you take anything besides Synthroid, the thyroid drug most often available.

Delivery

Delivery is not usually any different for a hypothyroid mother. I had an uncomplicated, planned C-section (my baby was completely breech—and hypothyroidism does slightly increase the risk that your baby will have a breech presentation), and my daughter, Julia, was born a healthy 8½ pounds.

What about the Baby?

You may worry that if you are hypothyroid or have an autoimmune disease that your baby will, too. It's rare, but it can happen. However, since thyroid disease typically doesn't appear until the second decade of life, it's not likely to be seen in infants. Congenital hypothyroidism appears in 1 per 4,000 or 5,000 newborns. If thyroid therapy is started during their first 3 months, most of these children will have normal intellectual development. Untreated, however, their hypothyroidism can lead to serious mental and physical impairment. In the United States, all newborns are required to be tested for low T4 levels; the test is typically done along with the heel stick for PKU (phenylketonuria). But you will want to double-check at the hospital or with your baby's pediatrician at his or her first posthospital visit to ensure that the thyroid test was performed.

Management of your thyroid condition after pregnancy, including challenges that some women have breastfeeding when on thyroid hormone replacement, are discussed at length in my book *Living Well with Hypothyroidism.*

PART FIVE

Living Well, Now and into the Future

15

Living Well with Hyperthyroidism: Creating Your Plan for the Future

One of the most important, difficult, confusing, and even controversial parts of dealing with Graves' disease and hyperthyroidism is choosing the right treatment for you. Among Europe's top endocrinologists, 84 percent recommend antithyroid drugs, followed by thyroidectomy (10 percent), and only 6 percent recommend radioactive iodine (RAI). If a first course of antithyroid drugs doesn't work, then 43 percent recommend surgery, 32 percent suggest another course of antithyroid drugs, and only 25 percent recommend RAI.

But the majority of practitioners in the United States push for RAI as the first course of treatment. How can you decide which way to go? The main thing is to understand your options. Many patients want to focus on approaches that allow enough time to see if their thyroid goes into remission on its own. Still others want time to really investigate and choose their approach before making a permanent decision.

Only you can decide which way to proceed, but the most important thing is to be informed and to work with a practitioner to guide you. In choosing your plan, there are probably four paths you can take (excluding surgery).

■ A Complete Alternative/Holistic/Nutritional Approach

This approach is certainly an option, but it needs to be followed with an experienced practitioner who can guide and monitor you. It will require patience and persistence because you aren't likely to get immediate results. You need to deal with symptoms, then explore the root causes of the condition, and work to resolve symptoms using a range of alternative and holistic approaches.

Some people have had success. In particular, Chinese medicine and the Johnson Nutritional Protocol (chapter 10) have anecdotally been reported as successful in some patients.

Pros

On the plus side, with an alternative approach you are recognizing the body's innate ability to heal and you're working on the root causes of the condition. You are not just covering up symptoms or getting rid of the gland—which is really a "kill the messenger" situation. Your thyroid is not your enemy. It's the underlying imbalance that is causing the thyroid to produce too much hormone. So treatment that focuses on identifying the imbalance presents the appealing possibility that you may not only resolve the condition—that is, go into remission—but perhaps even cure it.

You avoid the potential side effects from antithyroid drugs. You avoid permanently disabling a gland that has a critical role in your body. And you can potentially avoid a resulting lifetime of hypothyroidism and its related side effects and conditions. Despite assurances by many doctors, treating hypothyroidism with drugs is not simple. It requires subtle and responsive interaction with the patient to find the right drug and balance for optimal thyroid hormone replacement. Hypothyroidism also brings with it a very real likelihood of substantial weight gain, along with other symptoms that can include fatigue, hair loss, fertility problems, depression, and more.

One-third of patients may simply go into remission on their own. So a holistic approach allows your thyroid to return to normal without any permanent ramifications for you. Jeri is one patient who decided to see if alternative medicine might be the answer for her thyroid problems:

I decided to see a homeopath in September 2003. She changed my diet, took me off wheat, and I started eating a lot more protein to try and up the energy levels. She has treated me with antioxidants, omega-3 capsules, a progesterone cream, a vitamin B multicomplex, and Saint-John's-wort, and some homeopathic drops. It took about 3 months before I started feeling better. I've been feeling great. I still suffer with the anxiety every now and then, but I'm in therapy learning coping techniques. We also had to adjust the drops a few times, mostly to help get rid of the anxiety. I did blood tests in May 2004 and my thyroid is now normal.

Cons

On the downside, managing your condition naturally can take months or years before you achieve the desired results. It requires diligence and patience to pursue an often multifaceted approach. You may need to follow a time-consuming program of Chinese herbs, acupuncture, dietary changes, and stress-reduction techniques to get the results you need.

Also, it's not an option to pursue an all-natural medicine approach when you have severe or rapidly progressing symptoms, particularly when they're life-threatening. You simply may not have the time. In acute hyperthyroidism, where heart rate and blood pressure may be elevated and you are at risk of thyroid storm or vision loss from Graves' ophthalmopathy, medical intervention is needed. You don't have the luxury of the time needed to start off with an alternative or all-natural approach as your only treatment. If you are over 50, this approach can be riskier, since you may be at a far greater risk for atrial fibrillation if you are not aggressively and quickly treating hyperthyroidism.

■ An Integrative (Conventional Plus Alternative) Approach

An integrative approach combines the best of conventional medical treatment with alternative natural and holistic approaches. First, conventional medicines and/or foods/supplements/lifestyle changes are used to slow thyroid hormone production and reduce the initial symptoms of hyperthyroidism. Second, when symptoms are stabilized and treated—and are not life-threatening—longer-term efforts to use alternative and holistic approaches are initiated. Everything from the Johnson Nutritional Protocol to Chinese medicine to herbal treatments to various mind-body approaches may be tried to deal with the underlying causes of the condition, with the goal of curing the thyroid problem or at least reaching long-term remission.

Dr. Richard Shames feels that patients should absolutely consider this integrative approach, despite the push for a permanent treatment such as RAI or surgery:

> *Treatments—like RAI and surgery—that have been proven necessary for mostly the severe cases of hyperthyroidism are now used even for the mildest cases. Patients with no symptoms at all are even getting RAI, simply because they have a low TSH. Alternatives can be explored first in some cases.*

Pros
A natural, alternative medicine approach treats the actual disease, not just the symptoms, with the goal of remission or even a cure. You are not treating your thyroid gland as an enemy—you are

simply dealing with the ramifications of the excess thyroid hormone until you can determine a way to heal the underlying imbalances causing it.

You may be able to avoid permanent measures that disable your thyroid and leave you hypothyroid for life. Combining natural approaches may allow you to take a much smaller dose of prescription antithyroid medications. The greatest risk of serious side effects with antithyroid drugs is at higher doses; they are considered extremely safe at very low doses that many patients use as part of their integrative therapies.

The addition of antithyroid drugs to the mix may help reduce antibody levels and calm down the overactive immune reactions of Graves' disease. Since one-third of those diagnosed as hyperthyroid will have complete remission without any special treatment, this approach leaves open the possibility for remission, since you haven't permanently destroyed or disabled your thyroid.

Jo and her doctor chose not to destroy her thyroid permanently. She went on propylthiouracil (PTU), complemented by lifestyle change, for her hyperthyroidism treatment:

The plan is to get me stable and then continue on that dose for approximately 12 to 18 months, then wean me off the PTU slowly to see if I can achieve remission. If not, then back on the drugs and repeat all over again (and again and again until we get the desired result). As it is my immune system that is at fault, I am reluctant to have any (or all) of my thyroid removed . . . and my doctor agrees with that. We've had lots of discussion about general health and ways that I can add value to the PTU treatment by avoiding stress, stimulants, etc. I'm now quite an expert at recognizing when I'm on the way up and have made quite a few lifestyle changes to try to support my body in getting well again.

Holistic physician Dr. Carol Roberts also believes in using an integrative approach whenever possible for her hyperthyroidism patients:

As a holistic doctor, I like to approach chronic problems like Graves' disease with all the tools I have available to me. That includes herbs, homeopathic remedies (unique to the individual), and Inderal when necessary. The first treatment of conventional medicine is the beta-blocking agent Inderal, or propranolol. This drug can be lifesaving if a patient is in thyroid storm, or hyperthyroid crisis. All depends on the level of severity of the case. If the patient is not hypertensive or having cardiac symptoms, then it may be reasonable to treat with homeopathic remedies (under a qualified homeopath), or acupuncture, or herbal remedies. Obliteration of the thyroid is the very last resort. You can't get back a thyroid that's been burned or cut out. However, reversing disease is a tricky thing and takes great commitment on the part of the patient. Is she really ready to change? Only the patient can answer that. Does she have a mild or acute form, and which therapy is the best for her? She may have to stand up to her allopathic doctors and seek some out-of-the-box answers.

Cons

You must be an informed and empowered patient because you will need to find a practitioner who is willing to work with you medically, understanding that you are also pursuing natural and alternative options—not an easy proposition. You'll also need to find an alternative practitioner who is willing to be your partner in treating your Graves' disease or hyperthyroidism condition. Many practitioners are afraid of working with this condition because it does present life-threatening symptoms in rare cases.

If you are following a nutritional or herbal protocol on your own, you will need to become a bit of a scientist, carefully documenting your responses to various doses of supplements, herbs, foods, and so on. You will also need to go through quite a bit of trial and error with your program of approaches in order to find the right mix that controls or resolves your condition.

This option may not be for you if you have severe, rapidly progressing, or life-threatening symptoms.

■ An Antithyroid Drug Approach

The vast majority of Graves' disease and hyperthyroidism patients in Europe receive long-term antithyroid drug therapy for their condition. As discussed throughout this book, whereas RAI is the first choice in the United States, antithyroid drugs are used everywhere else, with RAI and surgery chosen only in those cases where antithyroid drugs simply aren't working.

Pros

The upside of using antithyroid drug treatment is that it does allow for adjustment up and down to meet the fluctuations in thyroid function that commonly take place in Graves' disease and hyperthyroidism. It also deals with the side effects of the condition without treating the thyroid like an enemy and destroying the gland itself.

The risk of developing side effects from antithyroid medications is very small: usually less than 1 percent have serious side effects, and they are almost always associated with very high doses in the first few weeks of treatment. For patients who are on these drugs over time, there's no evidence that they can't be taken safely for many years, even for a lifetime if necessary.

Antithyroid drugs can help reduce circulating antibody levels, which helps to calm down the immune system and relieve symptoms. Antithyroid treatment also allows the body to go into remission, which again is a possibility in one-third of patients. And, after remission, only 20 percent of Graves' disease patients treated with antithyroid drugs become hypothyroid after 20 years.

When Elizabeth became hyperthyroid, her doctor recommended RAI right away, but she did research and found an endocrinologist who supported her decision for antithyroid drug therapy:

I went on Tapazole and after 2 years tried to go off the drug, but my Graves' returned. Then after another 2 years, I went into remission, and I have been normal for about 3 years. How much of that remission had to do with perimenopause and/or an abatement of stress I will never know. I do know that it is hard to find doctors who are willing to take the alternative route.

According to endocrinologist Dr. Ken Blanchard:

The antithyroid drugs do have potentially serious dermatologic and bone marrow toxicity, but this is uncommon and usually occurs in the first few months of treatment. I have one patient in her late 50s who has elected to continue on Tapazole rather than submit to RAI treatment. As long as people are good pill-takers, this is a viable alternative. Mainly, it keeps the thyroid gland producing a good T4-T3-T2 mixture so that if the overall activity of the gland is controlled, the patient feels fairly well. I am not aware of serious problems with these drugs occurring after years of use. If a patient is limited to a physician who continues to believe that nobody needs T3, it is probably better to have that physician simply juggling antithyroid medications.

Endocrinologist Dr. Ted Friedman also works with antithyroid drugs. He feels that despite some concerns, they are still usually a better option than RAI:

*The advantage of antithyroid medications is that after treat-
ment, L-thyroxine treatment can be avoided in many patients, while the disadvantage is that some patients will
remain hyperthyroid when receiving medications. In contrast, after receiving radioactive iodine, most patients are
cured but require L-thyroxine treatment. Although most patients who become hypothyroid feel well after L-thyroxine
treatment, some patients never feel as well on L-thyroxine as
before treatment.*

Cons

One of the challenges with this treatment in the United States is
finding a doctor willing to work with you who isn't already sold on
the idea that you need an irreversible, permanent treatment such as
RAI or surgery. Many doctors are so steeped in the medical model
of RAI first that it can be a challenge to find one who is less aggressive about permanently disabling your thyroid.

You need to be disciplined about taking your pills regularly and
on time. If you're always forgetting to take medication, this may not
be a good option for you. Some people are also allergic to these
drugs. If you have terrible allergic side effects, you may be unable to
use long-term antithyroid therapy, in which case you may need to
pursue a treatment such as RAI or surgery if you have severe
Graves' disease or hyperthyroidism.

Finally, there is the risk, albeit small, of severe side effects such as
agranulocytosis. Side effects usually occur in the early weeks of
starting a drug in patients on high doses, but in very rare cases
agranulocytosis can be fatal.

▌ Radioactive Iodine (RAI) Treatment

As discussed throughout this book, many doctors in the United States feel strongly that the first-line treatment for Graves' disease and/or hyperthyroidism—even in the mildest, earliest forms—should be radioactive iodine—a permanent, irreversible treatment that almost always leaves you hypothyroid for life. If you are not well informed from the start, you can easily find yourself being shepherded into RAI fairly quickly without knowing your options.

Pros

The positive aspect of radioactive iodine is that it's a noninvasive technique—no surgery is required to permanently disable the thyroid. It effectively deals with hyperthyroidism in the majority of patients, making the thyroid unable to become overactive.

RAI is considered a relatively safe procedure, with a low risk of resulting conditions in the future such as cancer. In life-threatening cases of Graves' disease or hyperthyroidism, RAI is usually an effective and noninvasive treatment when antithyroid drugs simply won't control the condition. Hazel was one patient who decided on RAI, after researching the pros and cons, and considering her own health situation:

> It was not a hard decision for me to make. I was done having children, didn't like the risks of surgery nor the time I would have to be away from my family, and I was allergic to the antithyroid drugs, so I could no longer take them. I was given a larger than normal dose of RAI in order to kill the thyroid in one attempt instead of two or three. It worked! I began Synthroid and was stabilized in 4 months time (much shorter than expected). I was pleased with my RAI experience and easy stabilization on Synthroid. I have had my Synthroid ad-

justed only once. I am now taking two different strengths (alternating), since I fall somewhere between the two. I generally feel good most of the time.

Endocrinologist and author Dr. Ken Blanchard tends to favor RAI, but he has some caveats:

This is my choice in general simply because I know that I can do thyroid replacement in such patients that will truly reproduce normal physiology. This involves giving either pure T3 or thyroid extract in time-release capsules in addition to T4. If the patient is fairly isolated and the physician who will be treating that patient is known to believe nobody needs T3 because T4 turns into T3, they may well want to avoid RAI. The RAI patients fall at the far end of a spectrum in which their total body thyroid economy is running off the medication they are taking, as opposed to a person with an intact thyroid who needs a small amount of supplementation. When the former are treated with 100 percent T4, they often lead a miserable existence. When the latter are given relatively small amounts of T4, they are still producing the natural mixture for the most part and so the infusion of 100 percent T4 does not distort the peripheral T4-T3-T2 metabolism much.

Cons

RAI does not cure Graves' disease; it deactivates the symptom of Graves' disease—the overactive thyroid. Most patients become permanently hypothyroid after RAI, which means exchanging one chronic disease—hyperthyroidism—for another—hypothyroidism. If done early in the course of your condition, as is often the case in the United States, you may also be permanently disabling a thyroid that would have gone into remission in time.

RAI is known to worsen Graves' ophthalmopathy and may trigger an increase in autoimmune activity and antibodies. You may have temporary or permanent salivary gland damage after RAI, especially dry mouth syndrome. There is a very slight increase in your risk of thyroid cancer and ovarian cancer after RAI.

You cannot have RAI under any circumstances while pregnant, since it poses a risk to an unborn baby. If you want to get pregnant, you are cautioned to wait at least 6 months after RAI before you stop using birth control.

In her excellent book *Healing Options*, author and patient advocate Kate Flax summarizes her regrets about having RAI:

> *Even though I was seriously ill with Graves' disease, I was sorry, six months postdiagnosis, that I was seduced by the quick fix, irradiation, which was merely a momentary solution and not a long-term one. I focused on the absence of disease and not on my health and a positive state. I did become less agitated. I also stopped having a period for two months. I suffered mentally, physically, and spiritually before, during and after the radiation. The presuffering was not from my not wanting to forfeit a major gland in my body but feeling there were no other options. My goiter, although described to me by my endocrinologist as "quite small," was growing and I had made my decision out of fear.*

Tammy, a mother in her early thirties, also shares her regrets:

> *The reality of RAI began to seep in . . . no one had told me I couldn't be near my children for a week; no one had said I would lose my hair; no one had prepared me for those gut-wrenching heart palpitations; no one prepared me for what was to come in the weeks and months ahead. The weight gain, the anemia, the psoriasis, the vision changes, the problems with my digestive system, and the never-ending battle with reg-*

*ulating the replacement medication; the problems with my
heart arrhythmia. No one had prepared me for any of the en-
suing events—events that would drive a sane person nuts.*

According to thyroid expert Dr. David Brownstein, RAI should
be the last treatment of choice for Graves' disease:

*All other options should be exhausted before resorting to ra-
dioactive iodine. Radioactive iodine not only injures and destroys thyroid tissue, it injures and destroys any tissues where
iodine binds to, including breast, prostate, ovarian, testicular,
hypothalamic, and pituitary, as well as other glandular tissues. My experience has shown that there are much safer options for treating hyperthyroid symptoms including iodine
therapy, antithyroid medications, and surgery, if needed.*

■ Surgery

Surgical removal of all or part of the thyroid is the last-choice treatment in the United States, but it is the second choice after antithyroid drugs outside the United States.

Pros

The positives of surgery are that it is highly and rapidly effective
at eliminating large goiters, especially those that may interfere with
swallowing or breathing or that are cosmetically unacceptable.
Surgery does not increase the risk of or worsen Graves' ophthalmopathy, making it a safe choice for eye disease patients at any
course of their disease.

Surgery is safe for children and for pregnant women in their second trimester if antithyroid drugs are not controlling their hyperthyroidism. When Graves' disease and hyperthyroidism are severe,

surgery is very effective, with a relapse rate of less than 10 percent, versus as high as 40 percent for RAI in some patients.

In general, surgery is considered quite safe, and complications are rare if the thyroid surgeon is very experienced. Surgery has an almost immediate effect in reducing thyroid levels and resolving hyperthyroidism.

Cons

On the downside, surgery does not cure Graves' disease; it eliminates the gland that was under autoimmune attack.

Even after partial or subtotal thyroidectomy, most patients become permanently hypothyroid. Again, you are exchanging one chronic disease, Graves' disease/hyperthyroidism, for another, hypothyroidism, along with the various risks, symptoms, and side effects of an underactive thyroid.

While surgery is not typically done on a rush basis, if done too early in the course of your condition, you do risk permanently disabling a thyroid that might have gone into remission. Surgery presents a slight risk of parathyroid or nerve damage. There are not many experienced thyroid surgeons in the United States, and your risk of complications will be substantially higher if your surgeon is less experienced.

■ Recap Table

The following table summarizes some of the key considerations in comparing antithyroid drugs, RAI, and surgery:

Question	Antithyroid Drugs	Radioactive Iodine (RAI)	Surgery
How long will it take to see improvements?	2–4 weeks in most patients.	1–2 months for majority, some as long as 4 months.	1–2 weeks in most patients.
How likely is it that you'll have a relapse?	About 60–70%.	20% chance, depending on the dosage of RAI given.	No likelihood with full thyroidectomy, some chance with partial thyroidectomy.
How likely is it that you'll become hypothyroid?	10–15% after 15 years.	Very likely. How quickly depends on dose and other factors. 10–30% during first 2 years; 5% per year thereafter.	100% likelihood, with full thyroidectomy, some chance with partial thyroidectomy.
What are the risks?	Risk of minor side effects: 5%. Risk of major problems: less than 1%. Other dangers of long-term usage are unknown.	Hypothyroidism: 90% within 10 years. Other side effects: less than 1%. Other dangers decades after RAI are unknown.	Hypothyroidism is almost 100% likely. Less than 1% risk from anesthetics, surgery complications, nerve or parathyroid damage, hemorrhage,

(*continued*)

Question	Antithyroid Drugs	Radioactive Iodine (RAI)	Surgery
			swelling if you have an experienced surgeon. More risk with less experienced surgeon.
Safe when pregnant?	Yes— PTU.	Not under any circumstance.	Yes, during 2nd trimester.
Safe while breastfeeding?	Yes— PTU.	No. If breastfeeding, must "pump and dump" until radiation danger passes	Yes.
Safe when planning pregnancy?	Yes— PTU.	No. Wait 6 months after RAI.	Yes.
Safe with severe thyroid eye disease?	Yes.	May worsen eye problems, especially in smokers. Taking steroids before may help.	Yes.
Will this eliminate a very large goiter?	Not likely to.	Higher dose of RAI may eliminate, but can recur.	Yes.

Question	Antithyroid Drugs	Radioactive Iodine (RAI)	Surgery
Safe or appropriate during childhood?	Yes.	Controversial— some say safe, others say potential cancer risk.	Yes, but long-term hypothyroidism may be risk to children.

▮ Other Self-Care Efforts

There are a number of other self-care efforts that can and should be an important part of living well with Graves' disease and hyperthyroidism.

Monitor Remission

Some doctors and patient groups talk about RAI, surgery, or antithyroid drugs as the "cure" for Graves' disease or hyperthyroidism. This is not really true. Hyperthyroidism is a condition in which the thyroid is producing too much thyroid hormone. You can reverse or treat the condition and eliminate the excess thyroid hormone using drugs, RAI, or surgery, but that's not technically a cure.

Graves' disease is an autoimmune condition. Presently, there is no demonstrable medical cure for Graves' or most other autoimmune diseases. When we talk about curing Graves' disease, we are usually talking about long-term remission.

Some estimates indicate that a fourth to a third of all Graves' disease and hyperthyroidism patients go into remission. In remission the thyroid levels are normal—euthyroid—and antithyroid drugs are no longer required to maintain stable thyroid function.

Keep in mind that remission is not a static condition—it's a potentially fluctuating condition. If you do have a remission, you need to be vigilant about monitoring your symptoms and periodically have your thyroid levels checked for life.

Stop Smoking

You know it's bad for you. You know all the negative side effects. And now you know that it worsens Graves' disease, worsens Graves' ophthalmopathy, and increases your risk of relapse. And I'm not speaking as someone who doesn't know how incredibly hard it is to quit. I started smoking at 17 and went through my 20s and into my 30s smoking one to two packs a day. In fact, I blame my thyroid condition in part on the fact that I was such a heavy smoker.

I tried quitting with hypnosis, acupuncture, and stop smoking programs. Nothing worked for me. But after starting to show asthma symptoms and after getting married, I decided I *had* to quit. I worked with a therapist whose focus was on various brain wave patterns of addiction. She hooked me up to a brain wave machine to find out which particular things had the effect of creating alpha (relaxing) waves in me.

The therapist's idea was that people who are addicted to smoking are trying to change an "off" brain chemistry by self-medicating (perhaps not enough serotonin, etc., need the adrenaline). When you stop smoking, the brain goes into a theta pattern—agitated, irritated—and looks for a cigarette to return to alpha relaxation. The therapist wanted to find the other things that can be done to help get that alpha state going.

For some people, it is exercise, but it never had been for me, so I needed something else that worked. We tried a variety of different things—relaxation tapes, Mozart music, whale sounds, biofeedback, and so on. None of them worked until we came to needlework. Yes, crocheting and sewing, of all things, put my brain waves into an alpha pattern right away.

My doctor prescribed a mild tranquilizer, clonazepam, and said to

take one pill when things got truly difficult. I took about five pills total over a 1 month period. In the meantime, I crocheted . . . and crocheted . . . and crocheted, ending up with about six queen-size
granny square afghans in 4 months. I put down my crochet hooks
and haven't crocheted a stitch since—and haven't smoked a puff in
10 years.

There are many resources out there that can help: drugs, nicotine
delivery systems, nutritional supplements, support groups. Try
them all, and keep trying. Ultimately, I think the thing is to find support, and find that thing that helps you get your alpha pattern, then
go at it with a vengeance! Keep quitting until you get good at it!

Minimize Allergies

We know that allergies can become a significant trigger for worsening antibody levels and symptoms in patients with Graves' disease. So it's particularly important that you get good allergy
treatment, take a preventive antihistamine if necessary throughout
pollen and seasonal allergy times, and avoid foods that trigger allergic reactions.

Monitor for Possible Conditions

Be aware that having had Graves' disease/hyperthyroidism, you
are at increased risk of several conditions. Make sure that you are
periodically monitored and/or tested for:

- Ovarian cancer: Periodically ask for a CA-125 test, a
  blood test that can help identify if you're at increased risk
  for ovarian cancer.
- Osteoporosis: You should have periodic bone density testing.
- Heart disease: Since heart disease is more common in thyroid patients, blood work should monitor cardiac risk factors such as cholesterol, triglycerides, and homocysteine

levels. If heart disease is suspected, electrocardiograms, cardiac stress tests, and other tests, may be necessary for diagnosis.

Other Tips

In the course of talking to many people while writing this book, I was reminded of some miscellaneous pointers that can be of help to thyroid patients. When you are hyperthyroid, your symptoms such as increased heart rate and blood pressure can be dramatically worsened by taking anything that has a stimulant. Carefully read the labels on over-the-counter medicines. If the label says not to take if you have thyroid disease, listen! This is a particular concern for over-the-counter cold remedies that contain pseudoephedrine (e.g., Sudafed), which can quickly worsen your thyrotoxic symptoms. Also make sure you consult with your physician before having any numbing medicine such as procaine (Novocain), which may trigger a racing heartbeat.

There is a shortage of endocrinologists in the United States. Thus, it's sometimes very hard to get an appointment. If you have an endocrinologist and are starting antithyroid drug treatment, or you've had RAI or surgery scheduled, talk with the doctor's staff and book monthly appointments as far ahead as you can. This way, you can go in for regular monitoring of your thyroid levels. You may also want to ask the doctor for a number of undated lab slips to order blood work. If you are having symptoms and the doctor can't see you right away, you can go to a nearby lab, have the blood drawn, and have the results sent to your doctor for evaluation.

▌Into The Future

What is in store in the future for Graves' disease and hyperthyroidism treatment? Here is a recap of some of the most important developments.

Thyroid Arterial Embolization

One promising development on the horizon is a technique called thyroid arterial embolization. The blood supply to the thyroid is blocked as a way to disable the thyroid's hormone-producing capabilities. One study looked at thyroid arterial embolization as a treatment for Graves' patients and found that 64 percent of the patients returned to normal thyroid levels during the study period. At the end of a 27-month follow-up period, all but 2 of 24 patients remained in euthyroid remission; the 2 required antithyroid drugs to maintain normal thyroid levels. Overall, the researchers found that thyroid arterial embolization is an effective, minimally invasive, and safe method for the treatment of Graves' disease patients and may help those patients who can't or choose not to follow typical therapies such as oral medication, radioactive iodine, or surgery.

New Surgical Options

A variety of new and innovative surgical options are becoming increasingly available for thyroidectomy. Argonplasma resection avoids some of the common disadvantages of the typical thyroid surgery, including blood loss. An argon plasma coagulation system causes almost no bleeding and provides a very smooth resection line without any jaggedness to the incision. The technique typically results in minimal damage to remaining thyroid tissue, a shortening of the surgical time, and a shorter hospital stay.

Another important technique has been developed in Japan and is known as the laparoscopic breast incision, which results in minimal scarring for patients. It involves a half-inch-diameter incision on the breast of the patient, and the laparoscopic tube is inserted into that incision toward the neck to remove the thyroid. This is in contrast to the typical surgery, which usually leaves a scar of around 3 to 5 inches.

Alternative to Amiodarone

The drug amiodarone that is used to control dangerous heart arrhythmias frequently causes hyperthyroidism. A new drug called dronedarone is being researched. Apparently it is as effective as amiodarone but without serious side effects, particularly on the thyroid. Ask your doctor whether this new drug may be an option for you.

Color Flow Doppler Sonography (CFDS)

Color flow Doppler sonography (CFDS) is becoming an increasingly important way to evaluate the thyroid. Using Doppler color flow sonogram, many thyroid problems can be detected. It's thought that CFDS, a fast, noninvasive imaging procedure, may end up becoming a standard tool in all endocrinology departments for evaluation of hyperthyroid patients. It may replace the need for most radioactive uptake scans for hyperthyroidism diagnosis.

More Research into Causes

Researchers in the United Kingdom have actually discovered how the immune system attacks the thyroid in Graves' disease. Apparently, people with Graves' disease have certain genes that are mistakenly activated. Certain cells, which are programmed to die to prevent the thyroid from becoming too big, become the target of the immune system when they multiply, then don't die as preprogrammed. Researchers suggest that these findings point to possible treatments in the future to control the abnormal genes and even slow down or prevent the development of the disease.

Of course, more research is needed. Some of the topics that should be on the priority list for research include:

- Causes of Graves' disease
- Alternative medicine/nutritional/holistic treatments for Graves' disease and hyperthyroidism

- Long-term risks of radioactive iodine treatment, especially genetic risks, risks to children, risks of cancer, and so on
- Autoimmune process in Graves' disease

As a Graves' disease patient, one of the most important things that you can do is join the American Autoimmune Related Diseases Association (AARDA). AARDA is the only group in the United States that is making an unbiased and independent effort to collectively research and understand autoimmune diseases, looking for the risks, triggers, causes, and mechanisms behind autoimmune disease to ultimately find ways to prevent it, cure it, or fully treat it, rather than simply "manage" it, as is the case in many conditions.

AARDA's focus is to bring about collaboration in autoimmune research education and awareness. In this effort to get researchers to collaborate, as well as to promote education and public awareness about autoimmune diseases, AARDA has led the way. AARDA has also formed a national coalition of autoimmune patient groups, with 18 groups to date belonging to a coordinated, national advocacy effort.

AARDA publishes a helpful quarterly newsletter and sponsors various research efforts and functions. Annual membership for an individual is very affordable, and your support and research dollars go to the only national organization dedicated to autoimmune disease. To join, contact:

American Autoimmune Related Diseases Association
National Office
22100 Gratiot Ave. E.
Detroit, MI 48021
810-776-3900
E-mail: aarda@aol.com
Web site: http://www.aarda.org

■ Success Stories

Susan, a middle-aged Grave's disease patient who has had a successful recovery, shares her thoughts about how to live well:

1. *Take care of your body, mind, and soul. You cannot separate them.*
2. *Listen to your body and react accordingly. Ignoring the problem will not make it go away.*
3. *Never stop searching for the truth. Don't give up. Take control of the situation. If you are not happy with the results and the doctor, move on; find another doctor. Ask for help and advice.*
4. *Talk to as many people as possible about your condition. Somewhere in this world there is a good doctor who will believe in you and help you. Be persistent. Like my friend said, "Be like a dripping tap."*
5. *Read, read, read—knowledge is power and powerful.*
6. *Eat healthy, exercise, and minimize stress factors.*
7. *Once you're diagnosed, it is important to practice positive thinking. Surround yourself with positive people, music, beautiful things, everything that makes you happy and makes you feel relaxed. I have struggled to accept my chronic condition. I take long walks and learned to appreciate what I have and to make the best of what I have. I have learned to take care of myself at all levels and to reach out to those who are less fortunate than I am. It gives me a sense of worthiness. I use my experiences to help other people to get diagnosed. My attitude is: if you don't feel well, find someone else who is not happy and make their day!*
8. *If you want to conquer/control your conditions, become its friend, not its enemy. When you have a bad day, take*

it easy. When you have a good day, take it easy. Don't overdo it. I have learned to slow down and not to dance too fast.

9. *I have learned that you can tell the doctors what to do. It's your life, it's your health, it's your body, and you pay them to do it.*

10. *Don't let the doctor or people decide what's best for you, keep an open mind, look at all your options, then you decide.*

11. *Educate yourself and others about the thyroid/autoimmune diseases and their complications.*

When Esther's symptoms and blood tests indicated hyperthyroidism, she decided that she was not willing to give up or destroy her thyroid gland with RAI:

It seemed too severe as a first intervention. So I began taking Tapazole (25 mg), but because I believe in alternative medicine and the mind-body connection, I did many other things to support my healing. For example, I began weekly acupuncture treatments, also took Chinese herbs, and was placed on a special diet by my acupuncturist. Within 3 months I became hypothyroid and decided to go off the Tapazole and just continue with other alternative strategies. I did counseling to deal with stressful emotional issues, cut back on my workload, read everything I could about the thyroid, spoke with lots of people who had Graves', and became more reflective and spiritual.

For about a year, I was considered subclinically hyperthyroid. I had no symptoms, normal T3 and T4, but almost undetectable TSH. Then I had another stressful experience with a relationship and my T3 and T4 numbers started to rise, so I again began taking Tapazole (15 mg) at my endo's recommendation. I took Tapazole for 13 months, reducing the dosage to 10 mg, while learning how to relax more, be more patient, etc. Last December I took myself off the Tapazole and have been tested every 6–8 weeks since. So far my TSH and T3-T4 are still within the normal range. I have no symptoms and hope to remain in remission. I am fortunate to have an endo that supports my judgments and works with me as a partner. I see him every 8 weeks. I encourage people to use their thyroid condition to look at their lives and make whatever adjustments they can to facilitate their healing.

Wendy is a singer whose thyroid problem had threatened her livelihood, but who is finally living well.

Since my medication levels have been properly adjusted, I have been able to regain my performance levels. My recovery was so complete that in May 2004 I performed an extremely difficult classical solo vocal performance that I simply could not have done a year before. And for me, a major part of the quality of my life rests in music. I feel very blessed that these gifts have been restored to me and for everyone who has helped me along the way. Some days, I even think that my recovery has been a miracle! Just this past week, I received the latest test results, and they have now been stable for 6 months, so I'm not scheduled for another test for a year. I feel great! I continue on a combination T4/T3 regimen, and I feel really well. For the first time, I feel optimistic about the future!

▌ Keep in Touch

I encourage you to write me anytime with thoughts, ideas, comments about the book, or if you want to share your personal story or experiences with Graves' disease and hyperthyroidism. You can reach me by e-mail at mshomon@thyroid-info.com, or regular mail at P.O. Box 565, Kensington, MD 20895-0565.

Our education about thyroid disease doesn't stop here. This book is just one effort in what should be an ongoing search for answers, information, and new developments to help diagnose, treat, and even potentially cure hyperthyroidism. Every day, I review medical journals, news sources, Web sites, and conventional and alternative health resources, looking for information that can be of help to people with thyroid disease. Each month brings new developments in the search for conventional and alternative solutions for thyroid patients—information that can help you continue your efforts to live well with thyroid disease. I feature links to the best of this new information on the Web and summarize important information at my Web site: www.thyroid-info.com.

I also publish key information and news in my newsletter, *Sticking Out Our Necks*. Each issue features the land of advice you've found in this book—knowledge you won't find assembled in one place anywhere else. You'll read about the newest thyroid-related ideas in complementary and alternative medicine. You'll discover exciting new ideas for better diagnosis, treatment, symptom relief, overall health, and empowerment for people with thyroid problems. You'll find more tips that will help you effectively lose weight, stop hair loss, improve fertility, minimize allergies, and much more. Reader questions, stories, and letters will make you feel less alone in your journey on the road to living well with thyroid disease.

A free e-mail newsletter is available online. Sign up at www .thyroid-info.com, or order your print subscription by calling the order processing line toll-free at 888-810-9471.

Appendixes

APPENDIX A

Resources

The following resources can help you in finding the right practitioners and approaches to live well with Graves' disease and hyperthyroidism. If you come across out-of-date information and would like the updated information, please visit my Web site: http://www.thyroid-info.com. You'll find current listings for organizations and their contact information at the site, current Web site addresses, links to online sources where you can get more information about books that are mentioned, and other helpful resources.

New resources of interest to thyroid patients are also featured regularly in my patient newsletter, *Sticking Out Our Necks*.

Sticking Out Our Necks—The Thyroid Patient Newsletter

Sticking Out Our Necks is my newsletter designed to keep thyroid patients up-to-date on important thyroid-related health news—both conventional and alternative—that affects your ability to live well. I scour the health wires, medical journals, and alternative medicine sources in the United States and around the world looking for information that promises better diagnosis, treatment, and symptom relief for people with thyroid problems. Special articles look at the latest information on weight loss with hypothyroidism, up-to-the-minute news on the thyroid drugs and their manufacturers, your inspiring letters and testimonials about the solutions you are finding that help you live well, linkages between thyroid and allergies, thyroid and fertility, and much more.

A unique feature of *Sticking Out Our Necks* is the regular reporting on new developments in complementary and alternative medicine that have promise in dealing with all facets of thyroid disease as well as treatment for unresolved thyroid symptoms. Unlike other patient-oriented newsletters, *Sticking Out Our Necks* has no affiliation with pharmaceutical companies or patient groups. This leaves me free to be honest and up front, telling it like it is about thyroid drugs and treatments and pharmaceutical company politics that have an impact on *your* quality of life. Each issue features eight pages packed full of news and information similar to what you've found in this book—information that helps you live well. Free news highlights from *Sticking Out Our Necks* are available via e-mail and online. Visit my book and newsletter Web site at http://www.thyroid-info.com for more information.

Mary Shomon's Health Information

Mary Shomon's Thyroid-Info Web Site
http://www.thyroid-info.com
A comprehensive site featuring news, articles, interviews, and information on all facets of thyroid disease, including both conventional and alternative approaches to diagnosis and treatment. Not sponsored by any pharmaceutical companies, so you get thousands of pages of unbiased, patient-oriented information from the nation's leading thyroid patient advocate. Find chats, support groups, online forums, and more to help you in your effort to live well with thyroid disease.

Thyroid Top Doctors Directory
http://www.thyroid-info.com/topdrs
A directory of patient-recommended top thyroid practitioners from around the country and the world organized by state and country.

Thyroid Site at About.com
http://thyroid.about.com
Founded and managed by Mary Shomon, the Thyroid Site at About.com features hundreds of links to top sites on the net, a weekly newsletter, support community, and more.

Sticking Out Our Necks Print Newsletter
http://www.thyroid-info.com/subscribe.htm
A bimonthly 12-page print newsletter mailed directly to you that features key thyroid-related conventional and alternative information in an unbiased, patient-oriented format.

Order online, or write or call:
Sticking Out Our Necks/Thyroid-Info
P.O. Box 365
Kensington, MD 20895-0365
888-810-9471

Sticking Out Our Necks E-mail Newsletter
http://www.thyroid-info.com/newsletters.htm

A monthly e-mail newsletter featuring key thyroid-related news, developments, links, interviews, and more. To subscribe, visit the Web site, or e-mail thyroidnews@thyroid-info.com.

Living Well with Hypothyroidism: What Your Doctor Doesn't Tell You . . . That You Need to Know
By Mary J. Shomon
HarperCollins, 2005
http://www.thyroid-info.com/book.htm

There are more than 20 million Americans suffering from the mysterious and frequently undiagnosed symptoms of hypothyroidism—an underactive thyroid. Hypothyroidism affects more people in the United States than diabetes, yet it is far less recognized or understood. Endured by weary patients and ignored by doctors, the common warning signs of hypothyroidism—weight gain, moodiness, fatigue, hair loss, fertility or menstrual problems, muscle aches/pains—are all too often attributed to stress, depression, age, lifestyle, "female problems," or simply dismissed as "all in the patient's head." Even when diagnosed, hypothyroidism is frequently treated improperly, preventing millions from feeling and living well. As a frustrated patient with thyroid disease, I took matters into my own hands and began researching and writing about thyroid problems. The result was my first health book, *Living Well with Hypothyroidism: What Your Doctor Doesn't Tell You . . . That You Need to Know.* The book offers both information and motivation to help you recognize the symptoms, get diagnosed, obtain the right treatments—both conventional and alternative—and understand how to truly live well with hypothyroidism.

The 2005 release is a revised and updated edition of the first edition, which was published in 2000 and became a national bestseller with 20 printings. As in the first edition, I provide detailed information on the warning signs, symptoms, and risk factors for hypothyroidism, along with a checklist you can bring to the doctor. I review and explain a wide range of treatments from conventional to integrative to holistic and share my own struggles, as well as the experiences and advice from thousands of patients and doctors I've encountered.

The new edition of *Living Well with Hypothyroidism* answers questions that often go unanswered and features expanded coverage of:

- Huge controversies over the latest testing, diagnosis, and treatment methods
- Information about thyroid drugs that the drug companies don't want patients to know
- Soy foods, perchlorate exposure, environmental estrogens, and their little understood role in hypothyroidism
- Losing weight despite being hypothyroid
- Hypothyroidism during and after menopause and in seniors
- Infertility, pregnancy, and breastfeeding challenges with hypothyroidism
- Alternative therapies that doctors often don't understand or discuss, including nutrition, herbs, and mind-body approaches
- First-person findings and advice from my recent, exclusive survey of 1,000+ patients
- Advice on treating the hypothyroid child

The Thyroid Diet: Manage Your Metabolism for Lasting Weight Loss
by Mary J. Shomon
HarperCollins, 2004
http://www.GoodMetabolism.com

The Thyroid Diet is the first book to tackle the critical connection between weight gain and thyroid disease, offering a conventional and alternative plan for lasting weight loss. An undiagnosed thyroid condition may contribute to weight gain or may doom diets to failure for as many as 20 million Americans with metabolic slowdown due to a malfunctioning thyroid gland.

The Thyroid Diet, a *New York Times* and Amazon.com bestselling book, helps many previously unsuccessful dieters get diagnosed and treated—and proper thyroid treatment may be all that's needed to successfully lose weight. Even after optimal treatment, however, weight problems plague many thyroid patients. *The Thyroid Diet* identifies the many frustrating impediments to weight loss for those patients and offers conventional and alternative solutions to help. It discusses optimal dietary changes, including how a thyroid sufferer should focus on a low-glycemic, high-fiber, lower-calorie diet, optimal timing of meals for maximum hormonal impact, avoiding thyroid-damaging foods, helpful herbs and supplements, and more. It contains several different eating plans, food lists, and a set of delicious and healthy gourmet recipes.

With handy worksheets to use in weight-loss tracking and a special resource section featuring Web sites, books, and support groups, here is vital help for the millions of thyroid patients dealing with weight problems. The GoodMetabolism.com Web site features the latest diet and weight-loss news of interest to thyroid and autoimmune disease patients, including developments, links, interviews, and more. *A Weight Off My Mind* free e-mail newsletter features the latest news and developments to help you lose weight.

Living Well with Autoimmune Disease: What Your Doctor Doesn't Tell You . . . That You Need to Know

By Mary Shomon
HarperCollins, 2002
http://www.autoimmunebook.com

After numerous printings, *Living Well with Autoimmune Disease* has established itself as the definitive guide to understanding mysterious and often difficult-to-pinpoint autoimmune disorders such as thyroid disease, Hashimoto's thyroiditis, Graves' disease, multiple sclerosis, rheumatoid arthritis, Sjögren's syndrome, lupus, alopecia, irritable bowel syndrome, psoriasis, Raynaud's disease, and many others. This book offers a road map to finding both conventional and alternative diagnosis, treatment, recovery, and in some cases even prevention or cure! *Alternative Medicine* magazine has said, "*Living Well with Autoimmune Disease* should not only prove inspirational for those afflicted with these mysterious conditions, but also offers solid, practical advice for getting your health back on track."

Autoimmune Site/The Autoimmune Report E-mail Newsletter

http://www.autoimmunebook.com

A Web site and monthly e-mail newsletter that review the latest conventional and alternative medical journals to bring you breaking information on autoimmune disease treatments, including new drugs, diets, and supplements.

Living Well with Chronic Fatigue Syndrome and Fibromyalgia:
What Your Doctor Doesn't Tell You . . . That You Need to Know
   By Mary Shomon
   HarperCollins, 2004
   http://www.cfsfibromyalgia.com
   The book and Web site feature an integrative approach to diagnosis and
treatment of chronic fatigue syndrome (CFS) and fibromyalgia—two conditions that are more common in thyroid patients and that share similar
symptoms. While most books promote one particular theory and treatment
approach, *Living Well with Chronic Fatigue Syndrome and Fibromyalgia*
looks at the bigger picture by exploring a myriad of theories and treatment
options from conventional therapies such as medication and vitamins to alternative approaches including yoga and massage. The book and site feature descriptions of risk factors and symptoms as well as a detailed
checklist you can use to aid in self-evaluation and diagnosis with your
physician. *Living Well with Chronic Fatigue Syndrome and Fibromyalgia*
is the first book to provide a comprehensive, personalized plan for those
suffering with CFS and fibromyalgia.

Patient Organizations and Advocacy Groups—North America

Broda Barnes Research Foundation
   P.O. Box 110098
   Trumbull, CT 06611
   Phone: 203-261-2101, Fax: 203-261-3017
   E-mail: info@BrodaBarnes.org
   Web site: http://www.brodabarnes.org
   This organization was founded to advance the theories and approaches
begun by Dr. Broda Barnes during his career. If you're interested in finding
a doctor who applies the Barnes basal metabolism approach to diagnosing
thyroid disease or who works with natural thyroid treatment, you might
want to contact this group. Some people have reported finding excellent,
open-minded doctors through this organization. For a small fee, they'll send
you a package of informational articles and materials, and information on
doctors who practice using their approaches.

Thyroid Foundation of America
    One Longfellow Pl. Ste. 1518
    Boston, MA 02114
    Phone: 800-832-8321, Fax: 617-534-1515
    E-mail: info@allthyroid.org
    Web sites: http://www.allthyroid.org/
    http://www.tsh.org/
This is the main U.S. organization involved in thyroid education and outreach. Primarily run by doctors and medical interests, and funded in part by pharmaceutical companies, this organization stays fairly close to the official party line, but does offer decent conventional introductory information on thyroid disease.

American Foundation of Thyroid Patients
    4322 Douglas Ave.
    Midland, TX 79703
    Phone: 432-694-9966
    E-mail: thyroid@flash.net
    Web site: http://www.thyroidfoundation.org/
A patient founded this thyroid organization, which offers a newsletter and other support.

American Thyroid Patients
    Web sites: http://www.geocities.com/americanthyroidpatients
    http://health.groups.yahoo.com/group/americanthyroidpatients/
National clearinghouse for support groups and a burgeoning advocacy group for patients.

Thyroid Foundation of Canada/La Fondation Canadienne de la Thyroide
    797 Princess St., Ste. 304
    Kingston, ON K7L 1G1
    Phone: 613-544-8364, 800-267-8822 (in Canada), Fax: 613-544-9731
    E-mail: thyroid@limestone.kosone.com
    Web site: http://www.thyroid.ca/
Canada's thyroid education–related organization for patients.

American Autoimmune Related Diseases Association
   22100 Gratiot Ave. E.
   Detroit, MI 48021
   Phone: 810-776-3900
   E-mail: aardal@aol.com
   Web site: http://www.aarda.org/
   Information about more than 50 different autoimmune disorders, including Hashimoto's disease and Graves' disease. This Web site and organization provide general information about autoimmune disorders and profiles of specific diseases.

Professional Thyroid Disease and Endocrinology Organizations

Endocrine Society
   8401 Connecticut Ave., Ste. 900
   Chevy Chase, MD 20815-6817
   Phone: 301-941-0200, Fax: 301-941-0259
   E-mail: endostaff@endo-society.org
   Web site: http://www.endo-society.org/
   Professional organization focusing on endocrine diseases, including thyroid disease, primarily serving practitioners, but it also provides information to thyroid patients.

American Association of Clinical Endocrinologists
   1000 Riverside Ave., Ste. 205
   Jacksonville, FL 32204
   Phone: 904-353-7878, Fax: 904-353-8185
   Web site: http://www.aace.com
   The American Association of Clinical Endocrinologists (AACE) is a professional medical organization devoted to clinical endocrinology. The Web site sponsors an online Specialist Search Page at http://www.aace.com/directory, which allows you to identify AACE members by geographic location, including international options. A unique feature is the ability to select by subspecialty. Again, as a mainstream organization of endocrinologists, expect conventional approaches from these referrals.

Hormone Foundation
   8401 Connecticut Ave., Ste. 900
   Chevy Chase, MD 20815-5817
   Phone: 800-HORMONE
   Web site: http://www.hormone.org
   Fact sheets and information about hormones and hormonal conditions, including thyroid disease.

American Thyroid Association
   6066 Leesburg Pike, Ste. 650
   Falls Church, VA 22041
   Phone: 703-998-8890, Fax: 703-998-8893
   Patient Information: 800-THYROID
   E-mail: admin@thyroid.org
   Web site: http://www.thyroid.org
   Professional organization for practitioners that also provides information to thyroid patients.

Organizations and Advocacy Groups—United Kingdom

ThyroidUK
   32 Darcy Rd.
   St Osyth, Clacton-on-Sea
   Essex CO16 8QF
   United Kingdom
   Web site: http://www.thyroiduk.org/

British Thyroid Foundation
   P.O. Box 97
   Clifford, Wetherby
   West Yorkshire LS23 6XD
   United Kingdom
   Phone: 0113-392-4600
   Web site: http://www.btf-thyroid.org

British Thyroid Association
   http://www.british-thyroid-association.org/

Thyroid Eye Disease (TED)
    Solstice, Sea Rd.
    Winchelsea Beach, East Sussex TN36 4LH
    United Kingdom
    Phone: 01797-222-338
    E-mail: tedassn@eclipse.co.uk
    Web site: http://www.thyroid-fed.org/members/TED.html

Organizations and Advocacy Groups—Other

European Thyroid Association
    E-mail: euro-thyroid-assoc@rh.dk
    Web site: http://www.eurothyroid.com

Thyroid Australia
    P.O. Box 2575
    Fitzroy Delivery Centre
    Victoria 3065
    Australia
    Phone: +61-3-9561-2483, Fax: +61-3-9561-4798
    E-mail: support@thyroid.org.au
    Web site: http://www.thyroid.org.au/

Australian Thyroid Foundation
    P.O. Box 186
    Westmead NSW 2145
    Australia
    Phone: 02-9890-6962 (answering service), Fax: 02-9845-7287
    E-mail: thyroid@icpmr.wsahs.nsw.gov.au
    Web site: http://www.thyroidfoundation.com.au/

Thyreoidea Landsforeningen
    Lis Larsen, Strandkrogen 4 A
    3630 Jægerspris, Denmark
    Phone: 47-53-03-70
    E-mail: lis_l@get2net.dk
    Web site: http://www.thyreoidea.dk/

Schilddrusen Liga Deutschland e.V.
Postfach 800 740 65907
Frankfurt, Germany
Phone: 49-69-31-40-53-76, Fax: 49-69-31-40-53-16
Web site: http://www.thyrolink.com/sf-liga

Associazione Italiana Basedowiani e Tiroidei
c/o Centro Minerva 7
Via Mazzini 43100
Parma, Italy
Phone: 39-521-207771, Fax: 39-521-207771

Schildlierstichting Nederland
Bezoekadres: Postadres: Stationsplein 6
3818 LE Amersfoort
The Netherlands
Phone: 0900-899-88-66, Fax: 073-656-50-64
Web site: http://www.schildklier.nl/

Vastsvenska Patientforeningen for Skoldkortelsjaka
Mejerivalen 8
439 36 Onsala, Sweden
Phone: 46-30-06-39-12, Fax: 46-30-06-39-12

Thyroid Support Groups

Master List of Thyroid Patient Support Groups and Forums
http://www.thyroid-info.com/support
A listing of various support groups and forums, including my own various forums for thyroid patients, weight loss, hormones, and more. Because information changes so frequently for the various boards, groups, and chats, this will have the latest list of support groups.

Thyroid Support Groups—USA
Web site: http://health.groups.yahoo.com/group/Thyroid_Support_Groups-USA/
A place to sign up for local and regional online support groups, and to find out about in-person support groups in your area.

Alt.support.thyroid
  Usenet: alt.support.thyroid
  Web site: http://www.altsupportthyroid.org/
  The Usenet bulletin board for thyroid patients.

National Graves' Disease Foundation
  Box 1969
  Brevard, NC 28712
  Phone: 828-877-5251
  Web site: http://www.ngdf.org/

Thyroid Self-Testing/Order Your Own Thyroid Tests

Biosafe
  Phone: 800-768-8446, ext. 123
  Web site: http://www.thyroid-info.com/tshtest.htm
  Biosafe offers an FDA-approved self-test for TSH that you can do at home. Order the kit, receive it in the mail, use the easy self-test kit to get a finger prick of blood, and mail the kit back in to get results. In addition to TSH, Biosafe offers home test kits for prostate-specific antigen, diabetes, and cholesterol.

HealthCheckUSA
  Phone: 800-929-2044
  Web site: http://www.thyroid-info.com/tshtest.htm
  HealthCheck offers a full range of thyroid tests, including thyroid antibodies testing. You order your own tests, then get the blood work done at a local HealthCheckUSA-affiliated lab. Results are sent to you. In addition to various thyroid tests, HealthCheckUSA offers a large number of other tests, including heart disease testing, hormone panels, allergy testing, cholesterol tests, diabetes and blood sugar tests.

Finding Thyroid and Other Doctors, Verifying Credentials

Thyroid Top Docs Directory
  Web site: http://www.thyroid-info.com/topdrs
  A free state-by-state and international listing of top doctors for thyroid disease founded by Mary Shomon in 1997. Doctors are recommended by thyroid patients, and listings often feature detailed information on why the particular doctor was recommended. Many open-minded holistic doctors

and doctors who work with innovative therapies such as Armour and T3 are included. There are some truly excellent doctors on this list, and many of the practitioners featured in this book were found via the *Thyroid Top Docs Directory*.

Armour Thyroid/Thyrolar—Find a Prescribing Physician Database
Web site: http://www.armourthyroid.com/locate.html
A database of doctors who are open to prescribing Armour and/or Thyrolar.

Broda Barnes—Informational Packet
P.O. Box 110098
Trumbull, CT 06611
Phone: 203-261-2101, Fax: 203-261-3017
E-mail: info@BrodaBarnes.org
Web site: http://www.brodabarnes.org/educational_packets.htm
The informational package includes a listing of holistic referral physicians in your state.

American Association of Clinical Endocrinologists—Find an Endocrinologist Database
Web site: http://www.aace.com/memsearch.php
A source for conventional endocrinologists who are AACE members.

American Thyroid Association—Find a Thyroid Specialist Database
Web site: http://www.thyroid.org/patients/specialists.php3
A source for conventional thyroid doctors who are AACE members.

Thyroid-Cancer.net—Locate a Thyroid Cancer Specialist
Web site: http://www.thyroid-cancer.net/resources/findaspec.php3
A source for conventional thyroid cancer specialists.

Endocrine Surgeons/Membership List
Web site: http://www.endocrinesurgeons.org/members/members.html
A source for endocrine surgeons.

NY Thyroid Center—Surgeon Referrals
Phone: 212-305-0442, Fax: 212-305-0445
E-mail: surgery@columbia.edu
A source for finding conventional thyroid surgeons and specialists.

HealthyNet Find a Practitioner
Web site: http://www.healthy.net/scr/center.asp?centerid=53
Excellent resource for finding alternative, complementary, holistic, and herbal practitioners.

American Osteopathic Association
142 E. Ontario St.
Chicago, IL 60611
Phone: 800-621-1773, 312-202-8000, Fax: 312-202-8200
E-mail: info@aoa-net.org
Web site: http://www.aoa-net.org/
The American Osteopathic Association has state referral lists for osteopaths in all 50 states.

American Board of Medical Specialties "Certified Doctor" Service
Phone: 800-776-2378
Web site: http://www.certifieddoctor.org
This is an online service that allows you to browse for conventional doctors by specialty and locale and get certification info on individual doctors.

American Medical Association (AMA) "Physician Select"
Web site: http://www.ama-assn.org/aps/amahg.htm
The AMA's Physician Select program allows you to browse its database for AMA member doctors who are almost always conventional doctors. It lists medical school and year graduated, residency training, primary practice, secondary practice, major professional activity, and board certification for all doctors who are licensed physicians.

AIM—Administrators in Medicine "DocFinder" Service
Web site: http://www.docboard.org/docfinder.html

American Holistic Health Association
   P.O. Box 17400
   Anaheim, CA 92817-7400
   Phone: 714-779-6152
   E-mail: mail@ahha.org
   Web site: http://www.ahha.org
   The American Holistic Health Association offers an online referral to its holistic doctor members.

American Holistic Medical Association
   12101 Menaul Blvd., N.E., Ste. C
   Albuquerque, NM 87112
   Phone: 505-292-7788, Fax: 505-293-7582
   Web site: http://www.holisticmedicine.org/
   The American Holistic Medical Association publishes a referral directory of member MDs and DOs.

1-800-DOCTORS and Similar Services
   Many areas have telephone-based doctor referral services. For example, 1-800-DOCTORS allows you to call up and obtain information on doctors in your area. You can also find out which conventional doctors in the system match up to your health care program. 1-800-DOCTORS operates in a number of major markets, including Chicago; Washington, D.C.; Dallas/Fort Worth; Denver; Houston; Milwaukee; and Philadelphia; and many cities have similar services. Check your yellow pages.

Hospital Referrals
   If a hospital in your area has a referral service, this can be a decent source of information and referrals to doctors. If the hospital's reputation is good, the doctors typically are going to be of a better caliber. Some of the more sophisticated hospital referral services will offer educational and practice style information about doctors in their databases.

Doctor Ratings
   Find out if any of your local magazines rate doctors. *Washingtonian* magazine, for example, periodically asks doctors to pick other Washington, D.C./Maryland/Virginia–area doctors they'd most recommend in particular specialties and publishes the results. It's always a comfort to me to see a doctor to whom I've been referred appear on this list, although it doesn't always guarantee I'll *like* that doctor!

Best Doctors

Phone: 888-DOCTORS

Web site: http://www.bestdoctors.com

Best Doctors has a Family Doc-Finder at its Web site where for a small fee you can find recommended primary care physicians in your area. You'll find only conventional doctors via this service. Best Doctors also conducts specialized physician searches for rare, catastrophic, or serious illnesses. The specialized search costs $1,500—only called for in the direst situations—but it's worth knowing about if you find yourself seriously in need of a specialist or expert.

Medical Board Charges or Actions

You can find out if disciplinary action has ever been taken against your doctor or if charges are pending against him or her by calling your state medical board. A good list of all medical boards is found at http://www.fsmb.org/members.htm.

Drug Information

RxList

Web site: http://www.rxlist.com

A professional site featuring in-depth information on various drugs.

WebMD Drug Checker

Web site: http://my.webmd.com/medical_information/drug_and_herb

Consumer-oriented information on drugs and herbs.

Thyroid Drug Manufacturers and Web Sites

Tapazole, Levoxyl, and Cytomel

Jones Pharma, Subsidiary of King Pharmaceuticals, Inc.

501 Fifth St.

Bristol, TN 37620

Phone: 888-840-5370

Fax: 866-990-0545

Corporate Web site: http://www.kingpharm.com

Tapazole Web site: http://www.kingpharm.com/product_view.asp?id_product=47

Levoxyl phone info: 866-LEVOXYL (538-6995)

Levoxyl Web site: http://www.levoxyl.com

Tapazole is the brand name for the antithyroid drug methimazole. Levoxyl is a levothyroxine product. Cytomel is liothyronine, the synthetic form of triiodothyronine (T3).

Armour Thyroid, Thyrolar, Levothroid

Forest Pharmaceuticals
Professional Affairs Department
13600 Shoreline Dr.
St. Louis, MO 63045
Phone: 800-678-1605, ext. 7301, Fax: 314-493-7457
E-mail: info@forestpharm.com
Corporate Web site: http://www.forestpharm.com/
Armour Web site: http://www.armourthyroid.com
Thyrolar Web site: http://www.thyrolar.com
Levothroid Web site: http://www.levothroid.com

Armour Thyroid is a natural thyroid hormone replacement product. Thyrolar is the brand name for liotrix, a synthetic T4/T3 levothyroxine/liothyronine combination drug. Levothroid is a levothyroxine drug. (Note: Currently, Armour Thyroid and Thyrolar are not readily available outside the United States. If you are interested in these products in Canada or other countries, start by contacting the Broda Barnes Foundation, see page 364.)

Unithroid

Made by Jerome Stevens Pharmaceuticals
Distributed by Lannett Pharmaceuticals
Phone: 800-325-9994, ext. 4

Unithroid was the first levothyroxine drug approved by the FDA.

Westhroid/Nature-throid

Western Research Laboratories
21602 N. 21st Ave.
Phoenix, AZ 85027
Phone: 877-797-7997
Administrative phone: 623-879-8537, Fax: 623-879-8683
Web site: http://www.westernresearchlaboratories.com/

Westhroid is a cornstarch-bound, natural thyroid hormone product made from desiccated pig thyroid gland. Nature-throid is also made from desiccated pig thyroid gland, but since it is bound with microcrystalline cellulose, it is hypoallergenic. Patients can get a list of doctors in their areas who use these products by contacting the company directly.

Synthroid
Abbott Laboratories
100 Abbott Park Rd.
Abbott Park, IL 60064-3500
Phone: 800-255-5162
E-mail form: https://abbott.com/contact.cfm
Corporate Web site: http://abbott.com
Synthroid Web site: http://www.synthroid.com
Synthroid is the top-selling levothyroxine drug.

Compounding Pharmacies

Some compounding pharmacies that will service mail order prescriptions and have expertise in preparing thyroid drugs, including time-released T3, are listed here.

Village Green
5415 Cedar Lane
Bethesda, MD 20814
Phone: 800-869-9159
Prescriptions: 301-530-1112, Fax: 301-493-4671
E-mail: info@myvillagegreen.com
Web site: http://www.myvillagegreen.com

The Compounder Pharmacy
575 W. Illinois Ave.
Aurora, IL 60506-2956
Phone: 630-859-0333, Fax: 630-859-0114
E-mail: info@theCompounder.com
Web site: http://www.theCompounder.com

Some Helpful Thyroid-Related Web Sites

Thyroid-Info/Thyroid Information Central—http://www.thyroid-info.com
Home page for this book and for my monthly news report, *Sticking Out Our Necks*. You'll find thyroid news and information, personal thyroid stories, and more. The site has hundreds of comprehensive, up-to-date links to the Web's best resources on hypothyroidism, thyroid disease, and health information.

Thyroid Disease at About.com—http://thyroid.about.com
This is my thyroid disease Web site at About.com (formerly the Mining Company) where you'll find dozens of feature articles related to all facets of thyroid disease, in-depth annotated links to hundreds of the Web's best thyroid disease sites, and my popular thyroid bulletin boards and 24-hour-a-day chat room, where you can exchange information and support with other people with thyroid disease.

Thyroid History—http://www.thyroidhistory.net
Edna Kyrie's well-researched, comprehensive site features many articles covering thyroid disease and thyroid research going back to the 1900s.

Endocrineweb—http://www.endocrineweb.com
A large site developed by doctors with more in-depth information on thyroid disease. Conventional focus but good depth of information.

Thyroid Disease Manager—http://www.thyroidmanager.org
Full-length book offering detailed, highly conventional thyroid information with a medical tone and focus, primarily for doctors.

International League of Atomic Women—
http://geocities.com/hotsprings/sauna/9913/
A site for women who have had or who are considering radioactive iodine treatment.

Ithyroid.com—John Johnson's Thyroid Web Site—
http://www.ithyroid.com
Home page for John Johnson, patient advocate and researcher of nutritional protocols for Graves' hyperthyroism.

Elaine Moore's Web Site—http://www.elaine-moore.com/gravesdisease/
Home page for Elaine Moore, Graves' and autoimmune disease patient advocate and author of several excellent books on Graves' disease and Graves' ophthalmopathy.

Alt.support.thyroid—http://www.altsupportthyroid.org/
Patient-oriented information on the full range of thyroid issues.

Dr. Jacob Teitelbaum's Site—http://www.endfatigue.com
Discusses chronic fatigue syndrome, fibromyalgia, and the connection to thyroid problems.

Broda Barnes Research Foundation—http://www.brodabarnes.org
Features information on thyroid and adrenal conditions.

Hormone Foundation—http://www.hormone.org
Good conventional overview information on thyroid and other hormone problems.

American Thyroid Association—http://www.thyroid.org
Good conventional overview information on thyroid and other hormone problems.

Thyroid-Related Books

There are a number of conventional thyroid books written by doctors and health writers, and frankly I'm not even going to list them here at all. I find them sometimes condescending, too similar to each other, and consistent in presenting a narrow, conventional, doctor-oriented—instead of patient-oriented—view. Here are the books I do recommend that can be of help in covering certain aspects of thyroid disease or hypothyroidism.

Overview

Overcoming Thyroid Disorders
By David Brownstein, MD
Good information on holistic and hormonal approaches to thyroid treatment.

The Thyroid Solution: A Mind-Body Program for Beating Depression and Regaining your Emotional and Physical Health
By Ridha Arem, MD
Strongest in its discussion of brain fog, depression, loss of libido, weight gain, anxiety, and the need for T3. Interesting information on the relationship of thyroid disease to brain chemistry, and resulting depression, anxiety disorders, mood disorders, and other mental and emotional effects of hypothyroidism.

Thyroid Balance

By Glenn Rothfeld, MD

Valuable book covering the various issues that cause the thyroid to go out of balance, including some alternative focus.

Thyroid for Dummies

By Alan L. Rubin, MD

If you need a detailed conventional overview book on thyroid disease, this comprehensive book is the one. Note, however, that it is *very* conventional and does not discuss alternative, holistic, or complementary ways of diagnosing and treating thyroid conditions.

Graves'/Hyperthyroidism

Graves' Disease: A Practical Guide

By Elaine Moore and Lisa Moore

Excellent, comprehensive, and well-researched overview of Graves' disease and hyperthyroidism that offers conventional and alternative information on diagnosis and treatment.

Thyroid Eye Disease: Understanding Graves' Ophthalmopathy

By Elaine Moore

Excellent book covering the details of thyroid eye disease (TED) and Graves' ophthalmopathy.

Hypothyroidism

ThyroidPower: Ten Steps to Total Health

By Richard Shames, MD, and Karilee Halo Shames, RN, PhD

Puts some basics of hypothyroidism's causes, tests, diagnosis, and treatments into a 10-step program of information that can help patients get properly diagnosed and treated. Also extra focus on autoimmune disease.

What Your Doctor May Not Tell You about Hypothyroidism

By Kenneth Blanchard, MD

Published in 2004, this interesting and helpful book is by popular Boston-area thyroid expert Kenneth Blanchard, who documents his innovative approach to treating hypothyroidism using a specific combination of T4 and T3 drugs.

Solved: The Riddle of Illness
Stephen Langer, MD, and James F. Scheer

Langer, a follower of Broda Barnes's theories, has written what he calls the follow-up to Barnes's book. It looks at some nutritional and vitamin approaches for hypothyroidism. It still feels like the doctor telling the patient what to do and doesn't address in any depth the problems of getting a diagnosis, dealing with doctors, and dealing with depression. The book is at its best discussing supplements and nutritional approaches that might help hypothyroidism.

Hypothyroidism: The Unsuspected Illness
Broda Otto Barnes, MD

This book, published back in 1982, was written by the now-deceased Dr. Broda Barnes. It is considered the bible for alternative thyroid information and the use of basal body temperature in diagnosis. The book is still in print but not likely to be stocked in bookstores. It is, however, available by special order or at the Web's online bookstores. A fair amount of the information is outdated, but it is the first book to truly acknowledge the wide-ranging impact that the thyroid has on nearly every facet of health. Also, it doesn't talk down to patients or dismiss various health concerns.

Other Thyroid and Hormone Books

The Thyroid Diet
By Mary J. Shomon

Information on how undiagnosed thyroid disease may cause weight problems, how to maximize the ability to lose weight in a thyroid patient, and effective weight-loss approaches, including recommended supplements and recipes.

The Great Thyroid Scandal
By Barry Durrant-Peatfield, MD

Published in the United Kingdom, this book discusses some of the holistic approaches used by popular thyroid expert Dr. Barry Durrant-Peatfield before he stopped his active practice. Interesting discussion on adrenal support. Hones in on problems in the UK health care system.

Your Guide to Metabolic Health
By Drs. Gina Honeyman-Lowe and John C. Lowe
Excellent overview of hypometabolism, including hypothyroidism, and an integrative approach to help treat this multidisciplinary problem.

Iodine: Why You Need It, Why You Can't Live Without It
By David Brownstein, MD
Information on the role of iodine in thyroid disease and other health concerns.

The Hormone Heresy: What Women MUST Know About Their Hormones
By Dr. Sherrill Sellman
Helpful overview of hormones and the controversies surrounding the use of estrogen.

Complementary and Alternative Resources

Acupuncture

American Association of Oriental Medicine
5530 Wisconsin Ave., Ste. 1210
Chevy Chase, MD 20815
Phone: 301-941-1064, 888-500-7999, Fax: 301-986-9313
E-mail: info@aaom.org
Web site: http://www.aaom.org/
AAOM provides referrals to practitioners who are state licensed or certified by various respected certifying organizations. AAOM has an online state-by-state referral search for traditional Chinese medicine and acupuncture practitioners at http://www.aaom.org/referral.html.

National Certification Commission for Acupuncture and Oriental Medicine
11 Canal Center Plaza, Ste. 300
Alexandria, VA 22314
Phone: 703-548-9004, Fax: 703-548-9079
E-mail: info@nccaom.org
Web site: http://www.nccaom.org/

NCCAOM awards the title DiplAc to acupuncture practitioners who pass its certification requirements. You can get a list of diplomates of acupuncture in your state for a small fee.

American Academy of Medical Acupuncture
   4929 Wilshire Blvd., Ste. 428
   Los Angeles, CA 90010
   Phone: 323-937-5514
   E-mail: JDOWDEN@prodigy.net
   AAMA, which provides referrals, requires that its members, who are all physicians, undergo at least 220 hours of continuing medical education in acupuncture.

Accreditation Commission for Acupuncture and Oriental Medicine
   Maryland Trade Center #3
   7501 Greenway Center Dr., Ste. 820
   Greenbelt, MD 20770
   Phone: 301-313-0855, Fax: 301-313-0912
   This organization can verify which American schools of acupuncture and Oriental medicine have reliable reputations.

Acupuncture.com
   Web site: http://www.acupuncture.com
   Acupuncture.com offers a list of licensed acupuncturists by state.

Ayurveda

Maharishi Ayurveda Medical Center
   Phone: 800-248-9050, 800-255-8332, Fax: 719-260-7400
   Provides information on ayurveda as well as referrals to ayurvedic practitioners.

Herbal Medicine

It doesn't hurt to start with a good overview of herbal medicine. I highly recommend the book *Herbal Defense*, by Robyn Landis, with Karta Purkh Singh Khalsa, published in 1997. Landis has a Web site located at http://www.bodyfueling.com with a variety of herbal information. Khalsa's site is located at http://www.kpkhalsa.com.

Herb Research Foundation
 4140 15th St.
 Boulder, CO 80304
 Phone: 303-449-2265 (office), 800-748-2617 (voice mail), Fax: 303-449-7849
 E-mail: rmccaleb@herbs.org
 Web site: http://www.herbs.org/
 More information on herbal support specifically for thyroid function is available, along with memberships in the group.

Nutritional and Vitamin Therapy

Many people read up on the various vitamin therapies and treat themselves using vitamins and minerals. This is a very common form of self-care. If you choose to self-treat, I'd urge you to get a copy of two key books:

Prescription for Nutritional Healing
By James F. Balch, MD, and Phyllis A. Balch

I consider this book the ultimate reference source for information on various natural approaches to disease and health problems. Part One reviews nutrients, food supplements, and herbal supplements. Part Two reviews various disorders and recommended nutritional treatments. Part Three covers other remedies and therapies. Before you buy another vitamin or herb, get a copy of this book.

8 Weeks to Optimum Health
Andrew Weil, MD

Andrew Weil is alternative medicine's current guru and spokesperson. Dr. Weil's book outlines an excellent 8-week, step-by-step guide to building up and nourishing the mind, body, and spirit as well as restoring energy and resilience to the immune system. His recommendations range from adding various supplements to your diet to periodically going on a "news fast." Dr. Weil's suggestions are practical, doable, and surprisingly effective.

You can also see Dr. Weil's Web site, http://www.drweil.com, for an excellent Vitamin Advisor and database.

American Dietetic Association's Nationwide Nutrition Network
Phone: 800-366-1655
 Web database: http://www.eatright.org/Public/index_7684.cfm
 This organization offers referrals to registered dietitians and a searchable online database of registered dietitians.

Naturopathy

American Association of Naturopathic Physicians
 3201 New Mexico Ave. N.W., Ste. 350
 Washington, DC 20016
 Phone: 866-538-2267, 202-895-1392, Fax: 202-274-1992
 E-mail: member.services@Naturopathic.org
 Web site: http://www.naturopathic.org/
 This group offers a referral line, directory, and brochures that explain naturopathic medicine. I believe the fee for this directory is $5.

Manual Healing and Bodywork

National Certification Board for Therapeutic Massage and Bodywork
 8201 Greensboro Dr., Ste. 300
 McLean, VA 22102
 Phone: 800-296-0664, 703-610-9015, Fax: 703-610-9005
 Web site: http://www.ncbtmb.com/
 This organization provides names of bodywork therapists certified by the board.

American Massage Therapy Association
 820 Davis St., Ste. 100
 Evanston, IL 60201-4444
 Phone: 847-864-0123, Fax: 847-864-1178
 Web site: http://www.amtamassage.org
 This group offers only information on massage therapy and referrals to therapists who are members of AMTA.

Associated Bodywork & Massage Professionals
 1271 Sugarbush Dr.
 Evergreen, CO 80439-9766
 Phone: 800-458-2267, 303-674-8478, Fax: 800-667-8260
 E-mail: expectmore@abmp.com
 Web site: www.abmp.com
 This group is a referal source for qualified massage and bodywork practitioners.

Osteopathic Manipulation

American Osteopathic Association
142 E. Ontario St.
Chicago, IL 60611
Phone: 800-621-1773, 312-202-8000, Fax: 312-202-8200
E-mail: info@aoa-net.org
Web site: http://www.aoa-net.org/
The association has state referral lists for all 50 states and can provide additional information on osteopathic medicine.

Mind-Body Therapy

There are so many places you can look for mind-body practitioners— everything from psychotherapists to ministers to yogis to art therapists. Ask friends, check bulletin boards or publications at your local health food store, even local alternative health or alternative newsweeklies, for ideas on how to find a good mind-body therapist. For traditional mental health support, such as a psychologist, a counselor, or general support groups, contact:

National Mental Health Association
2001 N. Beauregard St., 12th Floor
Alexandria, VA 22311
Phone: 703-684-7722 (main switchboard), 800-969-NMHA (6642), TTY: 800-433-5959, Fax: 703-684-5968
Web site: http://www.nmha.org/
Provides referrals to state and regional mental health associations and resources.

National Mental Health Consumers Self-Help Clearinghouse
1211 Chestnut St., Ste. 1207
Philadelphia, PA 19107
Phone: 800-553-4KEY (4539), 215-751-1810, Fax: 215-636-6312
E-mail: info@mhselfhelp.org
Web site: http://www.mhselfhelp.org/
Offers articles and books on consumer-oriented and mental health issues; and a reference file on relevant groups, organizations, and agencies.

Canadian Mental Health Association
    8 King St. E., Ste. 810
    Toronto ON M5C 1B5
    Phone: 416-484-7750, Fax: 416-484-4617
    E-mail: national@cmha.ca
    Web site: webmaster@cmha.ca
    Provides referrals to regional mental health associations and resources.

For other types of referrals, some of these organizations can help:

Center for Mind/Body Medicine
    5225 Connecticut Ave., N.W., Ste. 414
    Washington, DC 20015
    Phone: 202-966-7338
    E-mail: center@cmbm.org
    Web site: http://www.cmbm.org
    A nonprofit educational organization dedicated to reviving the spirit and
transforming the practice of medicine.

American Chronic Pain Association
    P.O. Box 850
    Rocklin, CA 95677
    Phone: 800-533-3231, Fax: 916-632-3208
    E-mail: ACPA@pacbell.net
    Web site: http://www.theacpa.org
    This group manages a list of over 500 support groups internationally
and publishes workbooks and a newsletter.

Center for Attitudinal Healing
    33 Buchanan Dr.
    Sausalito, CA 94965
    Phone: 415-331-6161, Fax: 415-331-4545
    E-mail: Home123@aol.com
    Web sites: http://www.healingcenter.org
    http://www.attitudinalhealing.org
    Support groups throughout the nation for people with chronic or serious
illness.

Wellness Community
919 18th St. N.W., Ste. 54
Washington, DC 20006
Phone: 800-793-WELL, 202-659-9709, Fax: 202-659-9301
E-mail: help@thewellnesscommunity.org
Web site: http://www.thewellnesscommunity.org
Chapters throughout the nation offer support groups for people with chronic or serious illness.

Phylameana lila Désy—Reiki/Healing Expert
Web sites: http//www.spiralvisions.com
http://www.healing.about.com
Excellent resource for information on all facts of mind-body healing and wellness, including Reiki.

The Everything Reiki Book
By Phylameana lila Désy
This book offers an excellent and reader-friendly overview of Reiki, and is appropriate at any level of Reiki interest and knowledge.

Yoga

Yoga in Daily Life Center/US
2402 Mt. Vernon Ave.
Alexandria, VA 22301
Phone: 703-299-8946, Fax: 703-299-9051
E-mail: alexandria@yoga-in-daily-life-usa.com
Web site: http://www.yoga-in-daily-life-usa.com
Offers yoga information and an extensive online book, video/audio, and supplies store. I highly recommend the "Yoga Nidra" relaxation tapes, and I practice yoga at home using the beginner video.

Yoga Journal
2054 University Ave.
Berkeley, CA 94704
Phone: 800-I-DO-YOGA, 510-841-9200, Fax: 510-644-3101
Web site: http://www.yogajournal.com/
This bimonthly magazine also publishes a directory of yoga teachers and organizations. The Web site features an online directory of teachers.

YogaClass
   Web site: http://yogaclass.com/
   YogaClass offers free online yoga, relaxation, and breathing classes presented in RealPlayer video/audio format.

YogaSite's Directory of Yoga Teachers
   Web site: http://www.yogasite.com/teachers.html
   This is a decent online directory of yoga teachers.

General Alternative Medicine Referral Sources

   Here are multidisciplinary national referrals to alternative medicine practitioners.

American College for Advancement in Medicine
   Web site: http://www.acam.org
   This nonprofit medical society dedicated to educating physicians on the latest findings in complementary/alternative medicine has a searchable listing of ACAM physicians at its Web site.

HealthWorld Online's Professional Referral Network
   Web site: http://www.healthy.net/clinic/refer/index.html
   Offers referrals to practitioners of alternative and complementary medicine and integrative health care. Searchable referral databases for a variety of alternative modalities.

American Holistic Health Association
   Web site: http://www.ahha.org/
   This organization offers referrals to a variety of certified holistic practitioners. Go to "Resource and Referral Lists" from the home page.

Well Mind Association
   Phone: 301-774-6617
   Offers national referrals to over 700 alternative practitioners.

Alternative Medicine Content Web sites

Dr. Weil—http://www.drweil.com
   A searchable alternative medicine database, interactive vitamin advisor, and alternative practitioner index make this one of the Web's premier alternative medicine resources.

Alternative Medicine Magazine—http://www.alternativemedicine.com
Full-text archive of this popular, well-done alternative medicine magazine. Features several excellent articles on alternative treatment for hypothyroidism.

HealthWorld Online—http://www.healthy.net/
Home page for extensive information on complementary and alternative medicine options in health care, including excellent database of articles related to hypothyroidism.

Losing Weight with Thyroid Disease
Some recommended weight-loss sites and products include:

Good Metabolism/Thyroid Diet—http://www.goodmetabolism.com
Ediets Online—http://www.ediets.com
Physique Transformation—http://www.physiquetransformation.com
Weight Watchers—http://www.weightwatchers.com/
WebMD—http://my.webmd.com/health_and_wellness/food_nutrition
iVillage Fitness—http://diet.ivillage.com
MEDLINEPlus Weight Loss—http://www.nlm.nih.gov/medlineplus/weight lossdieting.html

Selected books and their Web sites include:

The Thyroid Diet—http://www.goodmetabolism.com
Mastering Leptin—http://www.masteringleptin.com
Fat and Furious/Loree Taylor Jordan—http://www.loreetaylorjordan.com
The Atkins Diet—http://atkins.com
The Zone Diet—http://www.zoneperfect.com/Site/Content/index.asp
The No-Grain Diet—http://www.mercola.com/nograindiet
Fat Flush Diet—http://www.fatflush.com
The South Beach Diet—http://www.southbeachdiet.com
Sugar Busters—http://www.sugarbusters.com
8 Minutes in the Morning—http://www.jorgecruise.com
Fat Tracker Daily Diary—http://www.thefattracker.com

For a detailed list of resources, support groups, diet systems, books, and Web sites, see *The Thyroid Diet: Managing Your Metabolism for Lasting Weight Loss,* by Mary J. Shomon, and visit the book's Web site, at http://www.GoodMetabolism.com.

Depression

These organizations can provide more information, referrals, and support groups for depression.

National Alliance for the Mentally Ill
    Colonial Place Three
    2107 Wilson Blvd., Ste. 300
    Arlington, VA 22201-3042
    Phone: 703-524-7600, Fax: 703-524-9094, TDD: 703-516-7227,
Member Services: 800-950-NAMI
    Web site: http://www.nami.org/

National Depressive and Manic Depressive Association
    730 N. Franklin St., Ste. 501
    Chicago, IL 60610
    Phone: 800-826-DMDA (3632)
    Web site: http://www.ndmda.org/

National Mental Health Association
    2001 N. Beauregard St., 12th Floor
    Alexandria, VA 22311
    Phone: 703-684-7722, 800-969-NMHA (6642), TTY: 800-433-5959,
Fax: 703-684-5968
    Web site: http://www.nmha.org

American Psychological Association (APA) Consumer Help Center
    Phone: 800-964-2000
    Web site: http://helping.apa.org

Pregnancy, Infertility, and Hypothyroidism

Taking Charge of Your Fertility, The Definitive Guide to Natural Birth Control and Pregnancy Achievement
    By Toni Wechsler, MPH
    I consider this book the bible for understanding the menstrual cycle, fertility, and the hormonal fluctuations that women experience. This is the book we all *should* have been handed before we had our first periods.

Sher-Brody Institute for Reproductive Medicine (SBI), Geoffrey Sher, MD
> 6719 Alvarado Rd., Ste. 108
> San Diego, CA 92120
> Phone: 619-265-1800, Fax: 619-265-4055
> E-mail: sbronymd@cts.com

Drs. Sher and Brody are pioneers in the field of infertility in the United States. Sher is author of *In Vitro Fertilization: The A.R.T. of Making Babies.* He has expertise in working with heparin and IVIG treatments for infertility in patients with antithyroid antibodies.

On the Web
> Pregnancy at About.com—http://pregnancy.about.com
> The InterNational Council on Infertility Information Dissemination, Inc.—http://www.inciid.org/
> Immunology/Pregnancy Loss—http://www.inciid.org/immune.html
> Fertility Plus—http://www.fertilityplus.org/

General Conventional Health Information—Central Web Sites

WebMD—http://my.webmd.com
> Well-organized and informative general medical site, including conventional and some alternative information.

Intellihealth—http://www.intellihealth.com
> High-quality, overall medical site sponsored by Johns Hopkins.

Mayo Health O@sis—http://www.mayohealth.org
> High-quality, overall medical/health site sponsored by the Mayo Clinic.

Sympatico HealthyWay—http://www.nt.sympatico.ca/healthyway
> Top-notch Canadian site offering medical information, community, and support on a variety of conditions.

About.com Health—http://home.about.com/health
> Collection of personal expert guide–managed sites on a variety of health topics and medical conditions.

Health/Medical News Web Sites

Medical Breakthroughs—http://www.ivanhoe.com

ScienceDaily: Health & Medicine News—
http://www.sciencedaily.com/news/health_medicine.htm

HealthScout—http://www.healthscout.com

Google Health News—http://news.google.com/news/en/us/health.html

Yahoo Health News—
http://news.yahoo.com/news?tmpl=index&cid=751

Medical Research Web Sites

National Library of Medicine's PubMed—
http://www.ncbi.nhn.nih.gov/PubMed
   This is the Web's premier medical research source, offering an easy searchable database of abstracts and journal references from major medical journals for more than 30 years.

Medscape—http://www.med.scape.com
   While primarily for health professionals, Medscape offers in-depth articles that explore the medical aspects of various issues, usually written in English that consumers can understand.

Journal of the American Medical Association (JAMA)—
http://www.ama-assn.org/public/journals/jama/jamahome.htm
   Key medical journal in the United States.

New England Journal of Medicine (NEJM)—http://www.nejm.org
   Key medical journal in the United States.

British Medical Journal—http://www.bmj.com
   Key medical journal in the United Kingdom. Features full text of many articles. Extensive coverage of hypothyroidism.

Health Magazines and Newsletters

Some of the best health magazines and newsletters for conventional and alternative health news include Dr. Andrew Weil's *Self-Healing* newsletter; *Alternative Medicine* magazine; *Prevention* magazine; *Dr. Julian Whittaker's Newsletter; Townsend Letter; Health* magazine; *Natural Health;* and *Men's Health.*

Key Thyroid Eye Disease/Graves' Ophthalmopathy Centers

Shiley Eye Center/Thyroid Clinic
UCSD Department of Ophthalmology
9500 Gilman Dr.
La Jolla, CA 92093-0946
Phone: 858-534-6290
Web site: http://eyesite.ucsd.edu/
The doctors at Shiley see patients from all over the country, and their clinic accepts most insurance plans.

Cleveland Clinic/Cole Eye Institute
Cleveland Clinic Foundation
9500 Euclid Ave., Mail Code i-20
Cleveland, OH 44195
Phone: 216-444-2020, 800-223-2273, ext. 42020
Web site: http://www.clevelandclinic.org/eye/contact/

Mayo Clinic/Ophthalmology Department
200 First St. S.W.
Rochester, MN 55905
Phone: 507-284-2744 (ophthalmology appointment desk),
507-284-2111 (central office)
Web site: http://www.mayoclinic.org/graves-rst/details.html

Doctors and Practitioners Who Contributed to This Book

Here's a list of many of the practitioners who contributed to this book and how you can contact them.

Kenneth R. Blanchard, PhD, MD
2000 Washington St.
Newton, MA 02462
Phone: 617-527-1810, Fax: 617-965-5524
Web site: http://www.kblanchardmd.com

David Brownstein, MD
4173 Fieldbrook
West Bloomfield, MI 48323
Phone: 248-851-3372
E-mail: info@drbrownstein.com
Web site: http://www.drbrownstein.com

Hyla Cass, MD
1608 Michael Lane
Pacific Palisades, CA 90272
Phone: 310-459-9866, Fax: 310-459-9466
E-mail: thyroid@cassmd.com
Web site: http://www.cassmd.com

David B. Granet, MD
Associate Professor of Clinical Ophthalmology
Director of Abraham Ratner Children's Eye Center
Shiley Eye Center
University of California/San Diego Department of Ophthalmology
9500 Gilman Dr.
La Jolla, CA 92093-0946
Phone: 858-534-6290
Web site: http://eyesite.ucsd.edu/

Theodore Friedman, MD
4727 Wilshire Blvd., Ste. 100
Los Angeles CA 90010
Phone: 310-335-0327
Web site: http://www.goodhormonehealth.com

Gina Honeyman-Lowe, DC
> Center for Metabolic Health
> 1007 Pearl St., Ste. 280
> Boulder, CO 80302
> Phone/Fax: 303-413-9100
> E-mail: MetabolicHealth@aol.com
> Web site: http://www.drlowe.com

Don O. Kikkawa, MD
> Professor of Clinical Ophthalmology
> Chief, Division of Ophthalmic Plastic and Reconstructive Surgery
> Shiley Eye Center
> University of California/San Diego Department of Ophthalmology
> 9500 Gilman Dr.
> La Jolla, CA 92093-0946
> Phone: 858-534-6290
> Web site: http://eyesite.ucsd.edu/

Nadia Krupnikova, MD
> Psychiatrist
> Clinical Assistant Professor of Psychiatry
> George Washington University
> Washington, DC
> Phone: 240-314-0691 (office)

Stephen Langer, MD
> General Preventive Medicine and Clinical Nutrition
> 3031 Telegraph Ave., Ste. 230
> Berkley, CA 94705
> Phone: 510-548-7384

Kate Lemmerman, MD
> Kaplan Clinic
> 5275 Lee Highway, Ste. 200
> Arlington, VA 22207
> Phone: 703-532-4892
> Web site: http://www.kaplanclinic.com

Leah Levi, MD
Clinical Professor, Department of Ophthalmology
Clinical Professor, Department of Neurosciences
Chief, Neuro-ophthalmology
Shiley Eye Center
University of California/San Diego Department of Ophthalmology
9500 Gilman Dr.
La Jolla, CA 92093-0946
Phone: 858-534-6290
Web site: http://eyesite.ucsd.edu/

John C. Lowe, MA, DC
Board Certified: American Academy of Pain Management
Director, Fibromyalgia Research Foundation
c/o Center for Metabolic Health
1007 Pearl St., Ste. 280
Boulder, CO 80302
Phone: 303-413-9100, Fax: 303-604-0773
E-mail: DrLowe@drlowe.com
Web site: http://www.drlowe.com

Joseph Mercola, DO
Optimal Wellness Center
1443 W. Schaumburg Rd.
Schaumburg, IL 60194
Phone: 847-985-1777
Web site: http://www.mercola.com

Carol L. Roberts, MD, ABHM
President-elect, American Holistic Medical Association
Wellness Works
1209 Lakeside Dr.
Brandon, FL 33510
Phone: 813-661-3662, Fax: 813-661-0515
Web site: http://www.wellnessworks.us/

Richard Shames, MD
Karilee Shames, PhD, RN
  Preventive Medicine Center of Marin
  25 Mitchell Blvd., Ste. 8
  San Rafael, CA 94903
  Phone: 866-468-4979, Fax 415-472-7636
  E-mail: ThyroidPower@aol.com
  Web site: http://www.ThyroidPower.com

Brian Sheen
  Executive Director
  Quantum Healing, Yoga and Meditation Center
  12 N.E. 5th Ave.
  Delray Beach, FL 33483
  Phone: 561-272-3733
  Web site: http://www.spiritgrowth.com

Jacob E. Teitelbaum, MD
  Medical Director
  Annapolis Center for Effective CFS/Fibromyalgia Therapies
  466 Forelands Rd.
  Annapolis, MD 21401
  Phone: 410-573-5389, Fax: 410-266-6104
  Web site: http://www.Vitality101.com, http://www.endfatigue.com

Cynthia White
  Aerobic Instructor/Personal Trainer
  Denton, TX
  Phone: 940-440-9130

Kenneth N. Woliner, MD, ABFP
  Holistic Family Medicine, LLC
  2499 Glades Rd., #106A
  Boca Raton, FL 33431
  Phone: 561-620-7779, Fax 561-367-9509
  E-mail: knw6@cornell.edu

Updates

If you have new resources you'd like to recommend for future updates, or if you know of updates to the information in this section, please drop me a line by e-mail at mshomon@thyroid-info.com, or regular mail at P.O. Box 565, Kensington, MD 20895-0565.

APPENDIX B

References

"Radiotherapy in thyroid eye disease: the effect on the field of binocular single vision." *Journal of the American Association for Pediatric Ophthalmology and Strabismus* 2002 April; 6(2): 71–6.

"Subclinical thyroid disease in patients with Parkinson's disease." *Archives of Gerontology and Geriatrics* 2001 November; 33(3): 295–300.

"The aftermath of orbital radiotherapy for Graves' ophthalmopathy." *Ophthalmology* 2002 Nov; 109(11): 2100–2107.

"The effect of methimazole pretreatment on the efficacy of radioactive iodine therapy in Graves' hyperthyroidism: one-year follow-up of a prospective, randomized study." *Journal of Clinical Endocrinology and Metabolism* 2001 August; 86(8): 3488–93.

"Thyroid tests for the clinical biochemist and physician: thyroid autoantibodies (TPOAb, TgAb and TRAb)." *Thyroid* 2003; 13(1): 45–56.

AACE Thyroid Task Force. "American Association of Clinical Endocrinologists Medical Guidelines for Clinical Practice for the Evaluation and Treatment of Hyperthyroidism and Hypothyroidism." *Endocrine Practice* 2002 November/December; 8(6): 457–69.

Abbassy et al. "Ultrasonographic and Doppler study of the thyroid gland in Graves' disease before and after treatment with antithyroid drugs." Endocr Pract 1997; 3(4): 225–230.

Abraham P., et al. "Antithyroid drug regimen for treating Graves' hyperthyroidism." *Cochrane Database of Systematic Reviews* 2004; (2): CD003420.

Ahmad et al. "Objective estimates of the probability of developing hypothyroidism following radioactive iodine treatment of thyrotoxicosis." *European Journal of Endocrinology* 2002 June; 146(6): 767–775.

Alexander, Erik. "High dose 131I therapy for the treatment of hyperthyroidism caused by Graves' disease." *Journal of Clinical Endocrinology and Metabolism* 87(3): 1073–1077.

Altea, M., et. al. "Long term effects of orbital decompression associated with glucocorticoids and radiotherapy in patients with Graves' ophthalmopathy." *Abstracts of the 30th Annual Meeting of the European Thyroid Association,* September 2004, Istanbul, Turkey, http://www.hotthyroidology.com/eta2004/download.php.

Amino N., et al. "Association of seasonal allergic rhinitis is high in Graves' disease and low in painless thyroiditis." *Thyroid* 2003 Aug; 13(8): 811–814.

Anil, C., et al. "Color flow Doppler sonography for etiological diagnosis of hyperthyroidism." *Abstracts of the 30th Annual Meeting of the European Thyroid Association,* September 2004, Istanbul, Turkey, http://www.hotthyroidology.com/eta2004/download.php.

Arem, Ridha. *The Thyroid Solution.* Ballantine Books, New York, 1999.

Atmaca, H., et al. "Thyrotoxic hypokalemic periodic paralysis: report of three cases." *Abstracts of the 30th Annual Meeting of the European Thyroid Association,* September 2004, Istanbul, Turkey, http://www.hotthyroidology.com/eta2004/download.php.

Azizi, F., et al. "Intellectual development and thyroid function in children who were breast-fed by thyrotoxic mothers taking methimazole." *Journal of Pediatric Endocrinology & Metabolism* 2003 Dec; 16(9): 1239–1243.

Balzs, C., et al. "Primary prevention of thyroid associated ophthalmopathy by pentoxifylline (PTX)." *Abstracts of the 30th Annual Meeting of the European Thyroid Association,* September 2004, Istanbul, Turkey, http://www.hotthyroidology.com/eta2004/download.php.

Balzs, C. S., et al. "High-dose intravenous immunoglobulin (IVIG) treatment of patients with post-partum relapsed thyroid associated ophthalmopathy (TAO)." *Endocrine Abstracts* 2002; 4: P95.

Barakate, et al. "Total thyroidectomy is now the preferred option for the surgical management of Graves' disease. *ANZ Journal of Surgery* 2002; 72(5): 321.

Bartalena, L. "Orbital radiotherapy for Graves' ophthalmopathy: Useful or Useless? Safe or Dangerous?" *Journal of Endocrinological Investigation* 2003; 26: 5–16.

Bartalena, L., et al., "Diagnosis and treatment of amiodarone-induced thyrotoxicosis (AIT) in Europe: results of an ETA Survey." *Abstracts of the 30th Annual Meeting of the European Thyroid Association,* September 2004, Istanbul, Turkey, http://www.hotthyroidology.com/eta2004/download.php.

Barton et al. "Influence of pre-treatment factors on outcomes following the use of high fixed dose radioiodine treatment for hyperthyroidism." *Endocrine Abstracts* 3: P277.

Ben-Skowronek, I., et al. "Transfer of Graves' disease following bone marrow transplantation." *Abstracts of the 30th Annual Meeting of the European Thyroid Association,* September 2004, Istanbul, Turkey, http://www.hot thyroidology.com/eta2004/download.php.

Benvenga, Salvatore, et al. "Usefulness of L-carnitine, a naturally occurring peripheral antagonist of thyroid hormone action, in iatrogenic hyperthyroidism: a randomized, double-blind, placebo-controlled clinical trial." *Journal of Clinical Endocrinology and Metabolism* August 2001; 86(8): 3579–94.

Bogazzi, F., et al. "Treatment with lithium prevents serum thyroid hormone increase after thionamide withdrawal and radioiodine (RAI) therapy in patients with Graves' disease." *Abstracts from the Goteborg, Sweden, Meeting, Hot Thyroidology,* European Thyroid Association, 2002.

Bonnema, S. J. "Propylthiouracil before 131I therapy of hyperthyroid diseases: effect on cure rate evaluated by a randomized clinical trial." *Journal of Clinical Endocrinology and Metabolism* 2004; 89(9): 4439–4444.

Bonnema et al. "Controversies in radioiodine therapy: the relation to ophthalmopathy, the possible radioprotective effect of antithyroid drugs and the use in large goitres." *European Journal of Endocrinology* 2002; 46(1): 1–11.

Brownstein, David, MD. *Overcoming Arthritis.* Medical Alternatives Press, Inc. West Bloomfield, MI. 2001.

Brunova, Jana, et al. "Hyperthyroidism therapy and weight gain." *Abstracts of the 84th Annual Meeting of the Endocrine Society,* June 2002.

Bryan McIver et al. "Lack of effect of thyroxine in patients with Graves' hyperthyroidism who are treated with an antithyroid drug." *New England Journal of Medicine* 1996 January 25; 334(4): 220–224.

Carella, C., et al. "Second generation TRAB assay in Graves' disease: different criteria of evaluation before and after a full course of methimazole treatment." *Abstracts of the 30th Annual Meeting of the European Thyroid Association,* September 2004, Istanbul, Turkey, http://www.hotthyroidology. com/eta2004/download.php.

Caron, P. J., et al. Three-month octreotide-LAR treatment in patients with Graves' orbitopathy: clinical results of a randomized, placebo-controlled, double-blind study." *Abstracts of the 30th Annual Meeting of the European Thyroid Association,* September 2004, Istanbul, Turkey, http://www.hot thyroidology.com/eta2004/download.php.

Ceccarelli, C., et al. "Spermatogenesis is impaired in hyperthyroidism." *Abstracts from the Goteborg, Sweden, Meeting, Hot Thyroidology,* European Thyroid Association, 2002.

Chen, Y. T., and Khoo, D. H. "Thyroid diseases in pregnancy." *Annals of the Academy of Medicine, Singapore* 2002 May; 31(3): 296–302.

Chikh, I., et al. "Compare radioiodine and surgical treatment efficacy of Graves' disease." *Abstracts of the 30th Annual Meeting of the European Thyroid Association,* September 2004, Istanbul, Turkey, http://www.hot thyroidology.com/eta2004/download.php.

Clark, J. D., et al. "Iodine-131 therapy of hyperthyroidism in pediatric patients." *Journal of Nuclear Medicine* 1995 March; 36(3): 442–445.

Cooper, David S. "Antithyroid drugs in the management of patients with Graves' disease: an evidence-based approach to therapeutic controversies." *Journal of Clinical Endocrinology and Metabolism* 2003; 88(8): 3474–3481.

Corapcioglu, D., et al. "Relationship between thyroid autoimmunity and *Yersinia enterocolitica* antibodies." *Thyroid* 2002 July; 12(7): 613–617.

Coulam, Carolyn B., and Hemenway, Nancy P. "Immunology may be key to pregnancy loss." InterNational Council on Infertility Information Dissemination, Inc., http://www.inciid.org, 1999.

Dale, J., et al. "Weight gain following treatment of hyperthyroidism." *Clinical Endocrinology.* 2001 August; 55(2): 233–239.

De Groot, Leslie. *Thyroid Disease Manager.* Online book, http://www.thyroid manager.org/.

Dereli, D., et al. "Orbital Gallium-67 scintigraphy in Graves' Ophthalmopathy." *Abstracts of the 30th Annual Meeting of the European Thyroid Association,* September 2004, Istanbul, Turkey, http://www.hotthyroidology. com/eta2004/download.php.

de Ronde, W., et al. " 'Hungry bone' syndrome, characterized by prolonged symptomatic hypocalcemia, as a complication of the treatment for hyperthyroidism." *Nederlands Fijdschrift Voor Geneeskunde* 2004 January 31; 148(5): 231–234.

Desy, Phylameana lila. *The Everything Reiki Book: Channel Your Positive Energy to Reduce Stress, Promote Healing, and Enhance Your Quality of Life.* Adams, MA, 2004.

Di Lelio, A., et al. "Treatment of autonomous thyroid nodules: value of percutaneous ethanol injection." *American Journal of Roentgerology* 1995 January; 164(1): 207–213.

Ditkoff, Beth Ann, and Lo Gerfo, Paul. *The Thyroid Guide.* HarperPerennial, New York, 2000.

Dralle, H., et al. "Morbidity after subtotal and total thyroidectomy in patients with Graves' disease: the basis for decision-making regarding surgical indication and extent of resection." *Zeitschrift fur arztliche Fortbildung und Qualitatssicherung* 2004 May; 98 (Suppl 5): 45–53.

Erbagci, I., et al. "Comparison of the intravenous methylprednisolone pulse therapy versus oral prednisone in patients with Graves' ophthalmopathy." *Abstracts of the 30th Annual Meeting of the European Thyroid Association,* September 2004, Istanbul, Turkey, http://www.hotthyroidology.com/eta2004/download.php.

Ertirer, M. E., et al. "Only thyroid volume seems to affect the time to achieve euthyroidism in hyperthyroid patients treated by radioiodine." *Abstracts of the 30th Annual Meeting of the European Thyroid Association,* September 2004, Istanbul, Turkey, http://www.hotthyroidology.com/eta2004/download.php.

Evans et al. "Thyroid peroxidase antibodies are not a surrogate for thyroid stimulating antibodies in the investigation of the etiology of thyrotoxicosis." *Endocrine Abstracts* 3 P294, 2003.

Fisher, Joseph. "Management of thyrotoxicosis." *Southern Medicine J* 2002; 95(5): 493–505.

Flax, Kate. *Healing Options: A Report on Graves' Disease Treatments.* Sally Breer, New York, 1998.

Floyd, John. "Thyrotoxicosis." Emedicine.com, June 21, 2002.

Ford, Gillian. *Listening to Your Hormones.* Prima Lifestyles, New York, 1997.

Friedman, Ted, MD. Various personal interviews. 2004.

Gaby, Alan "L-carnitine for hyperthyroidism—literature review and commentary." *Townsend Letter for Doctors and Patients,* October 2003.

Georgala, S., et al., "Pretibial myxedema as the initial manifestation of Graves' disease." *Journal of the European Academy of Dermatology and Venereology* July 2002; 16(4): 380.

George, Jake, and Patterson, Nancy. *Graves' Disease: In Our Own Words.* Blue Note Publications, Florida, 2002.

Glaser, Nicole, et. al. "Pediatric endocrinology: predictors of early remission of hyperthyroidism in children." *Journal of Clinical Endocrinology and Metabolism* 1997; 82(6): 1719–1726.

Glinoer, Daniel. "Thyroid regulation and dysfunction in the pregnant patient." Thyroid Manager, 2003, http://www.thyroidmanager.org/Chapter14/14-text.htm.

Gold, Jonathan. "Hyperthyroidism." Emedicine.com, May 26, 2004.

Goletti, O., Monzani, F., Lenziardi, M., et al. "Cold thyroid nodules: a new application of percutaneous ethanol injection treatment." *Journal of Clinical Ultrasound* 1994 March–April; 22(3): 175–178.

Gorman, C. A., Garrity, J. A., et al. "The aftermath of orbital radiotherapy for Graves' ophthalmopathy." *Ophthalmology* 2002 November; 109(11): 2100–2107.

Gotsch, Gwen. *The Womanly Art of Breastfeeding*. Torgus Publisher, Plume, NY, 1997.

Gruters, A. "Characteristic features of autoimmune thyroid disease in children." *Zeitschrift fur arzliche Fortbildung und Qualitatssicherung* 2004 May; 98 (Suppl 5): 67–71.

Guvener, N.D., et al. "Thyroid cancer in patients with hyperthyroidism." *Abstracts of the 30th Annual Meeting of the European Thyroid Association*, September 2004, Istanbul, Turkey, http://www.hotthyroidology.com/eta2004/download.php.

Habra, Mouhammed Amir, et al. "Medullary thyroid carcinoma associated with hyperthyroidism: a case report and review of the literature." *Thyroid* 2004; 14(5): 391–396.

Hashizume, K., et al. "Administration of thyroxine in treated Graves' disease. Effects on the level of antibodies to thyroid-stimulating hormone receptors and on the risk of recurrence of hyperthyroidism." April 4, 1991; 324(14): 947–953.

Hermida, J.S., et al. "Prevention of recurrent amiodarone-induced hyperthyroidism by iodine." *Arch Mal Coeur Vaiss* 2004 Mar; 97(3): 207–213.

Homsanit, M. et al., "Efficacy of single daily dosage of methimazole vs. propylthiouracil in the induction of euthyroidism." *Clinical Endocrinology* 2001 54(3): 385–390.

Huggins, Kathleen. *The Nursing Mother's Companion*, Harvard Common Press. Boston. 1999.

Hull, Janet. *Sweet Poison: How the World's Most Popular Artificial Sweetener Is Killing Us—My Story*. New Horizon Press. 2001.

Jayapaul, M., et al. "Recurrent painful unilateral gynaecomastia with relapsing hyperthyroidism." *Endocrine Abstracts* 2003; 6: OC3.

Kermani, Asra. "Toxic nodular goiter." Emedicine.com, May 23, 2002.

Kikkawa, D.O., et al. "Graded orbital decompression based on severity of proptosis." *Ophthalmology* 2002 July; 109(7): 1219–1224.

Krassas, G., et al. "Short-term body weight and body composition changes in hyper- and hypothyroid patients immediately after reaching euthyroidism." *Abstracts of the 30th Annual Meeting of the European Thyroid Association*, September 2004, Istanbul, Turkey, http://www.hotthyroidology.com/eta2004/download.php.

Krassas, G.E., et. al. "A prospective controlled study of the impact of hyperthyroidism on reproductive function in males." *Abstracts from the Goteborg, Sweden, Meeting, Hot Thyroidology*, European Thyroid Association, 2002.

Kvetny, J., et al. "Subclinical hyperthyroidism represents a condition with increased atherothrombotic risk." *Abstracts of the 30th Annual Meeting of the European Thyroid Association*, September 2004, Istanbul, Turkey, http://www.hotthyroidology.com/eta2004/download.php

Langer, Stephen. *Solved: The Riddle of Illness*. McGraw-Hill, Lincolnwood, IL., 2000.

Lee, Stephanie. "Hyperthyroidism." Emedicine.com, March 3, 2004.

Levin, Jeff. *God, Faith, and Health: Exploring the Spirituality-Healing Connection*. Wiley. New York. 2002.

Li, X. M., et al. "Clinical observation on xiehuo yangyin powder in treating 30 initial stage of toxic and diffuse goiter patients." *Zhongguo Zhong Xi Yi Jie He Za Zhi* 2003 November; 23(11): 829–831.

Lingvay, Ildiko. "De Quervain thyroiditis." Emedicine.com, January 7, 2002.

Livraghi, T., et al. "Treatment of autonomous thyroid nodules with percutaneous ethanol injection: preliminary results." *Radiology* 1994; 175: 827–829.

Lucas, A., et al. "Medical therapy of Graves' disease: does thyroxine prevent recurrence of hyperthyroidism?" *J Clin Endocrinol Metab* 1997 August; 82(8): 2410–2413.

Lumera, G., et al. "Unilateral Graves' orbitopathy: a case-control and retrospective follow-up study." *Abstracts of the 30th Annual Meeting of the European Thyroid Association*, September 2004, Istanbul, Turkey, http://www.hotthyroidology.com/eta2004/download.php.

Mandel, S. J., et al. "Radioactive iodine and the salivary glands." *PubMed 1: Thyroid* 2003 March; 13(3): 265–271.

Manifold, Craig. "Hyperthyroidism, thyroid storm, and Graves' disease." Emedicine.com, July 25, 2002.

Massart, C., et al. "A Clinical and biological model predictive of relapse after antithyroid drug treatment in patients with Graves' disease." *Abstracts of the 30th Annual Meeting of the European Thyroid Association,* September 2004, Istanbul, Turkey, http://www.hotthyroidology.com/eta2004/download.php.

Matawaran, Bien J., et al. "Obese hyperthyroidism among Filipino patients." *Abstracts of the 84th Annual Meeting of the Endocrine Society*, June 2002.

Menconi, F., et al. "Liver enzyme alterations in patients with Graves' ophthalmopthy treated with intravenous glucocorticoids: frequency and putative risk factors." *Abstracts of the 30th Annual Meeting of the European Thyroid Association*, September 2004, Istanbul, Turkey, http://www.hotthyroidology.com/eta2004/download.php.

Mestman, Jorge H. "Perinatal thyroid dysfunction: prenatal diagnosis and treatment." *Medscape Women's Health eJournal* 1997; 2(4).

Mladenova, G. G., et al. "Relationship of stressful life events and psychological disturbances to Graves' disease in children and adolescents." *Abstracts of the 30th Annual Meeting of the European Thyroid Association*, September 2004, Istanbul, Turkey, http://www.hotthyroidology.com/eta2004/download.php.

Moore, Elaine A. *Thyroid Eye Disease: Understanding Graves' Ophthalmopathy*. SaraHealthPress/Trafford Publishing, Canada, 2003.

Moore, Elaine A., with Lisa Moore. *Graves' Disease: A Praactical Guide*. McFarland & Company, Inc., North Carolina, 2001.

Murphy, E., et al. "The use of lithium as an adjunct to radioiodine therapy for thyrotoxicosis." *Endocrine Abstracts* 3 P303, http://www.endocrine-abstracts.org/ea/0003/ea0003p303.htm, 2003.

Nedreb, et al. "Predictors of outcome and comparison of different drug regimens for the prevention of relapse in patients with Graves' disease." *European Journal of Endocrinology* 2002 Nov; 147(5): 583–9.

Nedrebo, Bjorn G., et al. "Graves' disease: drug regimens and predictors outcome." *Abstracts of the 84th Annual Meeting of the Endocrine Society*, June 2002.

Nenkov, R. N., et al. "Argon plasma resection in thyroid surgery—practical applications, indications and advantages." *Abstracts of the 30th Annual Meeting of the European Thyroid Association*, September 2004, Istanbul, Turkey, http://www.hotthyroidology.com/eta2004/download.php.

Newman, Jack. *The Ultimate Breastfeeding Book of Answers: The Most Comprehensive Problem-Solution Guide to Breastfeeding from the Foremost Expert in North America*. Prima Publishing, Roseville, CA, 2000.

Nguyen, Phuong. "Autoimmune thyroid disease and pregnancy." Emedicine.com, April 9, 2002.

Osman, F., et al. "Atrial fibrillation predicts mortality in thyrotoxicosis." *Endocrine Abstracts, 21st Joint Meeting of the British Endocrine Societies*, April 8–11, 2002.

Panzer, C. "Rapid preoperative preparation for severe hyperthyroid Graves' disease." *Journal of Clinical Endocrinology and Metabolism* 2004 May; 89(5): 2142–2144.

Papadopoulou, F., et al. "Bone mineral density in patients with hyperthyroidism before and 5 years after the initiation of treatment." *Abstracts of the 30th Annual Meeting of the European Thyroid Association*, September 2004, Istanbul, Turkey, http://www.hotthyroidology.com/eta2004/download.php.

Parmar, M. S., et al. "Recurrent hamburger thyrotoxicosis," *Canadian Medical Association Journal* 2003 September 2; 169(5): 415–417.

Pijl, H., et al. "Food choice in hyperthyroidism: potential influence of the autonomic nervous system and brain serotonin precursor availability." *Journal of Clinical Endocrinology and Metabolism* 2001; 86(12): 5848–5853.

Pohl, P.P., et al. "Hypocalcaemic syndrome after Graves' disease surgery—complication or physiologic response." *Abstracts of the 30th Annual Meeting of the European Thyroid Association,* September 2004, Istanbul, Turkey, http://www.hotthyroidology.com/eta2004/download.php.

Porapioglu, D., et al. "Determination of the effect of propylthiouracil to radioiodine therapy in Graves' disease." *Abstracts of the 30th Annual Meeting of the European Thyroid Association,* September 2004, Istanbul, Turkey, http://www.hotthyroidology.com/eta2004/download.php.

Power, M.L., et al. "Diagnosing and managing thyroid disorders during pregnancy: a survey of obstetrician-gynecologists." *Obstet Gynecol Surv* 2004 August; 59(8): 572–574.

Qureshi, Mohammad N., et al. "Unusual case of recurrent thyrotoxic periodic paralysis caused by dietary potassium deficiency." *Abstracts of the 84th Annual Meeting of the Endocrine Society,* June 2002.

Raza, J., et al. "Thyrotoxicosis in children: thirty years' experience." *Acta Paediatrica* 1999 September; 88(9): 937–941.

Razvi, S., et al. "Low failure rate of fixed administered activity of 400 MBq 131I with pretreatment with carbimazole for thyrotoxicosis: the Gateshead Protocol." *Nuclear Medicine Communications* 2004 July; 25(7): 675–682.

Richards, Byron. *Mastering Leptin: The Leptin Diet, Solving Obesity and Preventing Disease, Second Edition.* Wellness Resources Book. Minneapolis. 2002.

Ringold et al. "Further evidence for a strong genetic influence on the development of autoimmune thyroid disease: the California twin study." *Thyroid* 2002 August; 12(8): 647–653.

Rivkees, Scott. "Editorial: radioactive iodine use in childhood Graves' disease: time to wake up and smell the I-131." *Journal of Clinical Endocrinology and Metabolism* 2004; 89(9): 4227–4228.

Roberts, H.J. "Aspartame disease: a possible cause for concomitant Graves' disease and pulmonary hypertension." *Texas Heart Institute Journal* 2004; 31(1): 105.

Roberts, H.J. "Aspartame and hyperthyroidism: a presidential affliction reconsidered." *Townsend Letter for Doctors & Patients* 1997 May; 86–8.

Rothfeld, Glenn, and Romaine, Deborah. *Thyroid Balance.* Adams Media, Avon, Mass.; 2003.

Rubin, Alan. *Thyroid for Dummies.* Hungry Minds, New York, 2001.

Santos, R. B., et al. "Propylthiouracil reduces the effectiveness of radioiodine treatment in hyperthyroid patients with Graves' disease. *Thyroid* 2004 July; 14(7): 525–530.

Segni, M., et al. "Special features of Graves' disease in early childhood." *Thyroid* 1999 September; 9(9): 871–877.

Seshadri, Krishna G. "Subacute thyroiditis." Emedicine.com, February 19, 2002.

Shames, Richard. Various personal interviews. 2004.

Shames, Richard and Karilee. *Thyroid Power: Ten Steps to Total Health.* HarperResource, New York, 2002.

Shomon, Mary J. *Living Well with Chronic Fatigue Syndrome and Fibromyalgia.* HarperCollins, New York, 2004.

Shomon, Mary J. *The Thyroid Diet: Manage Your Metablolism for Lasting Weight Loss.* HarperCollins, New York, 2004.

Simescu, M., et al. "Results of treatment with methotrexate (MT) and methotrexate combined with corticosteroid (C) on severe and moderate Graves' ophthalmopathy (GO)." *Abstracts of the 30th Annual Meeting of the European Thyroid Association,* September 2004, Istanbul, Turkey, http://www.hotthyroidology.com/eta2004/download.php.

Simonton, O. Carl. *Getting Well Again.* Bantam, New York, 1978.

Suher, M., et al. "Graves' disease in a renal transplant recipient." *Abstracts of the 30th Annual Meeting of the European Thyroid Association,* September 2004, Istanbul, Turkey, http://www.hotthyroidology.com/eta2004/download.php.

Susman, Ed. "ESC: less toxic drug controls atrial fibrillation: dronedarone could replace amiodarone, which has side-effects on other organs." *Medical Post* 2004 September 21; 40(35).

Swiatkiewicz, J., et al. "Neuromonitoring of the recurrent laryngeal nerve during thyroidectomy." *Abstracts of the 30th Annual Meeting of the European Thyroid Association,* September 2004, Istanbul, Turkey, http://www.hot thyroidology.com/eta2004/download.php.

Tada, H., et al. "Blocking-type anti-TSH receptor antibodies and relation to responsiveness to antithyroid drug therapy and remission in Graves' disease." *Clinical Endocrinology* 2003 April; 58(4): 403–408.

Terwee, et al. "Long-term effects of Graves' ophthalmopathy on health-related quality of life." *European Journal of Endocrinology* 2002 June; 146(6): 751–757.

Tigas, S., et al. "Is excessive weight gain after ablative treatment of hyperthyroidism due to inadequate thyroid hormone therapy?" *Thyroid* 2000 December; 10(12): 1107–1111.

Vaidya, Bijayeswar. "The genetics of autoimmune thyroid disease." *Journal of Clinical Endocrinology and Metabolism* 2002; 87(12): 5385–5397.

Varghese, B., et al. "The follow-up status of patients 10 years after treatment with radioactive iodine (RI) for hyperthyroidism." *Endocrine Abstracts* 2003; 3: P288.

Vaseghi, M., et al. "Minimally invasive orbital decompression for Graves' ophthalmopathy." *The Annals of Otology, Rhinology, and Laryngology* 2003; 112: 57–62.

Verive, Michael. "Hypokalemia." Emedicine.com, March 12, 2003.

Vestergaard, Peter. "Meta-analysis, smoking and thyroid disorders." *European Journal of Endocrinology* 2002 February; 146 (2): 153–61.

Volpe, R. "The pathogenesis of Graves' disease." *Endocrine Practice* 1995; 1(2): 103–115.

Vrca, V., et al. "Supplementation with antioxidants in the treatment of Graves' disease: the effect on the extracellular antioxidative parameters." *Acta Pharmaceutica* 2004 June; 54(2): 79–89.

Vrca, V. B., et al. "Supplementation with antioxidants in the treatment of Graves' disease: the effect on glutathione peroxidase activity and concentration of selenium." *Clinica Chimica Acta; International Journal of Clinical Chemistry* 2004 March; 341(1–2): 55–63.

Wakelkamp, I. M., et al. "Orbital irradiation for Graves' ophthalmopathy: Is it safe? A long-term follow-up study." *Ophthalmology* 2004 August; 111(8): 1557–1562.

Wechsler, Toni. *Taking Charge of Your Fertility: The Definitive Guide to Natural Birth Control, Pregnancy Achievement, and Reproductive Health* (revised edition), Quill, New York, 2001.

Weetman, Anthony P. "Graves' disease." *New England Journal of Medicine* 2000 October 26; 343(17): 1236–1248.

Weetman, A. P., et al. "Treatment of Graves' disease with the block-replace regimen of antithyroid drugs: the effect of treatment duration and immunogenetic susceptibility on relapse." *The Quarterly Journal of Medicine* 1994 June; 87(6): 337–341.

Weetman, A. P., et al. "Current management of thyroid-associated ophthalmopathy in Europe. Results of an international survey." *Clinical Endocrinology* 1998 July; 49(1): 21–28.

Wiersinga, W. M., "Epidemiology and prevention of Graves' ophthalmopathy." *Thyroid* 2002; 12: 855–860.

Woliner, Kenneth, MD. Various personal interviews. 2004.

Wood, Lawrence, et al. *Your Thyroid: A Home Reference.* Ballantine Books, New York, 1995.

Xiao, H., et al. "Arterial embolization: a novel approach to thyroid ablative therapy for Graves' disease." *Journal of Clinical Endocrinology and Metabolism* 2002; 87(8): 3583–3589.

Yen, Michael. "Thyroid ophthalmopathy." Emedicine.com, May 3, 2004.

Yeung, Jim and Sai-Ching. "Graves' disease." Emedicine.com, January 30, 2002.

Yilmaz, E., et al. "Determination of the effect of propylthiouracil to radioiodine therapy in toxic nodular goitre." *Abstracts of the 30th Annual Meeting of the European Thyroid Association,* September 2004, Istanbul, Turkey, http://www.hotthyroidology.com/eta2004/download.php.

Yim, C., et al. "The postpartum recurrence of Graves' disease and its contributing factors." *Abstracts of the 30th Annual Meeting of the European Thyroid Association,* September 2004, Istanbul, Turkey, http://www.hotthyroidology.com/eta2004/download.php.

Zargar, Abdul Hamid, et al. "Clinical and endocrine aspects of thyrotoxicosis and its cardiovascular complications." *Annals of Saudi Medicine* 1999; 485–487.

INDEX